Medical Science & the Law: The Life & Death Controversy

Medical Science & the Law: The Life & Death Controversy

Edited by Lester A. Sobel

Contributing editors: Seth Abraham
Raymond Hill, Chris Larson,
Stephen Orlofsky, Lauren Sass,
Barry Youngerman

Indexer: Grace M. Ferrara

Facts On File
119 West 57th Street, New York, N.Y. 10019

Medical Science & the Law: The Life & Death Controversy

Published by Facts on File, Inc.,
119 West 57th Street, New York, N.Y. 10019.

Library of Congress Cataloging in Publication Data
Main entry under title:

Medical science & the law.
(Checkmark books)
Includes index.
1. Medical laws and legislation—United States.
2. Medical ethics. I. Sobel, Lester A. II. Abraham, Seth. [DNLM: 1. Ethics, Medical. 2. Jurisprudence—United States. W32 AA1 M4]
KF3821.M42 344'.73'041 77-70130
ISBN 0-87196-286-1

9 8 7 6 5 4 3 2 1
PRINTED IN
THE UNITED STATES OF AMERICA

Contents

Page

INTRODUCTION 1
ABORTION 7
Basics of the Controversy 7
State Legislation 8
Opposing Views Argued 15
1973 Supreme Court Ruling Upholds Abortion Rights ... 20
'Right-to-Life' Proposals 25
Further Court Action 33
1976 Political Positions 37
Religious & Other Developments 39
BIRTH CONTROL 43
Public Policy & Controversy 43
Population Policy & Birth Rate 46
The Pill 51
Sterilization 56
Religion & Birth Control 57
Birth Control Dangers 58
EXPERIMENTING ON PEOPLE 61
Ethical & Legal Problems Vs. Need for Experimentation 61
Controversial Experiments 64
'Genetic Engineering' 71
THE MIND 77
Behavior Modification 77
Psychosurgery 83
Other Developments Involving Mental Problems & the Law 87

PROBLEMS OF DEATH 95
When Does Death Occur? 95
'Death With Dignity': The Senate Hearings 97
The 'Right to Die' & Mercy Killing 100
REGULATION 107
Government Policy 107
Laetrile Controversy 110
Action on DES 113
Ban on Cyclamates & Saccharin 115
Action on Amphetamines 118
Diabetes Drugs Curbed 120
Other FDA Actions & Powers 123
Other Developments 127
UNNECESSARY SURGERY 133
Congressional Report 133
INDEX 175

Introduction

PROBLEMS OF LAW AND MORALITY have vexed medical practitioners and society since the early days of civilization. the development of the healing arts and of the sciences connected with them has added to these problems. Such matters as the control of human fertility, the care of the dying, experimentation with living people and the use of questionable treatments have almost always transcended the sphere of medical science; they have long been recognized as involving religion, ethics, public policy and law.

The connection between medicine and law began to be defined as early as the third millenium B.C. in Egypt and Mesopotamia. In Egypt, it is said, this connection was personified by Imhotep (*circa* 2980-2900 B.C.), who was believed to have served simultaneously as chief justice and personal physician to Pharoah Zoser. Sumerian laws of the late third millenium and early second millenium B.C. were believed to have included ordinances on the payment of physicians and on punishment for unsuccessful medical treatment. These laws presumably were the inspiration for similar legislation in Hammurabi's Code of Laws (*circa* 1700 B.C.). Rome's *leges duodecim tabularum* (449 B.C.) provided that the fetus in *utero* had the same rights as a child already born to inherit its father's estate, and it gave the *pater familias* (the chief of a clan) the right to decide whether it was necessary to kill a seriously deformed child.

The Greek physician Hippocrates of Cos (*circa* 460-377 B.C.) is generally regarded as the "father of medicine." Hippocrates and his school produced major works on medical practice and medical law, and the so-called Hippocratic Oath is still the basic ethical guide for the medical profession.

The graduating physician, on taking the Hippocratic Oath, swears: ". . . I will prescribe regimen for the good of my patients according to my ability and my judgment and never do harm to anyone. To please no one will I prescribe a deadly drug, nor give advice which may cause his death. Nor will I give a woman a pessary to procure abortion. . . . In every house where I come I will enter only for the good of my patients, keeping myself far from all intentional ill-doing. . . . All that may come to my knowledge in the exercise of my profession or outside of my profession or in daily commerce with men, which ought not to be spread abroad, I will keep secret and will never reveal. . . ."

Religious qualms about abortion and birth control have played a major role in modern laws prohibiting or controlling such practices. Religion has also been one of the important factors in controversy involving the propriety of some modern scientific experimentation, especially in regard to research on human reproduction. But other considerations have also become increasingly important in the issue of how far medical science should—or should not—go.

Vice President Walter F. Mondale, then a Democratic Senator from Minnesota, pointed out to the U.S. Senate March 24, 1971 that it had become necessary "to consider and study the ethical, social and legal implications of advances in biomedical science and technology." Among developments motivating this concern, he said, were such breakthroughs as heart transplants, "the first successful test-tube fertilization of a human egg" and the prediction by Dr. James D. Watson "that we will soon see the day when a baby will be conceived in a test tube and placed in a woman who will bear the child." Mondale said:

> . . . Recent advances in biology and medicine make it increasingly clear that we are rapidly acquiring greater powers to modify and perhaps control the capacities and activities of men by direct intervention into and manipulation of their bodies and minds. Certain means are already in use or at hand—for example, organ transplantation, prenatal diagnosis of genetic defects, electrical stimulation of the brain. Others await the solution of relatively minor technical problems, while still others depend upon further basic reasearch. All of these developments raise profound and difficult questions of theory and practice, for individuals and for society. . . .
>
> . . . There have been major increases in the ability to detect genetic diseases, even in fetuses still unborn. By examining fetal cells present in fluid obtained from the wombs of pregnant women, diagnosis of diseases such as Mongolism are now being made. As treatment for most genetic diseases is not now available, the diagnosis is generally followed by abortion of the affected fetus.

. . . Major steps have been taken toward developing a technology of genetic engineering which might eventually be able to provide a cure for diseases such as hemophilia, cystic fibrosis or diabetes. . . .

But these welcome prospects are accompanied by others which are frankly disturbing. In other areas of genetic research, work has progressed which may soon make possible the asexual production of large numbers of identical humans, by a technique known as cloning. Work is also in progress to make possible the predetermination of the sex of unborn children.

Research into the nervous system and behavior proceeds at an accelerated pace. . . . New drugs offer possibilities both for novel therapies and for novel abuses. There has also been increasing experimentation with electrical stimulation and with selective destruction of certain areas of the human brain, in order to achieve desired behavioral changes.

In the area of clinical medicine, there has been considerable effort to resolve existing confusion concerning the definition of clinical death. This confusion is due to the fact that, thanks to medical progress, the traditional signs of life—heartbeat and respiration—can now be maintained almost entirely by machines. Since many human matters depend upon the distinction between a man alive and a man dead, the importance of resolving this dilemma cannot be overemphasized. . . .

While holding forth the promise of continued improvements in medicine's abilities to cure disease and alleviate suffering, . . .[recent scientific] developments also pose profound questions and troublesome problems. There are questions about who shall benefit from and who shall pay for the use of new technologies. Shall a person be denied life simply because he does not have enough money for an organ transplant?

There will be questions about the use and abuse of power. When and under what circumstances can organs be removed for transplanting? Who should decide how long a person is to be kept alive by the use of a machine? Exactly what constitutes informed consent for a prospective transplant donor or recipient? . . .

There will be questions about our duties to future generations and about the limits on what we can and can not do to the unborn. Is it ethical for man and wife, each carrying a gene for a serious hereditary disease, to procreate, knowing that their children have a significant chance of acquiring the disease? Should the law enjoin certain marriages or require sterilization for such eugenic consideration? What rights do unborn children have to protect them in experiments involving genetic engineering or test tube fertilization? . . .

. . . We shall face questions concerning the desirable limits of the voluntary manipulations of our own bodies and minds. Some have expressed concern over the possible dehumanizing consequences of increasing the laboratory control over human procreation or of the increasing use and abuse of drugs which alter states of consciousness.

We shall face questions about the impact of biomedical technology on our social institutions. What will be the effect of genetic manipulation or laboratory-based reproduction on the human family? . . .

We shall face serious questions of law and legal institutions. What will the predicted new-fangled modes of reproduction do to the laws of paternity and inheritance? What would happen to the concept of legal responsibility if certain genetic diseases were shown to predispose to antisocial or criminal behavior? What would be done to those individuals with such traits?

We should expect that some people will try to have certain particularly frightening technologies banned by statute. Should this be done? Could such prohibition be effective?

Finally, we . . . will face problems of public policy. We shall need to be informed of coming developments, of the promises they hold forth and the problems they present, and of public attitudes in these matters. We shall need to decide what avenues of research hold out the most promise for human progress. And we shall need to help devise the means for preventing undesirable consequences.

. . . As serious and as vexing as these practical questions may be, there is yet another matter perhaps more profound. The biomedical technologies work directly on man's biological nature, including those aspects long regarded most distinctively human. Thus, we should expect major challenges to our traditional image of man as this technology unfolds. The impact on our ideas of free will, birth, and death, and the good life is likely to be even more staggering than any actual manipulation performed with the new technologies. . . .

Sen. Edward M. Kennedy (D, Mass.) discussed the issue in the Senate Aug. 1, 1972. "Advances in modern medical sciences have lengthened the span and changed the quality and very meaning of human life," he said. "But at the same time, these advances have opened a Pandora's box of ethical, social and legal issues in areas such as heart transplants, artificial kidneys, test-tube babies, genetic intervention, behavior modification and experiments on human beings." Kennedy continued:

For example, recently a hospital has been sued for allegedly allowing a black laborer to die so that his heart could be used in a transplant operation. . . . [The case] illustrates the range of difficult questions which must be faced: When heartbeat and other vital signs can be maintained by artificial means, how is death to be defined? Under what circumstances may the organs of the deceased be used for transplant? Who should give permission for such transplant? Did racial considerations affect the decision to use this heart, as was alleged in the suit?

Medical science advances pose many other difficult ethical and social questions: . . .

Should retarded persons be segregated from members of the opposite sex? Should they be sterilized?

What are the ethical implications of test tube babies? What will happen to our population when men and women are free to determine the sex of their children? Or to fabricate babies with pre-established characteristics?

How should society regulate the use of behavior modification drugs and other techniques to control human behavior? How can we control the controllers?

How should the nation allocate scarce medical resources between organ transplants for a few individuals versus research and services which can help many?

Which individuals should receive the life and death benefit of artificial kidney facilities? How should we choose among those who need this help? . . .

The solutions to these sorts of problems cannot be found within science alone. As Dr. Jerome Wiesner said, 'Science is no substitute for thought.' These issues cannot be resolved by complex mathematical formulas or high speed computers.

> They fundamentally involve questions of ethics and social responsibility. To come to grips with them, we must focus the full range of human talent and imagination—from the natural and social sciences, the arts and humanities, religion and philosophy, and the professions of law, medicine and public service. We must draw on all the resources mankind has to offer; for after all it is the quality of man's life which is at stake. . . .

The problems brought up by Mondale and Kennedy are part of a many-sided topic that in recent years has been dubbed "bioethics." This "life and death" subject is much involved with the "right to life," a term used in opposition to abortion. But it is equally concerned with "the right to die" or "death with dignity," expressions that question the medical profession's right to prolong life by extraordinary means after all hope for recovery—or even for consciousness or lucidity—has gone. Bioethics is also involved in the controversies over medical, surgical and psychological experiments with living human beings, in the disputes over birth control and in the issue of recombinant DNA research, in which genetic material is transferred from one organism to another.

These issues are the subject of this book, which is intended to serve as a record of the "life and death" topics as controversy over them gathered momentum during the 1970s. The material that follows is based principally on the account presented by FACTS ON FILE in its weekly reports on world affairs. A conscientious effort was made to record all events without bias and to make this volume a balanced and accurate reference tool.

LESTER A. SOBEL

New York, N.Y.
August, 1977

Abortion

Basics of the Controversy

The controversy over abortion in the U.S. is largely viewed, rightly or wrongly, as a dispute between a religious viewpoint that insists on completely prohibiting the practice and a secular stand that abortion should be a private matter left to the option of women desiring abortions and their physicians.

Although opponents of abortion include Protestants and Jews (and probably atheists as well), the general view appears to be that Roman Catholics comprise the principal force working for a ban on abortion. This opinion apparently stems from the Vatican's repeated reaffirmation of its stand against abortion and birth control. The opinion prevails despite the refusal of many Catholics in public and private life to take part in "right to life" activity and despite frequent statements by Catholic political figures that they will obey the law—regardless of whether it is pro- or anti-abortion.

Strong anti-abortion laws had been the rule throughout the U.S. until the end of the 1960s, and it was said by authorities as late as the middle-1960s that there was little chance of change. But, as Prof. Gilbert Geis of the University of California noted in "Not the Law's Business?" (a monograph produced in 1972 for the National Institute of Mental Health), "the rapidity of alterations in public attitudes and official policies in regard to abortion has been extraordinary." By 1970 Hawaii had enacted a law permitting "abortion on demand," and other states seemed ready to follow.

"The enhanced vigor ... of the feminist movement played a very large role in the change," Geis asserted. Other factors, he said, included "Malthusian fears of over-population disaster," the increased ease of birth control methods and "the declining hold of theological orthodoxy on the minds and allegiances of Americans."

According to Geis, "it was a single sensational case, however, which thrust the abortion issue into public awareness. The case—that of Sherri Finkbine ... —involved the use by a pregnant woman of a drug, thalidomide, that appeared 'likely' to cause her to give birth to a deformed child. Once the issue had been raised, it was but a short polemical jump from matters of physical deformity to those of psychic aberration, and from concern with the baby's well-being to concern with the mother's. Inevitably ... the fundamental question appeared: Should the state have any right at all to dictate that the pregnant woman had to carry her child to term?"

(Mrs. Finkbine ultimately had an abortion in Sweden, where the fetus was found to be deformed.)

Definition. A "discursive" definition of the term "abortion" was prepared by the staff of the U.S. House Commerce Committee's Subcommittee on Health & the Environment. The definition:

abortion: termination of a pregnancy before the fetus has attained viability, i.e. become capable of independent extra-uterine life. Viability is usually defined in terms of the duration of pregnancy, weight of the fetus, and/or, occasionally, the length of the fetus. A recent inquiry by WHO [World Health Organization] revealed considerable variation in the definitions used in different countries. It has traditionally been assumed that viability is attained at 28 weeks of gestation, corresponding to a fetal weight of approximately 1000 g. This definition is based on the observation that infants below this weight have little chance of survival, while the mortality of infants above 1000 g. declines rapidly. A variety of different types of abortions is distinguished: early—less than 12 completed weeks of gestation; late—more than 12 weeks; induced—caused by deliberate action undertaken with the intention of terminating pregnancy; spontaneous—all abortions other than induced ones, even if externally caused, for instance by trauma or treatment of an independent condition; therapeutic—caused for the treatment of the pregnant woman.

British abortion law 'satisfactory.' Three British birth control authorities said Feb. 6, 1970 that Great Britain's controversial abortion law had operated satisfactorily during the 18 months since it had been enacted. The three experts—a sociologist, a family planner and a physician—recorded their joint opinions in The Lancet, a British medical journal.

The experts said the law had neither turned London into "the abortion capital of the world," nor had it driven up the rate anywhere close to that in Japan or East European nations. They agreed that the law was working "more satisfactorily, perhaps, than either its opponents or its advocates anticipated."

British health officials reported that 65,241 abortions were reported between the effective date of the act (April 27, 1967) and Oct. 28, 1969, when the figures were tabulated. Of these, about 47,127 were effected on the decisions of physicians who deemed that the operations were justifiable for either the mental or physical health of the pregnant women.

The officials also noted that despite predictions from the bill's opponents that single pregnant women would stream into London to take advantage of the law, less than seven of every 100 abortions were performed on women whose permanent residence was outside Great Britain.

State Legislation

Hawaii legislature legalizes abortions. The upper house of the Hawaii State Legislature Feb. 25, 1970 adopted a bill that would legalize abortions in Hawaii performed by licensed physicians or osteopaths in a hospital sanctioned by the state or the federal government. Gov. John A. Burns let the bill become law March 11 without signing it.

The new measure repealed Hawaii's 101-year-old statute that permitted abortions only if the woman's life was in danger. Under the new law, any woman who had lived in Hawaii for at least 90 days would be allowed to have an abortion within the first four or five months of her pregnancy simply because she did not wish to have a baby.

The eligibility clause permitting the operation only within the first four or five months of pregnancy was inserted after the Roman Catholic Church had waged a long struggle to block the passage of the new bill. The requirement was viewed by some Hawaii legislators as a compromise measure to secure the bill's passage.

The residency requirement was included after Hawaii's House of Representatives voted down the same bill which lacked any residency clause. The requirement was written in after a conference committee between members of both Houses.

State Sen. Vincent H. Yano, who played a key role in having the bill adopted, indicated that he and Gov. Burns agreed that any abortion should be left up to the individual mother and her physician. Opponents of the measure argued that the new law could create "an abortion mill" in Honolulu.

Administrators of hospitals in Hawaii reported a considerable rise in the number of abortion operations March 22.

At the Kapiolani Maternity and Gynecological Hospital in Honolulu, officials reported 46 abortions were performed in the first full week since the new law went into effect. Kapiolani administrators said this compared with a total of 70 abortions (under regulations of the old law) in a one-year period from 1968–1969. At Queen's Medical Center, the largest in Hawaii, 13 abortions were performed in the first week. This compared with the hospital's previous rate of about two a month.

Richard Davi, the chief administrator at Kapiolani, said the hospital could perform only 32 abortions a week because "we have so many other surgical cases to handle." Davi said that most of the women who had applied for abortions at Kapiolani appeared to be very young.

N.Y. also legalizes abortions. New York Gov. Nelson A. Rockefeller April 11, 1970 signed into law a controversial abortion reform bill that increased a woman's control over the medical termination of her pregnancy.

Under the new law, a woman and her physician could decide to terminate a pregnancy for any reason at any time up to the 24th week of pregnancy. After the 24th week an abortion could be performed only if the pregnancy jeopardized the woman's life. Under New York's old law, in effect since 1830, an abortion was permissible only to save a woman's life. The new law took effect July 1.

Stormy and emotional debate over the reform bill dominated nearly the entire session of the State Legislature. The State Senate voted March 18, 31–26, to replace the state's old law with what would have been the most liberal abortion reform bill ever passed in the U.S. Under the Senate version, there were no time limits on abortions, no residency requirements nor any provisions specifying how many times a woman could obtain an abortion. State assemblymen in the lower house predicted that the Senate version would not pass the Assembly unless some of those restrictions were written into the bill.

The Assembly March 30 rejected the Senate version of the bill, 71–73, three votes short of the 76 required for passage.

The bill was saved, however, when a Republican congresswoman in the early morning hours March 31 used a parliamentary maneuver to erase the unfavorable vote and table the bill for further discussion.

After a last-minute switch during a new roll call April 9, the Assembly passed a bill, 76–73, that would have removed all but one restriction on abortions in New York. The one provision written into the bill by the Assembly provided that an abortion could be performed for any reason up to the 24th week of pregnancy and after that only to save a woman's life. During the vote, Assemblyman George M. Michaels, an upstate Democrat, interrupted the roll call to announce that he was changing his "no" vote to "yes." "I realize, Mr. Speaker, that I am terminating my political career, but I cannot in good conscience sit here and allow my vote to be the one that defeats this bill." (Michaels failed to obtain the endorsement of his party for re-election April 19.)

The Senate voted 31–26 April 10 to accept the Assembly's version of the reform bill. The archbishop of New York, Terence Cardinal Cooke, issued an unsuccessful plea to Gov. Rockefeller on behalf of the Roman Catholic bishops of the state to veto the bill.

■ The Vatican published a message from Pope Paul VI Oct. 12 denouncing legalized abortion and euthanasia (mercy killing) as barbarism.

The letter was intended for a meeting of the International Federation of Catholic Medical Associations in Washington, D. C.

Vatican sources said the Pope's indictment of legalized abortion as counter to "centuries of civilization" clearly alluded to the new abortion law adopted in New York. The Pope said that "mercy killing" without the patient's consent was murder, with his consent was suicide.

Drop in deaths ascribed to new law—A former New York City health official said Oct. 12, 1971 that the liberalized abortion law had cut the city's maternal death rate by more than half since its inception.

Dr. David Harris, a former New York deputy commissioner of health, attributed the current low rate of two deaths for every 10,000 live births to the new, safe abortions which made criminal abortions unnecessary. The rate was the lowest in the city's history.

Harris made his report to the American Public Health Association, meeting in Minneapolis.

Harris said that through the years, abortion—mostly criminal abortions—had been the single leading cause of maternity-related deaths, accounting for about a third of such deaths each year.

According to medical figures, there were 15 abortion-related deaths in New York City in the first year the law was in effect. One year before the liberalized law was adopted, 24 deaths were tied to abortion-related causes.

Rockefeller for tightening abortion law—Gov. Rockefeller said April 25, 1972 that he favored amending New York's new abortion law by shortening the period during which a woman could legally obtain an abortion.

Rockefeller's remarks came amid renewed efforts by some organizations, predominantly Roman Catholic groups, to have the state legislature repeal the liberalized abortion law.

Under the liberalized law, a woman was allowed to have a legal abortion for any reason up to the 24th week of pregnancy.

Rockefeller recommended that the law be amended to reduce the 24-week period for permissible abortions to a 16-week limit. He said he believed "a modification in the present law is desirable" and if the legislature adopted such an amendment, "I will give it my approval."

Rockefeller vetoes repeal bill—Resisting pressure intensified by President Richard M. Nixon's intercession on the side of antiabortion forces, Gov. Rockefeller May 13, 1972 vetoed a bill that would have repealed New York's liberalized abortion law.

Rockefeller said: "I can see no justification now for repealing this reform and thus condemning hundreds of thousands of women to the dark age once again."

The repeal bill would have restored New York's old abortion law under which a woman could only obtain an abortion when her life was in jeopardy.

Rockefeller had been under pressure from the Roman Catholic Church and groups across the state which had organized under the "right-to-life" banner to sign the repeal bill.

The pressure was increased when the Archdiocese of New York released a letter from President Nixon to Archbishop Terence Cardinal Cooke expressing support for the campaign to repeal the liberalized law.

Rockefeller took note in his veto message that the state legislature was under heavy election-year pressure to repeal the reform law. He said he respected "the moral convictions of both sides" in the issue, but he added that "personal vilification and political coercion" surrounding the issue "raised doubts" that the legislature's votes "represented the will of a majority of the people of New York State."

Nixon had projected himself into the legislative fight in New York over abortion legislation by sending a letter to Cardinal Cooke enunciating his support for the repeal effort.

The text of Nixon's letter was released by the Archdiocese of New York May 6.

In his letter, Nixon said "I would personally like to associate myself with the convictions you deeply feel and eloquently express." Nixon called the drive of the antiabortion forces "truly a noble endeavor."

Following disclosure of Nixon's letter, there was a rising tide of criticism over Nixon's decision to intervene in a local issue. Rockefeller, who had tried to head off the repeal campaign by vowing that he would veto any antiabortion bill, was reported May 8 to be "very upset" over Nixon's letter. Rockefeller's office said "we are referring all calls [on Nixon's letter] to the White House on this."

The White House moved quickly to assuage emotions stirred by the President's letter.

John D. Ehrlichman, Nixon's top advisor on domestic affairs, said May 10 that the letter to Cooke was intended as private correspondence and was not meant to intentionally embarrass Rockefeller. Ehrlichman attributed the White House's decision to give the archdiocese permission to publicize the letter to "sloppy staff work."

N.Y. law upheld—The New York State Court of Appeals July 7, 1972 upheld the state's liberalized abortion law by rejecting an argument that fetuses were legal entities having constitutional rights.

That argument, made in a case brought by Prof. Robert M. Byrn of Fordham University, was dismissed by the court, 5–2.

Byrn had claimed that the law, enacted in 1970, violated the 14th Amendment of the Constitution, which held in part that no state shall "deprive any person of life, liberty or property without due process of law."

Judge Charles B. Breitel, writing for the majority, said "unborn children have never been recognized as persons in the whole sense." Acknowledging that some religions and philosophies might see a conceived child as a person, "it is not true, however, that the legal order necessarily corresponds to the natural order."

Wisconsin law invalid. A three-judge federal court ruled in Milwaukee March 6, 1970 that part of the Wisconsin law forbidding abortions was unconstitutional. According to the ruling, a woman could have an abortion on demand of an "unquickened" child. The judges defined unquickened to mean a fetus before the first recognizable stages of movement. In effect, the court's ruling liberalized Wisconsin's laws on abortion despite the fact that a coalition of conservatives and Roman Catholics had twice before beaten down attempts by liberals in the state legislature to ease the statutes on abortions.

The main opposition to the court's ruling was reported to have come from Roman Catholics, who comprised nearly 38% of the state's population. They were in great part responsible for turning back an attempt by liberals in the legislature to have a liberalization of Wisconsin's abortion laws in January.

The Most Rev. William E. Cousins, archbishop of Milwaukee, said "our reaction [to the court's decision] must be one of disappointment and dismay." He said the ruling was "clearly against a generally acknowledged principle that a fetus has a right to life."

One of the community groups which opposed the court's ruling was the Wisconsin Citizens Concerned for the Unborn, a group that received strong backing from the Roman Catholic Church. The association denounced the decision as a "disaster" and demanded an immediate appeal.

State Rep. Kenneth Merkel, a member of the John Birch Society, said that the decision "was typical of the sickness that is contagious in our federal courts. . . ."

An appeal of the decision was dismissed by the Supreme Court on procedural grounds Oct. 12.

Vermont law voided after repeal effort loses. After bitter debate, Vermont's State Senate March 18, 1970 killed a bill that would have repealed the state's 124-year-old abortion statutes. The 20–10 vote came after the Senate March 17 voted 15–14 to give the measure preliminary approval.

Nearly two years later, however, the state Supreme Court ruled unanimously Jan. 14, 1972 that the old antiabortion law was unconstitutional.

The law, which was enacted in 1846, permitted a doctor to perform an abortion only if a woman's life was in danger.

The court upset a lower court decision which dismissed a request by a welfare recipient for a declaratory judgment to block prosecution if she obtained an abortion.

Michigan law unenforceable. Michigan State Judge Clarence A. Reid Jr. ruled March 31, 1970 that the state's abortion law was unenforceable because of its vagueness. Reid dismissed the charges against a Detroit physician and his wife who were charged with conspiracy to commit an illegal abortion. Reid said he found the language incorporated in the state law that permitted a physician to terminate a pregnancy only when "necessary to preserve life" so vague as to deny the accused due process of law under the 14th Amendment of the U.S. Constitution.

Michigan rejects liberalization—In the Nov. 7, 1972 elections, Michigan voters defeated a proposal to liberalize abortion. The vote followed an intensive campaign that the two sides agreed would have national implications.

Pro-abortion forces in Michigan had succeeded in getting the issue on the ballot by having 300,000 persons sign petitions calling on the voters to override legislative refusal to liberalize a tough abortion law on the books since 1846. In its last four sessions, the legislature had failed to reach agreement on abortion reform.

Under the proposed law, physicians licensed by the state could terminate pregnancies at the patient's request during the first 20 weeks of pregnancy in a hospital, state-owned clinic or similar facility. Existing law allowed abortions only when a woman's life was in danger.

Virginia enacts liberalized law. Gov. Linwood Holton of Virginia signed into law during the week of April 5, 1970 a new and liberalized state abortion bill that was approved during the opening weeks of the 1970 legislative session. The new law would allow therapeutic abortions if the continuation of the pregnancy was "likely to result in the death of the woman or substantially impair the mental or physical health of the woman." The new law also provided for abortions if pregnancy resulted from rape or incest. The new law revised a 123-year-old statute that permitted abortions only if the life of the mother was endangered by continued pregnancy. The revision went into effect June 26.

Alaska liberalization vetoed. Gov. Keith Miller of Alaska April 18, 1970 vetoed a bill that would have given Alaska a reform abortion law almost without restrictions. Miller, a Methodist, said his decision to veto the measure was based on "the right to life."

He also said he disagreed with those who said he should not allow his personal convictions to influence his decision. "Any man who does not follow his personal convictions in conducting state business," he said, "is not worthy of the office of governor." Miller based a third objection to the bill on what he termed the bill's serious legal deficiencies.

The measure, passed by both houses of the legislature the week of April 13, would have allowed abortions to be a matter between the mother and her physician while the fetus was incapable of sustaining life independent of the mother, generally regarded to be until the 26th week of pregnancy.

Maryland liberalization vetoed. Maryland Gov. Marvin Mandel May 26, 1970 vetoed a liberalized abortion bill that would have erased all state restrictions on abortions. The bill was sent to the governor's office after it passed the General Assembly March 31.

Mandel emphasized that he had vetoed the bill on legal rather than ethical grounds. He said he was particularly concerned that the bill contained no residency requirements, that an unmarried minor girl could have an abortion without parental consent, and that the bill failed to include any time limit on when an abortion could be performed.

Mandel's veto could not be overridden by the General Assembly because 1970 was an election year for the legislature. The state constitution provided that a new legislature could not overturn the veto of a previous administration.

The veto left in effect a law enacted in 1968 that permitted abortions up to the 26th week of pregnancy in cases involving rape or incest, where there was a likelihood of a deformed baby or when the pregnancy endangered the mental or physical health of the mother.

Texas abortion law held invalid. A three-judge federal panel in Dallas declared Texas' abortion statutes unconstitutional June 17, 1970 on the ground that they abridged the right of women to choose whether they wanted to have children.

The three U.S. judges said in their decision that the fundamental right of a single woman or a married couple to choose whether to have children was protected by the Ninth through Fourteenth Amendments. The judges acted on a suit brought by a pregnant, unmarried woman, a married couple, and a physician facing two charges of criminal abortion.

Texas law held that any person instrumental in causing an abortion with the woman's consent could be jailed for two to five years. Murder charges could be filed, under the state's statute, when death occurred during an abortion attempt.

The judges ruled that the Texas laws were "overbroad" and "vague" and did not properly define for doctors what constituted criminal abortion liability.

Minnesota law held valid. A Minnesota district court judge Nov. 20, 1970 upheld as constitutional the state's 77-year abortion law in a test case involving a physicians's deliberate violation of the statute. The judge gave the defendant, a woman gynecologist, a suspended sentence for violating the law.

In handing down the verdict, Judge J. Jerome Plunkett praised Dr. Jane Hodgson for her "forthrightness and courage" in testing the statute. He also said that she could "take solace from the esteem" in which fellow physicians held her.

Dr. Hodgson, 55, was convicted Nov. 19 of violating the abortion law and Judge Plunkett sentenced her Nov. 20 to 30 days in jail but suspended it pending the outcome of an expected appeal.

Dr. Hodgson had admitted performing an abortion on a woman who had contracted German measles early in her pregnancy. (Medical evidence had shown that the illness increased the risk that a baby would be born deformed.) Under Minnesota law, an abortion was permitted only when the life of the mother was in danger.

Illinois ruling overturned. The Illinois Supreme Court Jan. 27, 1972 vacated a lower court ruling that would have permitted a 15-year-old girl who had threatened to kill herself the right to have an abortion.

By a 4–3 vote, the court threw out the ruling of a Cook County circuit court judge who said the girl could have an abortion because of her suicidal tendencies.

N.J. law voided. A federal court in Trenton, N.J. Feb. 29, 1972 invalidated New Jersey's 122-year-old abortion law. The law was held unconstitutional on the grounds that it was vague and an invasion of privacy.

In a 2–1 decision, the court held that the wording of the law "provides not a glimmer of notice" as to what one could or could not do. The New Jersey statute had prohibited abortions performed "without lawful justification."

The court added that the application of the law had not been clear. Some courts had found that it allowed abortions only to save the life of the mother, while prosecutors had agreed not to take action against abortions needed to safeguard the mother's life or her health.

The court added that the law also "chills" doctors' exercise of their constitutionally-guaranteed free speech rights and violated their 14th Amendment rights to "freely practice" the profession of their choice. On the issue of privacy, the court held that the constitutionally protected "right of privacy" extended to abortion and that the reasoning behind the laws prohibiting abortions was not "compelling enough" to justify the invasion of that right. In a key passage of the decision, the court said that "we hold that a woman has a constitutional right of privacy cognizable under the 9th and 14th Amendments to determine for herself whether to bear a child or to terminate a pregnancy in its early stages, free from unreasonable interference by the state."

Connecticut abortion laws upset. A panel of three federal judges in New Haven, Conn. struck down as unconstitutional April 18, 1972 Connecticut's 112-year-old statute prohibiting abortion.

In a 2-1 decision, the court held that the state could no longer prevent a woman from deciding "whether she will bear a child."

According to one report, Connecticut's abortion reformers interpreted the ruling to mean that the state would no longer be able to prohibit doctors from performing abortions, or preventing women from having abortions, or stop persons counseling in favor of abortion.

Under the stricken laws, abortions were permitted in Connecticut only to protect the life of the mother.

Judge J. Edward Lumbard, of the 2nd Circuit U.S. Court of Appeals, writing for the majority, said: "what was considered to be due process with respect to permissible abortions in 1860 is not due process in 1972."

Concurring with Lumbard was District Judge John O. Newman. The dissenter was District Judge T. Emmett Clarie.

The old law was replaced by a new one enacted in May.

The new law, which was stronger than the one it replaced, allowed an abortion only when the "physical" life of the mother was threatened. The law was worded in that manner to prevent physicians from performing abortions to preserve what doctors said was the mother's mental health.

But the new law was also struck down as unconstitutional. The three-judge U.S. court in Hartford ruled Sept. 20, 2-1, that the law abridged the rights of a woman "to privacy and personal choice in matters of sex and family life."

In the September ruling, Judges Newman and Lumbard rejected the state's contention that a fetus was a legal person entitled to constitutional rights. Judge Claire objected that the majority view represented federal judicial intrusion into the legislative sphere.

The U.S. Supreme Court Oct. 16 granted Connecticut a stay of the ruling voiding the new law. The stay would keep the new law in force until the High Court decided on its constitutionality.

The court's 8-1 ruling, with Justice William O. Douglas dissenting, came two weeks after Justice Thurgood Marshall refused to grant the stay. After Marshall's ruling Oct. 3, Connecticut succeeded in having the full court take up the stay question.

Florida liberalization. Gov. Reubin Askew April 13, 1972 signed into law Florida's liberalized abortion bill.

Under the new statute, abortions would be permitted to protect a mother's life or health, in case of rape or incest or if it seemed certain that the mother would give birth to a retarded or deformed child.

California birth rate down. A University of California demographer said July

28, 1972 that California's five-year-old liberalized abortion law was curtailing the state's birth rate and also beginning to reduce the number of children on welfare.

Kingsley Davis said "the facts clearly show that rates are down for both legitimate and illegitimate births and among both blacks and whites." Davis, chairman of the International Population and Urban Research Center at the Berkeley campus, made his claims at a hearing on family planning and illegitimacy by a state social welfare board.

Davis told the board that California births declined by 11.5% from 1970 to 1971. The nationwide birth rate dropped 6%. According to Davis, abortions in California rose in 1970 to 65,000, nearly quadruple the number in 1969.

Some of new law ruled too vague—The California Supreme Court held Nov. 22 that certain requirements in the state's abortion law were too vague to enforce, clearing the way for women to obtain hospital abortions on demand.

Among the provisions ruled unconstitutionally vague was a requirement that abortions be approved by local hospital committees. The court also said the medical criteria for an abortion were unconstitutionally vague.

The court's 4–3 decision meant that a woman in the first 20 weeks of her pregnancy could obtain a legal abortion if it were performed by a licensed doctor in an accredited hospital. The judgment for an abortion would now rest solely with the woman and her doctor.

Pennsylvania abortion law vetoed. Pennsylvania Gov. Milton J. Shapp Nov. 30, 1972 vetoed an antiabortion bill that would have been among the nation's strictest. In vetoing the bill, Shapp termed it "so restrictive that it is unenforceable."

Under the bill, an abortion could be performed only when a panel of three hospital-based physicians decided that the continued pregnancy would endanger the life of the mother.

The bill was sent to Shapp's office Nov. 20 after the House of Representatives backed it, 127–50. Shortly after Shapp vetoed the bill, the House failed to override his action by 34 votes.

A three-judge federal panel ruled in Pittsburgh that Pennsylvania's medical assistance program for welfare recipients unconstitutionally discriminated against recipients who chose to have abortions, it was reported May 8, 1974.

The ruling voided state regulations requiring agreement by two doctors that a woman's life would be endangered by giving birth, evidence of rape or incest, or evidence of potential infant deformity before a welfare recipient could receive state reimbursement for an abortion.

Opposing Views Argued

AMA liberalizes abortion stand. A liberalization of its stand on abortion was approved by the American Medical Association (AMA) at its 119th annual convention, held in Chicago in June 1970.

Over objections lodged by Roman Catholic doctors, the AMA voted for the first time in its 123-year history June 25 to allow doctors to perform abortions for social and economic as well as medical reasons. The AMA voted 103 to 73 to consider abortions ethical if the following conditions were met:

(1) The physician was properly licensed to practice medicine; (2) the operation was performed in a hospital accredited by public health organizations; (3) two other physicians were consulted on the case.

After the vote, Dr. Gino Papola, president of the 6,000-member National Federation of Catholic Physicians, said he intended to resign from the AMA. He urged the nation's 35,000 other Catholic doctors to do the same.

The next annual AMA convention took place in Atlantic City, N.J. June 20–24, 1971. Addressing delegates June 21, Dr.

Robert H. Barter reported that his panel on abortions had found they were "acceptably" safe when done in the first three months of pregnancy in an accredited hospital or clinic. The panel also found that in any abortion complications could arise that would make the operation in a doctor's office unwise.

Nixon vs. unrestricted abortion. President Nixon said April 3, 1971 that he regarded abortion as "an unacceptable form of population control" and therefore had ordered the Defense Department to abandon its year-old liberalized abortion policy and to conform with state laws.

The President's statement, released from the Western White House in San Clemente, Calif., confirmed an April 2 report that he had directed the Pentagon to make its policy on abortions at military bases throughout the U.S. conform with the laws of the states in which the bases were situated.

Nixon's April 3 statement on abortion was believed to have been his first on the issue. In it he said he could not reconcile "unrestricted abortion policies, or abortion on demand" with his "personal belief in the sanctity of human life." He said the "sanctity of human life" included the life of "the yet unborn."

The directive which the President struck down had enabled the wives of servicemen to obtain abortions more easily than under state regulations, which were generally more restrictive. According to military sources, the wife of a serviceman could obtain an abortion on the recommendation of a military doctor and one consultant. Most states had a more difficult procedure.

In his statement, the President said that if a particular state restricted abortions, "the rule at the military base hospital are to correspond to that law."

Military officials had said that the liberalized abortion policy, which was ordered into effect July 31, 1970, was designed to standardize abortion procedures throughout the armed services and not necessarily to make it easier for servicemen's wives to obtain abortions.

Statistics released by the Defense Department Oct. 15 showed that abortions at military hospitals had dropped sharply after Nixon's statement.

In the first nine months of fiscal 1971—while the exemption was still in effect—abortions at military base hospitals averaged 423 a month. In the last three months of fiscal 1971 following the President's cancellation of the exemption, abortions averaged 121 a month.

D.C. abortion law upheld. The Supreme Court, by a 5–2 vote April 21, 1971, upheld the constitutionality of a 70-year-old District of Columbia law that permitted abortions only to protect the life and health of the mother. It was the court's first decision on the constitutionality of abortion laws.

The opinion, by Justice Hugo L. Black, reversed the November 1969 ruling of a U.S. judge who held that the D.C. statute was unconstitutionally vague.

The court held that the statute was not vague. But Black in his opinion used what was regarded as qualifying language that was expected to limit enforcement of the D.C. law and others like it.

Black said "health includes psychological as well as physical well-being," a distinction not made in the D.C. law. He also declared that in future abortion prosecutions the government would have to prove not only that an abortion took place, but that the woman's life or health was not in danger.

(Officials of an abortion clinic in Washington, indicating that the decision gave them considerable latitude to perform legal abortions, said April 21 that their clinic would continue to perform them.)

Black was joined by Chief Justice Burger and Justices Blackmun, Harlan and White. Justice Stewart dissented, declaring that if a licensed physician performed an abortion the law should accept that the woman's health made it necessary. In another dissent, Justice Douglas agreed with the federal judge who said that the law was unconstitutionally vague.

Justices Brennan and Marshall did not participate in the decision because they felt that the court lacked jurisdiction to hear the case upon direct appeal from a lower district court.

In the original case, Dr. Milan Vuitch, a Washington physician, was indicted under the D.C. anti-abortion statute. The law was declared unconstitutional and the indictment quashed by Federal District Judge Gerhard A. Gesell, who held that the law's language was too vague. Writing that the word health provided "no clear standard to guide either the doctor, the jury or the court," Gesell dismissed the case. The Justice Department appealed directly to the Supreme Court, charging that Vuitch operated an "abortion mill," without taking into account the patient's health.

Public for liberalization. A federal study made public Oct. 27, 1971 indicated that half the public was in favor of liberalized abortion law. Two years previously, survey data indicated that 85% of the nation opposed liberalizing the laws governing abortions.

The new statistics were released by the Commission on Population Growth and the American Future, for which the nationwide survey was made. Seventeen hundred adults were questioned for the survey.

One of the study's questions concerned the circumstances under which an abortion should be allowed. Of those questioned, 50% said the decision should be made by the persons involved and their doctor; 41% said abortions should be allowed only in certain circumstances; the remaining 9% had no opinion.

Similar responses were recorded for a second question; "Do you think abortions should be permitted where the parents already have all the children they want?"

Among the other findings reported by the commission were:

- Nearly 80% of those interviewed said they favored voluntary sterilization. In a 1966 survey 64% approved of it.
- More than half thought the government should try to slow down population growth and to promote the development of smaller cities to better distribute the population.
- More than half thought people should limit the size of their family even if they could afford more children.

64% back liberalized abortion laws—A Gallup Poll published Aug. 24, 1972 showed that 64% of the U.S. public favored full liberalization of abortion laws.

According to the latest poll, 56% of Roman Catholics now believed that abortion should be a matter for decision solely between a woman and her doctor.

The Gallup survey also showed that 73% of those questioned believed that birth control services and information should be made available to teen-agers.

The Gallup findings were based on personal interviews in June with 1,574 persons.

Study on abortion impact. An unpublished report by the Population Council's associate director claimed that even if all 50 states legalized abortion, it would have little impact on the nation's population growth.

But Dr. Christopher Tietze, who wrote the report for a presidential panel, said the nationwide legalization of abortions could curb the rate of illegitimate births in the U.S.

Tietze's report was disclosed in a Jan. 5, 1972 United Press International dispatch. Teitze based his projections on the number of legal abortions performed in New York City since mid-1970. In his report, Tietze estimated that 1,630,000 women would want abortions in the first year of nationwide legalized abortions on request. He predicted, however, that the birth rate would decline only about 1.5 per thousand population, a decrease of 300,000–350,000 births nationwide in the first year. The government had estimated the 1971 birth rate at 17.4 per thousand population, near a record low.

Tietze said the legalized abortions would have little impact on the birth rate, possibly because as many as 80% of the women seeking abortions would have them performed illegally if necessary to end their pregnancies.

Bar Association backs abortion. The issue of abortion was taken up by the American Bar Association's House of Delegates at the ABA midyear meeting held in New Orleans Feb. 7–8, 1972.

One of the surprises of the session Feb. 7 was the House of Delegates' approval of a uniform statute to permit women to obtain abortions "upon demand." The House of Delegates, traditionally a conservative body on social issues, approved the abortion proposal with only 30 dissenting votes.

The proposal had been drafted by the National Conference of Commissioners on Uniform State Laws, a legal group seeking to reduce disparities among state laws.

Under their proposal, abortions could be performed by physicians upon demand only within 20 weeks of the onset of pregnancy. After that, abortions would be permitted only to preserve the expectant mother's mental or physical health, or if the fetus was gravely deformed, or if the pregnancy was the result of incest or rape.

This proposal was more liberal than any of the abortion laws at that time on the books in all states except New York and Hawaii, where abortion on demand was in effect.

Abortion use widespread. A report prepared by the United Nations' Population Division, made public March 19, 1972 indicated that abortion might be the commonest form of birth control in the world.

The report said that "as the evidence accumulates, many have come to feel that abortion may be the single most widely used method of birth control in the world today. It appears to be common in many countries, whether legalized or not."

The 162-page report noted: "In the countries where data of good quality have been analyzed, the death rates among women undergoing legal abortions have been very low."

Catholics use birth control—A report published in the Jan. 5, 1973 issue of Science magazine by the 1970 National Fertility Study showed that 68% of white, married Catholic women aged 18–34 were using birth control methods proscribed by their church.

The defection rate was greatest among younger Catholic women (74% for those 30 and younger), although the use of birth control methods other than rhythm had increased from 30% in 1955 and from 51% in 1965 for the entire age group.

College educated women showed the largest measure of nonconformity with church teachings—between 1965 and 1970, their use of birth control increased from 40% to 65%.

The New York Times had reported Dec. 30, 1972 that the fertility study appeared to confirm previous reports released in May 1972 indicating that the average family size for Catholic women had declined from 3.45 children in 1965 to 2.75. The national figures showed a decrease from 2.57 to 2.35 children.

Liberalized abortion laws urged. The Commission on Population Growth and the American Future, whose members were appointed by President Nixon to look into population growth problems, formally recommended March 16, 1972 that all states liberalize their abortion laws and permit women to obtain abortions on request.

The commission called for the government to fund abortion services and urged that health insurance plans be tailored to cover the cost of abortions.

While the commission had been set up to study population growth, it based its latest recommendations entirely on other grounds.

For the most part, the panel based its report on the view that "all Americans regardless of age, marital status or income shold be entitled to avoid unwanted births."

The panel also assailed the "various prohibitions against abortion throughout the U.S.," asserting that they "stand as obstacles to the exercise of individual freedom: the freedom of women to make difficult moral choices based on their personal values, the freedom of women to control their own fertility, and finally, freedom from the burdens of unwanted childbearing."

The commission also linked a reduction in the number of illegal abortions to a decrease in maternal mortality and a decline in illegitimacy.

Using New York as a guidepost, where one of the nation's most liberal abortion laws was in effect, the commission pointed out that the maternal mortality ratios there dropped by two-thirds the year after abortion became available on request.

The panel noted that in 1971, New York City experienced the lowest ratio of maternal deaths since the city started keeping records.

According to the commission, the liberalized New York abortion law also exerted a downward influence on the city's illegitimacy rate.

Nixon rejects panel's proposals—President Nixon May 5 formally rejected the commission's proposals that all states greatly liberalize their abortion laws and make available contraceptive devices for teenagers

In a written statement, Nixon said that the panel's report notwithstanding, he still regarded abortion as "an unacceptable means of population control." He added that he did not support what he called "unrestricted abortion policies."

Nixon also rejected the panel's proposal for states to make contraceptive devices and other family planning services widely available to minors. He said "such measures would do nothing to preserve and strengthen close family relations."

Nixon said he would place his trust in the American people themselves. He said he believed they would make "sound judgments that are conducive both to the public interest and to personal family goals."

Mail running against abortion—The Commission on Population Growth and the American Future disclosed May 10 that mail it was receiving was running at the rate of 5-1 against a proposal that states liberalize their abortion laws.

According to a United Press International report, some of the opposition to the panel's proposal appeared to be organized. Some expressed their disapproval on form letters. Others sent anti-abortion letters they said had been distributed in churches.

Bishops condemn panel proposal—Calling abortion an "unspeakable" crime, 240 of the nation's Roman Catholic bishops April 13 condemned the commission's recommendation that abortion laws be liberalized.

The bishops also rejected the panel's suggestion that the quality of American life would be enhanced by diminished population growth.

The bishops said the use of abortions to eliminate unwanted children rested on "an immoral and dangerous principle." The bishops added: "experience has already taught us that our social problems" would not be solved "merely by a population decrease, but require a change of heart and a reordering of priorities for the entire nation."

The bishops reiterated their stand against abortions at the end of their 3-day spring meeting in Atlanta. No vote or stand was taken, outside of the abortion action.

No 1972 abortion planks. Neither of the major political parties mentioned abortion in the platforms adopted for the 1972 Presidential election campaign. The Democratic National Convention's Platform Committee June 27 rejected proposals to include a call for legalized abortions.

1973 Supreme Court Ruling Upholds Abortion Rights

State bans voided. In a landmark decision handed down Jan. 22, 1973, the Supreme Court ruled, 7–2, that a state may not prevent a woman from having an abortion during the first six months of pregnancy. The ruling invalidated abortion laws in Texas and Georgia and, by implication, did likewise to laws in 44 other states.

Writing for the majority, Justice Harry A. Blackmun based the ruling on a constitutional right to privacy but rejected the plaintiffs' plea for abortion on demand. Justices Byron R. White and William H. Rehnquist, President Nixon's most recent appointee, dissented, charging that the majority had used "raw judicial power" in deciding a controversial legislative issue according to its own preferences.

The decision was criticized by Roman Catholic leaders, and praised by family planning and women's liberation spokesmen.

Blackmun denied the contention of Texas and Georgia that the unborn fetus was a "person" endowed with due process rights under the 14th Admendment, and noted that most restrictive abortion laws had not been imposed until the second half of the 19th century.

On the other hand, the opinion said, "the 14th Amendment's concept of personal liberty and restrictions upon state action" guaranteed a privacy right that included "a woman's decision whether or not to terminate her pregnancy." By interfering with the decision, the state could harm the pregnant woman medically or psychologically, or could "force upon the woman a distressful life and future" and bring "a child into a family already unable, psychologically and otherwise, to care for it."

But Blackmun specifically denied that the woman's right was absolute, since "a state may properly assert important interests in safeguarding health, in maintaining medical standards and in protecting potential life." After the first three months of pregnancy, during which time "mortality in abortion is less than mortality in normal childbirth," the state may intervene to protect the health of the woman, by licensing and procedural rules. However, the court barred state residency laws, or procedural obstacles, such as requirements that the woman's physician obtain the approval of committees of doctors.

In the last 10 weeks of pregnancy, Blackmun ruled, when the fetus "presumably has the capability of meaningful life outside the mother's womb," the state "may go so far as to proscribe abortion during that period except when it is necessary to preserve the life or health of the mother."

The Texas law, like those of 30 other states, had barred all abortions except when the woman's life was in danger. The Georgia statute, passed in 1972, based on the American Law Institute model penal code and similar to laws in 14 other states, allowed abortions when a doctor concluded that a woman's life or health was in danger, that the fetus might be born deformed or that the pregnancy had resulted from rape. Both states had been sued by pregnant women seeking abortions.

Blackmun, in reading the decision to the court, noted that most state legislatures were in session, and could write new laws in accordance with the ruling. Only New York, Alaska, Hawaii and Washington had abortion laws liberal enough to meet the court's criteria.

In a dissent supported by Rehnquist, White said the ruling meant "the people and the legislatures of the 50 states are constitutionally disentitled to weigh the relative importance of the continued existence and development of the fetus on the one hand against a spectrum of possible impacts on the mother," which White characterized as "convenience, family planning, economics, dislike of children, the embarrassment of illegitimacy, etc." White said the court was "interposing a constitutional barrier to state efforts to protect human life" while "investing mothers and doctors with the constitutionally protected right to exterminate it."

Although President Nixon had publicly opposed liberalized abortion, three of his four court appointees—Blackmun, Chief

Justice Warren E. Burger and Justice Lewis F. Powell Jr.—voted to upset the Texas and Georgia laws. Nixon's directive barring abortions in military hospitals did not appear to be affected by the ruling, which did not impose a governmental responsibility to perform requested abortions.

Roman Catholic cardinals Terence Cooke of New York and John Krol of Philadelphia issued statements denouncing the ruling. Cooke said he hoped opponents of abortion would "do all in their power to reverse this injustice."

Dr. Alan F. Guttmacher, president of Planned Parenthood, Inc. welcomed the ruling but said "the three-month limit on unregulated abortions" imposed hardships "on the young and the poor who most often need an abortion after the 12th week." He said genetic defects in a fetus may not become apparent until late in a pregnancy. Officials of Zero Population Growth asked opponents of abortion "to work hard with us to improve access to contraception, thus eliminating the need for most abortions."

The court Feb. 26 unanimously refused to reconsider its Jan. 22 ruling, and it dismissed, without granting a hearing, a suit arguing that fetuses had a right to life. It held that the suit involved no "substantial federal question."

Anti-abortion amendment introduced. Sen. James L. Buckley (R, N.Y.) and five co-sponsoring senators May 31 introduced in the Senate a constitutional amendment prohibiting abortions except to save the life of the mother.

The amendment, designed to circumvent the Supreme Court decision striking down abortion laws, defined life as beginning when the fertilized ovum implanted itself on the wall of the uterus, a period usually four-seven days after fertilization. Under this definition, "morning after" pills would be considered contraceptive, and therapeutic treatment given to women immediately after rape would be legal.

Co-sponsors of the amendment were: Mark Hatfield (R, Ore.), Wallace F. Bennett (R, Utah), Carl T. Curtis (R, Neb.), Milton R. Young (R, N.D.), Harold Hughes (D, Iowa) and Dewey F. Bartlett (R, Okla.). All sponsors except Buckley and Bartlett were Protestants.

Controversy over decision. The Supreme Court decision was debated widely by advocates and opponents of liberalized abortion. One of the exchanges of opinion took place in the U.S. House of Representatives July 16, 1973. Rep. Lawrence J. Hogan (R, Md.), speaking for the antiabortion view, said:

New York State is a good example of what has been happening during the past few years. In 1970 the New York State Legislature passed a very liberal abortion law. After only 2 years the legislature reversed itself and repealed the liberalized law only to have it vetoed by Gov. Nelson Rockefeller.

In the 1972 election two States held referendums on whether not to liberalize their abortion laws. In both North Dakota and Michigan the voters overwhelming rejected the liberalized abortion laws. The results of the referendums on liberalized abortiton laws were as follows: Michigan, yes, 39 percent, no 61 percent; and North Dakota, yes, 23 percent no, 76.5 percent.

So, in retrospect we see that, despite the strong efforts made by proabortion groups across the country and despite the wide publicity given to so-called liberalized attitudes toward abortion, the pendulum was clearly swinging the other way—against liberalized abortion laws. My own State of Maryland refused, on a number of occasions, to make it easier to get an abortion.

On January 22, 1973, the Supreme Court ignored what the voters had been saying, ignored the rights of States to regulate abortion, ignored the scientific facts and created a new "right to privacy" and held that unborn babies can be destroyed up until the moment of birth in every State of the Union.

Many are under the misconception that the court decision allows abortion only during the early stages of pregnancy. The decision is far more sweeping than that. Let us take a look at exactly what the court decision says:

During the first 3 months of pregnancy, the State may neither prohibit nor regulate abortion. It is "left to the medical judgment of the pregnant woman's attending physician." In other words, the woman and her physician for no reason whatsoever, can decide to destroy the unborn child.

From the end of the first 3 months to viability—"viability is usually placed at about 7 months or 28 weeks, but often occurs as early as 24 weeks—the State may not prohibit abortion but may "regulate the abortion procedure in ways that are reasonably related to maternal health." No consideration is given to the health of the unborn child, only to the mother.

"For the stage subsequent to viability," the State may regulate and even proscribe, abortion "except where it is necessary, in appropriate medical judgment, for the preservation of the or health of the mother." The health of the mother includes, "psychological as well as physical well being," and "the medical judgment may be exercised in the light of all factors—physical, emotional, psychological, familial, and the woman's age—relevant to the well-being" of the mother. In other words if, a day before normal birth a woman decides that her "emotional" or "psychological" well-being would be impaired by the birth of the child, the child can be destroyed.

In other words, during the first 6 months of pregnancy there are no restrictions whatsoever on the performance of abortions, only minor regulations that can be established by the States as to the procedures that can be used, and during the last 3-month period the decision leaves so many doors open that any woman who wants an abortion will be able to get one.

I was badly shaken by the Supreme Court decision in January. I have been fighting abortion for some time because I cannot accept that it can be right—that it can be legal—to end one human life for the convenience of another human being. I wish every Member of Congress would take the time to see photographs of what the unborn child, the so-called fetus, looks like. Seeing the perfectly formed human features no one can logically challenge the obvious fact that this is a human being. It can be nothing else. So when we talk of abortion we should weigh the rights of this other human being as well as the rights of the mother. The Supreme Court did not do this.

On January 30 I introduced a constitutional amendment, House Joint Resolution 261, which would overturn the Supreme Court's decision on abortion. It is a simple amendment that would guarantee the right to life of the unborn child "from the moment of conception."

My amendment also addresses itself to the frightening trend that antilife forces are now pushing for euthanasia in the same way in which they pushed for abortion a few years ago. Therefore, section 2 of my constitutional amendment says:

> Neither the United States nor any State shall deprive any human being of life on account of illness, age, or incapacity. . . .

It is also noteworthy that since the Supreme Court decision in January, 11 States, the House of Representatives of Montana, and the Senate of West Virginia have passed memorial resolutions urging the Congress to enact a constitutional amendment to overrule the Court's abortion decision.

The States of Maine, Minnesota, Oklahoma, Utah, and West Virginia, Idaho, Louisiana, Maryland, Montana, Nebraska, New Jersey, North Dakota and South Dakota ask Congress to adopt an amendment to the Constitution to protect the unborn.

Certainly, for such a significant number of States to have already responded, it should clearly indicate to Congress that the people of the United States expect Congress to face up to this issue and do something about it.

More than 32 Members of the House have sponsored constitutional amendments on the question of abortion in the House and eight Members of the other body have also sponsored constitutional amendments. . . .

I think it is a tragedy that the Supreme Court, too, ignored all of our legal history. From the beginning of our legal history, the unborn child had certain legal rights which the legal system protected.

The child in the womb could inherit. If a father left a will which said that "I leave my estate to my children at the time of my death," a child in the womb not yet born inherited equally with the other born children. A child in the womb who was injured had the right to bring suit in tort for injury done to him before birth. He had the right to have a guardian appointed to bring suit against his father for support. He had a whole spectrum of human rights which were callously thrown out the window by the Supreme Court on January 22 when the most basic human right of all, the right to life itself, was destroyed.

At the same time, the Supreme Court created out of thin air the right to privacy, the right of privacy to allow a woman to say, "I can do anything with my body that I want."

Mr. Speaker, that is a fallacy. None of us have a right to do with our body what we want. We do not have the right to inject drugs into our body; we do not have the right to use our body for prostitution; we do not have the right to take a part of our body, our fist, and slam it into another's face, because it interferes with the rights of another human being. And that is all we are talking about in opposing abortion, the rights of another human being.

A woman cannot exercise her rights in such a way that she interferes with the rights of that other human being, the unborn child.

That is all we are talking about. We want to restore the human scale where this precious life is given some recognition, some value in the eyes of the law so it is not cast aside on some phony "right to privacy" that was just invented last January. . . .

Rep. Angelo D. Roncallo (R, N.Y.) warned that the abortion decision "has given added impetus to "segments of our society" prepared to dispose of "human life . . . if it is unwanted or somehow differs from an ill-defined norm." He held that "this demeaning, strictly pragmatic approach to life as a direct result of the Supreme Court decision can be measured. . . . . [A]t a recent meeting of the American Medical Association, Dr. Joseph P. Donnelly noted that there were more abortions last year in New York City than live births." He continued:

As an Episcopal priest, the Reverend Charles Patrick Carroll, so correctly told the AMA's Conference on Medicine and Religion:

> Medicine right now is without an ethic. The moment that you do what the patient demands, you open yourself to do what the state demands. If you can take life so glibly in the first two trimesters, what is to prevent you, please tell me, from taking it at any point in the spectrum? . . .

The abortion culture that has grown in the United States since the Supreme Court decision extends far beyond the abortion issue itself. All human life is being threatened by this pragmatic approach to research and medicine. In their never-ending quest for data, regardless of its significance, regardless of its availability through other means, researchers are filling their journals and computers without consideration for the humanity of their unwitting subjects. . . .

Doctors are aborting babies on demand, researchers are taking many of these human lives and performing the most bizarre experiments on them while a heart still beats in their tiny breasts. Others withhold penicillin from a group of black men suffering from syphilis so that the effects of this mind-crippling killer can be studied in detail. The retarded are given hepatitis to see why others have become infected. Now euthanasia once again rears its ugly head in our midst.

These people obviously cannot give their own informed consent, nor can it be given by others to the harm of the subject involved. As far back as 1944, in Prince against Massachusetts, a Federal Court held that:

> Parents may be free to become martyrs themselves, but it does not follow that they are free to make martyrs out of their children. . . .

Rep. Bella Abzug (D, N.Y.), supporting the Supreme Court decision, held that the remarks made by those opposing it "reflect a view that one does not have to recognize the fundamental constitutional right of privacy of a woman over her body and over her decisions." She said:

The fact is that the courts have been moving in the direction of finding, correctly, that matters concerning sex, family, and marriage are indeed matters of privacy and matters to be determined by the parties involved. This right of privacy has the protection of the 1st and 9th amendments and cannot be legislated against under the 14th and 5th amendments.

Much argument is being made here that there is no right of privacy—that in fact this right was sort of made up by the Supreme Court to cover abortion. This is legal and constitutional nonsense. In Roe against Wade, the Court said:

The Constitution does not explictly mention any right of privacy. In a line of decisions, however, going back perhaps as far as *Union Pacific R. Co.* v. *Botsford,* 141 U.S. 250, 251 (1891), the Court has recognized that a right of personal privacy, or a guarantee of certain areas or zones of privacy, does exist under the Constitution. In varying contexts the Court or individual Justices have indeed found at least the roots of that right in the First Amendment, *Stanley* v. *Georgia,* 394 U.S. 557, 564 (1969); in the Fourth and Fifth Amendments, *Terry* v. *Ohio,* 392 U.S. 1, 8–9 (1968), *Katz* v. *United States,* 389 U.S. 347, 350 (1967), *Boyd* v. *United States,* 116 U.S. 616 (1886), see *Olmstead* v. *United States,* 277 U.S. 438, 478 (1928) (Brandeis, J. dissenting); in the penumbras of the Bill of Rights, *Griswold* v. *Connecticut,* 381 U.S. 479, 484–485 (1965); in the Ninth Amendment, *id.,* at 486 (Goldberg, J., concurring); or in the concept of liberty guaranteed by the first section of the Fourteenth Amendment, see *Meyer* v. *Nebraska,* 262 U.S. 390, 399 (1923). These decisions make it clear that only personal rights that can be deemed "fundamental" or "implicit in the concept of ordered liberty," *Palko v. Connecticut,* 302 U.S. 319, 325 (1937), are included in this guarantee of personal privacy. They also make it clear that the right has some extension to activities relating to marriage, *Loving* v. *Virginia,* 388 U.S. 1, 12 (1967) procreation, *Skinner* v. *Oklahoma,* 316 U.S. 535, 541–542 (1942), contraception, *Eisenstadt* v. *Baird,* 405 U.S. 438, 453–454 (1972); *id.,* at 460, 463–465 (WHITE, J., concurring), family relationships, *Prince* v. *Massachusetts,* 321 U.S. 158, 166 (1944), and child rearing and education, *Pierce* v. *Society of Sisters,* 268 U.S. 510, 535 (1925), *Meyer* v. *Nebraska, supra.*

And the Court went on to hold:

This right of privacy, whether it be founded in the Fourteenth Amendment's concept of personal liberty and restrictions upon state action, as we feel it is, or, as the District Court determined, in the Ninth Amendment's reservation of rights to the people, is broad enough to encompass a woman's decision whether or not to terminate her pregnancy. . . .

Either the gentleman from Maryland (Mr. HOGAN) or one of the other Members who participated in this special order indicated that more than 1.3 million abortions took place in 1972. Indeed yes, 1.3 million abortions and probably more took place in 1972 and I would venture to say that they have taken place in that number for many years before and will continue to take place in that number for many years to come. There is a great deal of hypocrisy in this House on the part of those who act as though they did not know this prior to the decision; and who would like to hear no more of it; and would further like to ban abortions by legislating against them. The fact of the matter is that abortions do take place and will take place.

The Supreme Court decision, by eliminating abortions from the criminal statutes, will now make it possible for abortions to be performed under safe medical conditions and not in the back alleys of the past which have crippled and taken the lives of many women. . . .

You are entitled to your personal religious and moral views but they are irrelevant to this Supreme Court decision.

For example, one has a right to free speech. I am sure the Members will recognize that. They may not like what one is saying when one is expressing that right of free speech. But if it is a valid exercise of free speech one cannot interfere with that right. Your remedy is to have the free choice not to listen.

The same thing goes with the subject of abortion. You cannot choose whether or not you want an abortion because you all happen to be men. But there are women in this country who may choose not to have abortions, and indeed that is their right. Nothing in this decision coerces abortion. But those who object to abortion have no right to prevent others from exercising their valid constitutional right to have an abortion. Their remedy is to have the free choice not to have an abortion.

Rep. William J. Keating (R, Ohio) asserted that "the basic right to life has been challenged by the court." He added:

Modern science in the last decade has brought us a spectrum of knowledge about fertilization and early development that we only guessed at previously in history. In a book written by Dr. and Mrs. J. C. Wilke they discuss the scientific data on the beginning of human life.

Dr. and Mrs. Wilke point out that we now know that the sperm contributes 50 percent and that the egg contributes 50 percent of the new life. The sperm contains the genetic code of the father, and has no life or continuing function beyond the sole goal of its existence, that is, fertilization. The ovum contains the genetic code of the mother and is unquestionably part of her body. It has no other function than to be fertilized and, if it is not, it will die.

When, however, at fertilization, the 23 chromosomes from the sperm join the 23 chromosomes from the ovum, a new being is created. Never before in the history of the world nor ever again will a being identical to this one exist. This is a unique being, containing within itself a genetic package, completely programmed for and actively moving toward adult human existence. It has, by any standard, a life of its own and in no way is part of the mother or the father.

At first the medical profession calls this new, unique being a fertilized ovum and soon thereafter a zygote. Nothing will be added to this being the moment of fertilization and its ultimate death as an old person. It is all there in toto at the moment of conception, merely not fully developed.

Today we stand on the threshold of deciding whether or not we tolerate a new morality where the guarantees of the Declaration of Independence, the 14th amendment to the Constitution, and the previous traditions of our Juden-Christian heritage do not apply to all human life.

When, for example, the Court states that the unborn are not recognized by the law as "persons in the whole sense," and when, further, it uses as a precondition for legal protection the test whether one has the capability of meaningful life, one begins to question what the logical next step will be to this type of logic....

Lawsuits have already begun in nine States to compel hospitals to perform abortions. There have already been decisions handed down in Massachusetts and New Jersey. In Green Bay, Wisc., a doctor has brought suit against a private Methodist institution to allow him to perform abortions there.

In my district, the Cincinnati Enquirer had an article quoting the executive director of the Cincinnati chapter of the American Civil Liberties Union as saying that she was preparing letters to General, Bethesda North, Jewish, Providence, Our Lady of Mercy, and St. George hospitals to find out what their abortion policies are and whether they have changed with the Supreme Court decision.

The ACLU spokesman stated that if the hospitals had restrictive policies on abortion that are not in line with the Supreme Court decision that they would be liable for a suit.

It now seems that the same people who were working for liberalized abortion laws are now the same ones who are taking the hospitals to court to force the institution to perform abortions and are the leaders of efforts for sterilization and euthanasia.

In Florida, Dr. Russell Sackett, author of the "death with dignity" bill, has stated that—

> Florida has 1,500 mentally retarded and mentally ill patients, 90% of whom should be allowed to die.

The Supreme Court decision allows for the killing of the developing child in the womb of the mother; the Florida bill allows the killing of the mentally ill.

What we have witnessed with the cases of sterilization in Alabama, with the Supreme Court decision on abortion, and with the increased discussion of euthanasia is the Federal Government determining who shall have the right to life and the right to give life and who shall not have these rights....

Other Supreme Court rulings. Among other 1973 Supreme Court decisions involving the abortion issue:

The court June 4 upheld, 9–0, a lower court ruling rejecting an argument that abortions should not be covered by Medicaid, as the practice would interfere with the rights of a living, but unborn child.

The Supreme Court Nov. 12 upheld, by declining to accept for review, an Arkansas Supreme Court ruling that the state's abortion law was constitutional to the extent that it could bar laymen from performing abortions.

'Right-to-Life' Proposals

Hearings on amendments. The Senate Judiciary Constitutional Amendments Subcommittee held hearings March 6–7, 1974 on two proposed constitutional amendments aimed at rescinding the 1973 Supreme Court decision upholding a woman's right to decide whether or not to have an abortion. An amendment offered by Sen. Jesse Helms (R, N.C.) would guarantee, without exception, the right to life at the instant of conception. The other amendment, offered by Sen. James Buckley (R-Conservative, N.Y.), would allow abortion only when a reasonable medical certainty existed that the mother's life would be endangered by the continuation of the pregnancy.

Testifying before the subcommittee March 6, Buckley expressed a desire to restore the "traditional understanding" of the 14th Amendment, which he construed as the right to life. "It matters not, under my amendment," he said, "whether one is come to full term in a mother's womb." Buckley opposed abortions after rape but favored establishment of professionally-staffed treatment centers for rape victims.

Rep. John M. Zwach (R, Minn.), sponsor of an abortion amendment in the House, told the panel March 6 that framers of the Declaration of Independence said all men were "created equal," not that they were born equal.

John Cardinal Krol, archbishop of Philadelphia and president of the U.S. Catholic Conference, told the subcommittee March 7, "The right to life is not an invention of the [Roman] Catholic church or any other church. It is a basic human right which must undergird any civilized society." Humberto Cardinal Medeiros, archbishop of Boston, testified that the Catholic church opposed abortion, even to save the mother's life.

Rabbi J. David Bleich, who spoke for the Rabbinical Council of America and orthodox Judaism, said March 7 that fetal life was entitled to all the safeguards afforded all members of society.

Appearing in opposition to the amendments was Rep. Bella Abzug (D, N.Y.), who warned March 6 that the amendments "would impose a particular religious or moral ethic upon a nation that at its inception . . . rejected any dogma or creed as mandatory for all."

Colgate University professor Barbara McNeal testified March 7: "Should a male dominated [Catholic] religious hierarchy determine the moral posture and legal status of the opposite sex when the woman in question is caught up in a dilemma no man can fully understand? . . . A church that proclaims celibacy to reflect the highest levels of excellence and that takes the dimmest possible view of scientific methods of birth control is not in a logical position to impose its view on abortion on the remainder of the citizenry."

Rabbi Balfour Brickner, who as a representative of the Union of American Hebrew Congregations appeared as a spokesman for reform Judaism, testified March 7 that he interpreted Judaic law to mean that the fetus was not a person until it was born. Brickner said abortion was not wrong.

Rep. Abzug said in her testimony:

I am opposed to compulsory abortion. I am opposed to compulsory sterilization. I am also opposed to compulsory pregnancy.

Under the Supreme Court decision, no woman anywhere in the United States can be forced to have an abortion. Neither can she be forced to have a baby. She is free to decide, under certain limittaions specified by the Supreme Court, whether she should give birth to a child.

Man and woman are equal in the act of conception, but after that single act has occurred, it is the woman's body that carries and nurtures the embryo and the fetus.

It is the woman who experiences the physical and psychological changes of pregnancy.

It is the woman who has the discomforts and sometimes the medical complications that accompany pregnancy.

It is the woman who feels the pain of childbirth. It is the woman who may have the postpartum depression.

And in our society it is the woman who bears the major responsibility of caring for and raising the child and who often must leave school or her work to do so.

Childbearing and childraising is a great experience for most women. For some it is not. For some it is sometimes. The point is that it is a totally individual experience, the most highly personal process in a woman's life. . . .

Each year, before the Supreme Court decision was handed down, physicians had to treat about 350,00 women suffering from complications arising from illegal abortions. Each year, it has also been estimated some 400 to 1,000 women died as a result of illegal, out-of-hospital abortions. Sometimes months of intensive care would be required to save a woman's life.

In contrast, the experience in New York State which has had legalized abortion for more than three years shows a decline in deaths associated with abortions, a decline in the maternal death rate, a steep decrease in the number of infant deaths, and a striking decline in the numbers of women hospitalized due to botched abortions.

The New York experience has also shown a 25 percent decline in the birthrate between 1970 and 1972, a 12 percent decline in the number of out-of-wedlock births, and a 56 percent decline in the rate of newborn infants left for placement or simply abandoned in the hallways, doorsteps and other places.

A report by Planned Parenthood Federation of America, issued December 10, 1973, which I would like to submit along with other documents as part of my testimony, says:

"Elimination of dangerous illegal abortion removed the main single case of maternal deaths. And women for whom childbirth would be a high risk—the very young, women who have had many previous pregnancies or are nearing menopause, and women with medical handicaps—now have an alternative. Of course, availability of abortion alone doesn't account for declines in the National Maternal Mortality rates. Effective use of contraception is another factor. In fact, the New York evidence suggests that contraceptive practice improved markedly, perhaps related to the contraceptive counseling provided by facilities performing abortions."

As a result of the legalization of abortion in some states, more women have been able to procure abortions during the first 12 weeks of pregnancy, the safest period. A one-year study of almost 73,000 abortions performed in hospitals in five states showed that 75 percent took place during the first 12 weeks of pregnancy and less than three percent took place after the 20th week. The study shows that late abortions have been mostly frequent among women under the age of 18, mothers of six or more children, black women, and patients in public hospitals. These are the women who as a result of legalization of abortion now have the personal security of access to safe procedures and to contraceptive counseling.

Perhaps the most significant finding in the Planned Parenthood report was that "about seven in ten of the legal abortions of New York residents would have taken place anyway—most of them illegally—in the absence of the new law. In other words, the primary impact of legalizing abortion is to make safer, less expensive and more open a procedure which would have taken place anyway."

Those who would overrule *Roe v. Wade* (410 U.S., 113 (1973)) would ignore our experience with the practical consequences of attempting to prohibit abortion and the benefits we have seen in terms of improved maternal and infant health resulting from legalized abortion. Those who would impose a ban on abortion in the name of protecting the rights of the unborn would deprive recognized citizens of their rights under the First Amendment, which guarantees secular supremacy, and their Constitutional right to privacy.

In its decision, the Supreme Court held: "This right of privacy, whether it be founded in the Fourteenth Amendment's concept of personal liberty and restrictions upon state action, as we feel it is, or, as the District Court determined, in the Ninth Amendment's reservation of rights to the people, is broad enough to encompass a woman's decision whether or not to terminate her pregnancy." (410 U.S. at 153).

The court went on to discuss the hardships a state could impose upon a pregnant woman by denying her this choice:

"Specific and direct harm medically diagnosable even in early pregnancy may be involved. Maternity, or additional offspring, may force upon the woman a distressful life and future. Psychological harm may be imminent. Mental and physical health may be taxed by child care. There is also the distress, for all concerned, associated with the unwanted child, and there is the problem of bringing a child into a family already unable, psychologically and otherwise, to care for it. In other cases . . . the additional difficulties and continuing stigma of unwed motherhood may be involved. All these are factors the woman and her responsible physican necessarily will consider in consultation." (410 U.S. at 153).

The Court also held that although the right of personal privacy includes the abortion decision, "this right is not unqualified and must be considered against important state interests in regulation." It said a state may properly assert important interests in safeguarding health, in maintaining medical standards, and in protecting potential life. "At some point in pregnancy," the court continued, "these respective interests become sufficiently compelling to sustain regulation of the factors that govern the abortion decision." . . .

The core of these amendments is the concept that the zygote, embroyo or fetus is a human being indistinguishable from humans who have been born. The significance of birth itself might be wiped out by these amendments, with staggering implications for our society. Both amendments seek to define the unborn as a person. Helms would stretch this definition to the "moment of conception," and the Buckley amendment more circuitously speaks of "unborn offspring at every stage of their biological development." In attempting to write language into the constitution which determines when a human being becomes a human being, the authors of both amendments rush in where wiser persons have feared to tread.

The Supreme Court decision says on this point: "We need not resolve the difficult question of when life begins. When those trained in the respective disciplines of medicine, philosophy and theology are unable to arrive at any consensus, the judiciary, at this point in the development of man's knowledge, is not in a position to speculate as to the answer."

Yet if these amendments were adopted, the courts would be involved in unending speculation on this very question. Does Senator Buckley's phrase about every stage of biological development take us back to the sperm and the egg? It very well might. When does the "moment of conception" referred to by Senator Helms take place? Does it begin with fertilization or the process of implantation in the uterus, which occurs some five to eight days after the process of fertilization has been completed? And how could one possibly ascertain that legally? The state of pregnancy itself cannot be determined with certainty until some three weeks after implantation has occurred.

There can be no sensible or generally accepted legal determination of what the Supreme Court called in its decision "this most sensitive and difficult question." It pointed out that there has always been strong support for the view that life does not begin until live birth. This was the belief of the Stoics and it appears to be the predominant, though not the unanimous, attitude of the Jewish faith. It is the belief widely held by large segments of the Protestant community. Common law held that abortion performed before quickening—the first recognizable movement of the fetus *in utero,* appearing usually from the 16th to the 18th week of pregnancy—was not an indictable offense. Physicians often focus upon the point at which the fetus becomes "viable", that is, sufficiently well developed to live outside the mother's womb, albeit with artificial aid. Aristotle held a three-stage theory of life, in which the vegetable stage was reached at conception, the animal stage at animation, and the rational stage soon after live birth. St. Augustine, who made a distinction between *embryo inanimatus,* not yet endowed with a soul, and *embryo animatus,* at one point expressed the view that human powers cannot determine the point during fetal development at which the critical change occurs.

These theories of "mediate animation" and ensoulment held sway throughout the Middle Ages and the Renaissance in Europe and was official Roman Catholic dogma until the 19th Century. The belief that life begins from the moment of conception is now the official view of the Catholic Church and it is also held by many others on moral rather than religious grounds.

One can respect the right of the Catholic Church and many other sincere and earnest Americans to hold this belief without writing it into the basic secular law of our land. Indeed, if the Buckley and Helms views were to be accepted as mandates, we would have to call upon medical science to develop electronic spies or other devices, possibly placed within the body of the woman, to determine precisely when the sperm fertilized the egg, when the egg attaches itself to the wall of the uterus, and so forth. This would, of course, be the utimate invasion of privacy, but one can ask what is the point of making a constitutional reference to the "moment of conception" without considering how that is to be determined.

The Supreme Court decision held that a fetus is not a person within the meaning of the Fourteenth Amendment. It noted that those sections of the Constitution which refer to "person" have application only postnatally. "None indicates, with any assurance," said the Court, "that it has any possible prenatal application."

In view of this firm high court decision, the Bucley and Helms amendments are intended to change the constitution and to confer some uncertain measure of personhood upon the zygote, embryo or fetus in accordance with their vague definitions.

As a lawyer, I can assure you that if either amendment were added to the Constitution, our entire system of laws would become a chaotic mess and the only ones who would benefit would be the army of fetal protection lawyers that would undobutedly rush to the courts with thousands of mischievous lawsuits. . . .

We are all concerned with the right to life. We must also be concerned with preserving the essence of our democratic society which allows all viewpoints to flourish and compete for support.

Those who agree with Senators Buckley and Helms are perfectly free to model their own lives on these precepts. They are also free to state their views publicly, to argue, to seek to persuade other Americans of the rightness of their morality or dogma. But they have no right to demand that all Americans conform to their particular beliefs.

And they have given us no reason to believe that a ban on abortions would be any more workable than a ban on sexual intercourse. The only result would be to turn women unwillingly into lawbreakers.

Women's groups vs. amendments. Rep. Ronald V. Dellums (D, Calif.) inserted in the Congressional Record March 12, 1974 letters in which women's groups opposed the proposed antiabortion amendments.

Alice Travis, as chairperson of the Women's Caucus of the California Democratic Council (CDC), said in a Feb. 25 letter to Dellums that the CDC remained "diametrically opposed to any governmental infringement" on the "right of a woman to have an abortion on demand."

Sue Wimmershoff-Caplan, president of the Professional Women's Caucus, told Dellums in a Jan. 22 letter:

> **We are convinced that the right of every woman to control her reproductive processes is an elementary Constitutional Right upon which all of her other efforts and aspirations toward equality are based. We would like you to know that at our annual convention held in New York City at the end of September, 1973, the following resolution was adopted:**
>
> **Since control over our bodies is the very cornerstone of any equality for women, passage of the so-called "Right to Life Amendment" to the Constitution, which is now in the Judiciary Committee of the United States House of Representatives, would be an unmitigated disaster to the cause of women in the United States. It is an anomaly indeed, that while we still lack a Constitutional Amendment giving equal protection to women, we are now faced with the very real prospect of passage of a Constitutional Amendment granting greater rights to the fetus. Accordingly, defeat of the proposed "Right to Life Amendment" now in the Judiciary Committee in the House of Representatives in the United States Congress is imperative.**

Dellums July 18 inserted in the Congressional Record a July 11 letter in which Black Women Organized for Action (BWOA) expressed concern at a proposed antiabortion amendment that read:

> **"Neither the U.S. nor any state shall deprive any human being (from the moment of) conception of life without due process of law; nor deny any human being from the moment of conception, within its jurisdiction the equal protection of the law. Neither the U.S. nor any state shall deprive any human being of life on account of illness, age or incapacity."**

The BWOA letter continued:

> **BWOA recognized several problems with this amendment sponsored by Senator Mark Hatfield (Oregon) and Senator James Buckley (New York):**
>
> **1. Rape victims who conceive a child will be forced to bear the child.**
>
> **2. Danger to a mother's life will no longer be sufficient grounds for abortion.**
>
> **3. Abortion will be defined as murder.**
>
> **4. Women will not have free choice to make personal decisions on the abortion question.**
>
> **Black Women Organized for Action *does not* support this proposed amendment to the Constitution for Black women who are poor or who must depend upon public health facilities may resort to illegal abortion and jeopardize their life and health.**

Dellums, often a spokesman for black views in Congress, said in a statement in the July 18 issue of the Record that he considered it "the basic human right of each women to decide when to acquire a legal abortion." Dellums' statement continued:

> **The medically administered abortion, which has long been used by more affluent Americans, alters a natural process of the female body just as the vasectomy does the male. To illegalize abortion would only serve to impose further hardships on America's poor, in addition to thwarting medical advancement.**
>
> **Abortion as a right, not a privilege, should be available to every woman in this country without restriction by law or constitution amendment. For if this Congress opts to enact such legislation, a past era of quackery, self-induced abortions, and abortions at exorbitant fees will be reawakened.**
>
> **A wide array of individuals and organizations have taken a principled stand to support each woman's option to legally abort. However, at times opponents to legal abortion raise cries of "genocide" to support their position. During the turbulent sixties, some black organizations used the genocide argument to denounce a woman's right to legal abortion. Despite the rhetoric of such an argument, the fact remains that to legally deprive women of that right is immoral, insane, and unjust.**
>
> **Since then black organizations have taken a turn in thought. Given their plight in this country, blacks forsee potential dangers if abortion is illegalized.**

'Operation Avalanche.' Rep. Donald M. Fraser (D, Minn.) told Congress July 16, 1974 that a recent "sharp increase in antiabortion form letters" to Congress members had been organized by the Committee of Ten Million, "a national pro-life organization" headquartered in Glendale, Calif. Fraser inserted in the Congressional Record of July 17 a copy of "a cover letter to 18,000 bishops and pastors" that was written by Gilbert Durand, national chairman of the committee. The letter said in part:

1. Operation Avalanche will force enactment of the Human Life Amendment in 1975.

2. Operation Avalanche will deliver 10 million anti-abortion letters to Congress during the week of July 4, 1974.

3. Operation Avalanche will automatically organize 20,000 local pro-life *political action* groups. There are more groups than the Democratic and Republican Parties have, combined.

4. Operation Avalanche will elect a pro-life Congress.

5. Operation Avalanche will force state ratification of the Human Life Amendment by July 4, 1976.

"We consider the passage of a pro-life constitutional amendment a priority of the highest order."

"In all of this, well-planned and coordinated political organization by citizens at the nation, state and local levels is of highest importance."

"Our system of government, requires citizen participation, and in this case, there is a moral imperative for political activity."

The words are clear, deliberate and authoritative. They are the words of the National Council of Catholic Bishops, meeting in plenary session last November. Why this unprecedented pronouncement on the part of the American hierarchy?

Four reasons: (1) because of the gravity, frequency and legality of abortion in the United States today; (2) because a Human Life Amendment is the only means by which the state can discharge its paramount obligation—the protection of the God-given right to life itself; (3) because political organization and activity are the only available means of obtaining such a protective amendment; and (4) because under our system of government *all* citizens are obliged to vote and to work politically for a government responsive to the demands of justice.

If this moral obligation applies to *all* citizens, it particularly applies to pastors. It should be noted that abortion destroys not only the natural life of the child, but also the supernatural life of the mother. When we oppose abortion we are not only making a dutiful response to the obligations of justice, but are performing both corporal and spiritual works of mercy—noble acts of charity.

Now that it is clear what needs to be done, the question remains: how best to do it? For months the Committee of Ten Million has worked on this problem. Its carefully considered solution is entitled *Operation Avalanche*.

Operation Avalanche is a serious, realistic and uniquely effective response to the Bishop's recitation of what needs to be done. It is our best means of discharging our moral responsibilities in this election year—this crucial year.

Operation Avalanche will *quickly* organize 20,000 local pro-life political action groups—a splendid follow-up to the Bishop's suggestion. It will unleash 10 million letters on the Congress in one week. Its power will force enactment of the Human Life Amendment.

Ford for amendment. A White House spokesman indicated Sept. 5, 1974 that Gerald R. Ford, who had succeeded Richard Nixon as President, favored a constitutional amendment permitting states to decide whether or not to allow abortions. Characterizing this stance as consistent with past Ford positions on abortion, the spokesman also pointed to Ford's opposition to a 1972 Michigan referendum to permit abortion on demand.

Betty Ford, the President's wife, said at a Sept. 5 news conference that her views on abortion were "definitely closer" to those of Vice President-designate Nelson A. Rockefeller than Sen. James Buckley (R-Conservative, N.Y.). (As governor of New York, Rockefeller had favored abortions; Buckley was the sponsor of a constitutional amendment to prohibit abortions.)

The White House subsequently issued a statement that the views of the President and Mrs. Ford were not far apart. Their essential concern, the spokesman said, was that there must be a remedy in cases of serious illness or criminal attack.

Bans on federal-paid abortions lose. The Senate Sept. 17, 1974 approved an amendment to the fiscal 1975 Health, Education and Welfare (HEW)-Labor Department appropriations bill prohibiting use of federal funds to pay for abortions or abortion referrals, except to save the lives of mothers.

A similar, but more restrictive anti-abortion amendment to the House version of the HEW-Labor appropriations bill had been defeated in the House June 27, and the Senate proposal was eliminated in joint conference committee before the two houses of Congress passed the appropriations bill Nov. 26.

The Senate amendment's sponsor, Dewey F. Bartlett (R, Okla.), indicated that the funding cutoff was aimed at the HEW Medicaid program, which he said had helped to pay for abortions in at least 14 states. Opponents of the Bartlett measure contended that it would discriminate against poor women, who, unlike higher income women, could not afford abortions except with the assistance of Medicaid.

Sen. James Buckley, supporting Bartlett's stand, told the Senate:

One thing that has marked debate on this subject in this country, and one that I think does no credit to the medical profession in this country, is that the attitude has somehow been allowed to gain currency that an abortion, so long as it is performed legally, in some sanitary clinic, by a licensed physician, is safe. Yet, the overwhelming evidence that has been gathered from jurisdictions in Europe and in Japan and elsewhere, where legalized abortion has been permitted for a period of years, is that it is an unsafe procedure under the best circumstances. Therefore, I suggest that, as a matter of policy, we should not encourage the use of Federal funds to pay the cost of elective abortion.

I should like to support what I have just said in a few statements quoted from material that has been introduced to the hearings that are now going on with respect to an amendment to prohibit abortions except when necessary to save the life of the mother.

I should like to quote, for example, from a statement by Doctors Thomas Hilgers and Robert Shearen, in testimony presented to the Minnesota State Legislature. In that testimony is this flat statement:

In the majority of countries, including New York State, a woman is more likely to die from legal abortion than she is if she were to carry the pregnancy to term. This is in contradiction to what proponents of abortion would have us believe. It must be emphasized that these figures are for legal abortions done by licensed physicians in fully-accredited medical facilities.

The following year the Senate April 10, 1975 rejected, by 54–36 vote, an amendment to a health measure that would have prohibited federal funding of abortions under the Medicaid program for the poor.

Sen. Bartlett said HEW spent more than $40 million for 270,000 abortions in 1973, contended that the federal government had adopted a policy of encouraging abortions despite the national controversy surrounding the issue. "If this amendment is passed into law," Bartlett said, "we can eliminate those programs whose purpose is the taking of human life."

Opponents of the amendment, on the other hand, avoided the emotional side of the issue and maintained that the amendment was illegal, vaguely written and unfair to women too poor to afford abortions without Medicaid.

Sen. James Buckley supported the amendment:

Those who oppose this amendment suggest that it is discriminatory. They say that it would discriminate against the poor. The well-to-do can afford abortions, they tell us, but the poor need Government funds.

There are two points that should be raised about such a charge. First, it is simply not true that denying tax dollars for practices held to be rights by Supreme Court decisions is discriminatory. The taxpayer is under no obligation to fund with his money any and all rights. Traditional congressional policy prohibits this Federal financing, a policy which was first explicitly stated in the Family Planning Act of 1970 and reiterated in the first session of the 93d Congress by the enactment into law of an amendment proscribing the use of foreign aid funds for abortion. Both Houses of Congress are repeatedly on record as opposing Government funds for abortion.

The issue of Federal funding is wholly distinct from the constitutional question decided by the Supreme Court on January 22, 1973. It by no means follows from the fact that a woman is now legally permitted to seek an abortion, that the Federal Government is constitutionally or otherwise obligated to pay for it. It is apparent that abortion is now being promoted as a new-found panacea to certain social and economic problems. Several years ago, the arguments favoring liberalized abortion were couched almost exclusively in terms of the woman's "right to privacy." In the past few years, especially since the Supreme Court's ruling, the arguments for abortion have acquired a new and ominous focus, one that emphasizes the social, economic, and political utility of abortion. Abortions in general and publically funded abortions in particular, are now being advanced as a socially "progressive" and "enlightened" solution to the problems of poverty and welfare. When abortions are openly defended on the explicit grounds that they help to limit the welfare population and reduce publice expenditures, I submit we are traveling rapidly down a road that will subject all human life, born or unborn, to the risks of some social planner's cost/benefit calculus. This reduces itself to the simple argument that the way to eliminate people's problems is to eliminate people.

The second point that should be raised is quite simply that the obvious intent of this amendment is not discriminatory. I point out this abvious fact only because it seems to me that it does not contribute to rational debate to set up strawmen. The amendment is not discriminatory in intent; it will not be discriminatory in practice. It seeks to reaffirm a principle already written into law in two cases and one agreed to in other cases in votes in the Congress.

It is my hope that the debate over this issue will not become bogged down in irrelevant issues. The issue is clear and precise: Should tax dollars be used to fund abortions? The question has been asked here before. The answer has always been the same, and that answer is "No." . . .

Sen. Bob Packwood (R, Ore.) inserted in the Congressional Record a study by Morton Rosenberg, legislative attorney of the Library of Congress. According to Packwood, Rosenberg's study indicated that "statutory restriction of the use of federal and state funds for abortions" was unconstitutional. Rosenberg concluded:

The amendment under question would deny federal funds for the performance of abortions in any trimester. The provision would apply to any current law authorizing funds for such a purpose. Perforce, it would apply to the federal Medicaid program and would create a situation where pregnant indigent women who choose to carry their pregnancies to term would receive pre-natal and delivery benefits but indigent pregnant women who elect to terminate their pregnancies by abortion, for a reason other than to preserve their lives, would be denied financial assistance for this purpose. Such women would then have to either seek alternate ways or means to abort or carry to term.

Under such circumstances, and in the light of present decisional law, the federal government, faced with a suit testing the constitutionality of the provision, would be confronted with the following constitutional principles and guidelines:

(1) A woman's decision whether or not to terminate her pregnancy by abortion is a fundamental constitutional right.

(2) The government may not condition the receipt of a statutory benefit upon the forfeiture of a constitutional right.

(3) The constitutionality of a provision infringing upon a constitutional right will be measured by the compelling governmental interest standard under which the government must sustain the burden of showing that a challenged provision is justified by a legitimate governmental interest.

(4) In the past, courts, including the Supreme Court, have rejected moral repugnance, cost, desire to discourage, and administrative convenience, as insufficiently compelling or legitimate to sustain governmental action restrictive of a constitutional right.

In view of the foregoing, it appears that by eliminating abortion as one of the medical services that may be rendered indigent women under the Medicaid program, while at the same time continuing to allow all other medical services for pregnant women, the subject provision would be very likely to be held by the courts to create an invidious classification which restricts the fundamental right of women in that class to decide whether to have abortions. If this is indeed the prospect, the provision would conflict with the Supreme Court's decisions in *Roe* and *Doe* and lower court rulings interpreting those cases, and other Supreme Court rulings in analogous contexts, and would therefore be held to violate the equal protection standards of the Fifth Amendment.

In 1976, Congress Sept. 30 passed a controversial Labor-HEW bill containing a provision, approved by President Ford, that barred the use of federal funds disbursed through Medicaid for most abortions.

Both chambers had approved the bill's spending levels in August. The bill had not cleared Congress then because the House and Senate had disagreed on abortion. The House wanted a provision barring outright the use of the bill's funds to pay for or promote abortions; the Senate would not agree to such a provision. The final version incorporated a provision, worked out in a House-Senate conference committee, that barred use of the funds to pay for abortions "except where the life of the mother would be endangered if the fetus were carried to term."

Opponents of the abortion curb charged that it was discriminatory and unconstitutional because it would effectively deprive poor women of the right to an abortion. Supporters of the curb contended that the government should not fund operations that were considered immoral by a substantial percentage of citizens. (The New York Times Sept. 16 cited official HEW figures which showed that in 1975 between 250,000 and 300,000 women had received abortions that were paid for by Medicaid.)

Antiabortion proposals rejected. The Senate Judiciary Subcommittee on Contitutional Amendments Sept. 17, 1975 rejected eight proposed amendments to the Constitution that would have prohibited or restricted the right to abortions. The amendments ranged from one completely outlawing abortion to another that would have allowed each state to determine its own stand on abortion. The votes followed 18 months of subcommittee hearings on the controversial issue.

Sen. Birch Bayh (D, Ind.), chairman of the subcommittee, said after the votes, "I think the committee has spoken, at least for the duration of this Congress."

In 1976, the Senate voted April 28, by 47–40, to table another in a series of proposed constitutional amendments that would have outlawed abortions. While the vote was technically on a procedural question—whether the proposed amendment should be debated on the Senate floor—Jesse A. Helms (R, N.C.), the amendment's sponsor, said that a vote to table would be regarded as a vote for abortions.

The amendment sponsored by Helms would have barred all abortions, including those for women who had been raped or whose lives were endangered by pregnancy. Thirty-two Democrats and 15 Republicans voted in favor of the tabling motion; 20 members of each party voted against it.

Further Court Action

Stay on Medical abortion funds refused. The Supreme Court Nov. 8, 1976 refused to stay a lower-court order barring the federal government from withholding Medicaid funds for elective abortions. The lower-court order—issued Oct. 22 by Judge John F. Dooling Jr. in U.S. District Court in Brooklyn, N.Y.—had been sought by Planned Parenthood, the New York City Health and Hospitals Corp. and other parties. They had brought suit after Congress incorporated a ban on Medicaid funding for abortions in the fiscal-1977 appropriations bill for the Department of Health, Education and Welfare.

The stay, which would have barred the use of Medicaid funds for abortions while the case was under appeal, had been requested by Sen. James L. Buckley (R-Cons., N.Y.), Rep. Henry J. Hyde (R, Ill.) and others. Hyde was the sponsor of the aid-cutoff amendment to the HEW funding bill.

The Planned Parenthood suit had contended that the cut off on abortion funds discriminated against poor women by effectively denying them their constitutional right to an abortion.

HEW and the Justice Department had defended the law but did not endorse the request for a stay. In a communication to the Supreme Court concerning the request for the stay, the departments said they believed Dooling's ruling was "erroneous and [would] be reversed on appeal."

The Supreme Court ruling did not touch on the basic question of whether the Hyde amendment was constitutional. However, the ruling insured that federal Medicaid funding for abortions would continue until, or unless, the district court ruling was overturned on appeal.

The high court rejected the stay request in a one-sentence statement that did not record the views of individual justices.

(The following year the Supreme Court June 29, 1977 vacated, without comment, Dooling's 1976 decision that barred Congress from cutting off Medicaid funds for electrive abortions.)

1972 ruling on Medicaid reaffirmed—A three-judge U.S. District Court in Brooklyn March 10, 1976 had reaffirmed a decision it had handed down in 1972 barring the state from denying Medicaid reimbursements for voluntary abortions.

The state Social Services Department had appealed the district court's 1972 ruling to the U.S. Supreme Court, which had sent the case back to the lower court for reconsideration.

The lower court's 1972 ruling had been limited to the question of indigent women. The 1976 ruling broadened the issue to include all women, regardless of economic status. Also, for the first time, the state was prevented from withholding Medicaid reimbursements from women having abortions for other than health reasons.

Court orders elective abortions. The New Jersey Supreme Court ruled, 6–1, Nov. 17 that private, nonsectarian hospitals receiving government funds could not refuse to perform elective abortions. "Moral concepts cannot be the basis of a nonsectarian, nonprofit eleemosynary [charitable] hospital's regulations where that hospital is holding out the use of its facilities to the general public," Associate Justice Sidney M. Schreiber wrote in the majority opinion.

The decision overturned a ruling by Justice Herbert Horn of state Superior Court, who in October 1974 had upheld the regulations of three hospitals barring elective but not therapeutic abortions at their facilities.

The current ruling was in a suit originally filed on behalf of two South Jersey women, both on welfare, who had been denied elective abortions at the three hospitals named as defendants in the suit. The hospitals were Bridgeton Hospital, Salem County Memorial Hospital in Mannington and Newcomb Hospital in Vineland.

Since the three hospitals were tax-exempt and received financial support from the federal and state governments, Justice Schreiber reasoned, they were effectively "quasi-public institutions" that "must serve the public without discrimination." He added that there was "no valid distinction which justifies permission to utilize hospital facilities and equipment for therapeutic but not elective abortions."

The new decision altered the operational meaning of New Jersey's "conscience law" providing that no hospital would be subject to legal liability for refusing to perform elective or therapeutic abortions. To continue to follow this interpretation would be contrary to federal court decisions establishing the "constitutional right to an abortion during the first trimester. . . ," Schreiber said.

The decision affected at least 80 hospitals. It did not address itself to the right of hospitals run by religious organizations to refuse to perform abortions, nor did it clarify a staff doctor's individual right to withhold abortion services.

State funding not mandatory. The Supreme Court June 20, 1977 held, 6–3, that states and localities were not constitutionally required to fund elective abortions for indigent women. The decision, which came on separate cases in Pennsylvania, Connecticut and Missouri, was regarded as a major victory for the right-to-life movement.

The Missouri case, *Poelker v. Doe,* involved a campaign by St. Louis Mayor John H. Poelker to prevent abortions at his city's public hospitals. In an unsigned opinion, the Supreme Court, reversing a lower court ruling, held that the Constitution did not "forbid a state or city, pursuant to democratic processes, from expressing a preference for normal childbirth, as St. Louis has done."

Justice Lewis F. Powell Jr. wrote for the majority in both the Pennsylvania and Connecticut cases. The issue in the Pennsylvania case, *Beal v. Doe,* was whether the state could deny public funds for elective abortions without violating the federal Social Security Act. Powell, rejecting a lower court ruling, wrote that "encouraging normal childbirth" was an "unquestionably strong and legitimate interest" of any state and that there was nothing in the wording of the Social Security Act that would make the pursuit of that interest "unreasonable."

In the Connecticut case, *Maher v. Roe,* the high court reversed a lower court ruling that had found the state's bar on Medicaid-funded elective abortions beyond the first three months of pregnancy in violation of a poor woman's right to equal protection of the laws. (Connecticut continued to supply Medicaid funds for childbirths.) Powell wrote, "The state may have made childbirth a more attractive alternative, thereby influencing the woman's decision, but it has imposed no restriction on access to abortions that wasn't already there."

Powell said, "The indigency that may make it difficult—and in some cases, perhaps, impossible—for some women to have abortions is neither created nor in any way affected" by state regulations. The issue of whether the federal government itself legally could limit Medicaid funds for abortions was not addressed.

Powell rejected the argument that the withholding of Medicaid funds for abortions was an act of unlawful discrimination against the poor. "An indigent woman desiring an abortion," he contended, did not belong in "the limited category of disadvantaged classes" entitled to constitutional protection. Powell claimed the majority was not "unsympathetic to the plight" of such women and that its decisions in these cases signaled "no retreat" from the court's landmark 1973 rulings.

Justices William J. Brennan Jr., Harry A. Blackmun and Thurgood Marshall each issued sharp dissenting opinions. Brennan said the present rulings "seriously eroded the principles" of the 1973 decisions. Blackmun, the author of the 1973 majority opinions, called the present action "punitive and tragic" and said it would be an "invitation" for public officials under pressure from the right-to-life movement "to approve more such restrictions."

Marshall characterized the majority decisions as "vicious" and said they would "have the effect of preventing nearly all poor women from obtaining safe and legal abortions." He contended that the rulings would have a disproportionate effect on nonwhite women, those most dependent on Medicaid for health care.

The Supreme Court June 27 also vacated decisions of lower federal courts that had invalidated New York State and South Dakota restrictions on the use of Medicaid funds for elective abortions. The court also refused to review a New Jersey Supreme Court decision voiding bans placed on elective abortions by some nonprofit hospitals in that state.

Women's abortion rights extended. The Supreme Court, ruling on several cases in which abortion laws of Missouri and Massachusetts were contested, held, 6–3, July 1, 1976 that states could not require a woman to obtain her husband's consent before having an abortion. The court also ruled, 5–4, that states could not adopt a hard-and-fast requirement that women under the age of 18 get parental consent for an abortion. The court did say, however, that some form of state regulation for minors seeking abortions might not be unconstitutional.

In its landmark 1973 ruling, the court had affirmed the right of women to abortions during the first six months of pregnancy. (States were allowed to place certain restrictions—designed to protect the health of the pregnant women—on abortions during the second trimester). The 1973 ruling, however, had not resolved a number of issues related to abortions, of which consent by parents or husband was one.

A Missouri law, enacted in 1974, placed a number of curbs or legal requirements in those areas that the 1973 decision had left open. The court ruled on each as follows:

- Upheld unanimously a requirement that a woman give written "informed consent" in advance of an abortion.
- Upheld unanimously the state's right to require doctors to keep detailed records of abortions, so long as the requirement was not "abused or overdone" by state officials.
- Struck down, 6–3, a prohibition against employing "saline amniocentesis" after the first 12 weeks of pregnancy. The procedure was the most commonly used method of effecting abortions after the first trimester.
- Upheld unanimously the definition of fetal "viability" as the stage of development "when the life of the unborn child may be continued indefinitely outside the womb by natural or artificial life-supportive systems." The 1973 ruling allowed states to ban abortions of viable fetuses.
- Struck down, 6–3, a requirement that doctors performing an abortion endeavor to save the life of the fetus just as if the intention were that it be born alive.
- Ruled that doctors had standing to challenge in court laws barring use of Medicaid funds for elective abortions, because of their own interest in the matter (by a 9–0 vote) and because they could press the interests of their patients (by a 5–4 vote).

In the ruling on spousal consent for

abortions, Justice Harry A. Blackmun, writing for the majority, said, "The obvious fact is that when the wife and the husband disagree . . . only one of the two marriage partners can prevail. Since it is the woman who physically bears the child and who is the more directly and immediately affected by the pregnancy . . . , the balance weighs in her favor."

Dissenting from the ruling were Justices Byron R. White and William H. Rehnquist and Chief Justice Warren E. Burger. The same bloc formed the minorities in the other rulings, except for the one regarding the legal standing of doctors contesting medicaid laws. In the ruling on parental consent, they were joined by Justice John Paul Stevens.

The parental consent issue appeared in cases both from Missouri and Massachusetts. The Missouri statute was voided on this requirement, with the court reasoning (in Blackmun's words) that "the state does not have the constitutional authority to give a third party an absolute, and possibly arbitrary, veto over the decision of the physician and his patient . . . . Any independent interest the parent may have in the termination of the minor daughter's pregnancy is no more weighty than the right of privacy of the competent minor mature enough to have become pregnant."

The court, however, unanimously refused to uphold a federal court in Massachusetts that had struck down a section of a Massachusetts law that required parental consent for abortions by unmarried minors. The court noted that the law made an exception for minors who went to court and convinced the judge that there was good reason for an abortion. Therefore, the court held, the law might be interpreted in such a way as to "avoid or substantially modify" a constitutional challenge. The federal court should have waited to see whether the state courts interpreted the law in that light before ruling on it, the high court held.

The cases from which the rulings emerged were: Planned Parenthood of Missouri v. Danforth (74-1151), Danforth v. Planned Parenthood (74-1419), Singleton v. Wulff (74-1393), Bellotti v. Baird (75-73) and Hunerwadel v. Baird (75-109).

(The Supreme Court Jan. 15, 1975 had rejected an appeal by the state of Pennsylvania to reinstate the state's new abortion law, which restricted the right to an abortion by requiring a woman to obtain her husband's consent or her parents' approval if she were under 18. The law, which had been enjoined by a lower court pending further review, also banned use of public funds for abortions.)

Other Supreme Court decisions. Among other rulings of the high court:

■ Ruling Jan. 13, 1975, the Supreme Court unanimously affirmed a decision of a lower court that had overturned a Lousiana law that allowed the revocation of a doctor's license because he had performed an abortion before the Supreme Court legalized most abortions in January 1973.

■ The court June 16 held as an unconstitutional infringment on the freedom of the press a Virginia law—since amended—making it a misdemeanor to publish an advertisement for an abortion service operated in a state where abortions were legal.

■ The court Nov. 11, in a 9–0 opinion, warned state courts that they had "misinterpreted" the 1973 Supreme Court ruling legalizing abortion if they permitted persons who were not physicians to perform abortions. The high court said it had set aside anti-abortion laws as they applied to doctors but that it "did not go so far" as to immunize non-doctors.

State courts in Connecticut and Minnesota had applied the 1973 decision to protect non-physicians from prosecution, while New Jersey and Michigan courts had held that anti-abortion laws still applied to non-doctors.

■ The court Dec. 1, 1975 upheld a ruling permitting a private hospital that was government-funded to bar a doctor from performing abortions.

The Supreme Court March 1, 1976 declined to review a lower court decision allowing private hospitals that received federal funds to refuse to perform abortions and sterilization operations.

■ The Supreme Court Nov. 29, 1976 also upheld a decision of a lower court striking down an Indiana law that required abortions during the first trimester to be performed in a hospital or licensed health facility. The lower court found the bar to abortions in doctors' offices "clearly unconstitutional" in light of the Supreme Court's 1973 abortion decision. In upholding the ruling, the high court did not hear arguments or issue an opinion. Justice Byron R. White, in a dissent joined by Chief Justice Warren E. Burger and Justice William H. Rehnquist, objected to the summary treatment of the case by the court. White also contended that the 1973 high court bar to state interference in abortions during the first trimester should not be so interpreted as to prohibit regulations for health or safety.

■ The high court Jan. 25, 1977 affirmed without comment the decision of a lower court that barred Indiana officials from enforcing a state law that required minors seeking abortions in the first 12 weeks of pregnancy to get parental permission.

The court May 23 also affirmed a lower federal court decision voiding a Connecticut law requiring minors committed to the state's care to obtain the written consent of a state official before getting an abortion.

1976 Political Positions

In the 1976 Presidential election campaign, Republican President Gerald R. Ford and his successful Democratic challenger, Jimmy Carter, expressed their personal dislike of abortion.

Ford explains on TV. In a television interview with Walter Cronkite of CBS Feb. 3, President Ford stated his "moderate" position on the abortion issue, that he did not believe "in abortion on demand," did not agree with the Supreme Court decision of 1973 nor think that a constitutional amendment was "the proper remedy."

He favored "some flexibility." There were instances, such as rape or illness of the mother, he said, when abortion should be permitted.

The court decision, which struck down laws against abortion, "went too far," in his opinion, as did a constitutional amendment as a solution.

If there had to be action on the issue, Ford said, "it ought to be on a basis of what each individual state wishes to do under the circumstances."

He gave assurance that even though he disagreed with the Supreme Court decision, he would uphold the law as defined by the court.

If the constitutional amendment approach were taken, he preferred that it provide the states with more authority to restrict abortion than they had under the 1973 court ruling.

Party platforms. In its 1976 platform, the Democratic Party said:

> We fully recognize the religious and ethical nature of the concerns which many Americans have on the subject of abortion. We feel, however, that it is undesirable to attempt to amend the U.S. Constitution to overturn the Supreme Court decision in this area.

The Republican platform said:

> The question of abortion is one of the most difficult and controversial of our time. It is undoubtedly a moral and personal issue but it also involves complex questions relating to medical science and criminal justice. There are those in our party who favor complete support for the Supreme Court decision which permits abortion on demand. There are others who share sincere convictions that the Supreme Court's decision must be changed by a constitutional amendment prohibiting all abortions. Others have yet to take a position, or they have assumed a stance somewhere in between polar positions.
>
> We protest the Supreme Court's intrusion into the family structure through its denial of the parents' obligation and right to guide their minor children. The Republican Party favors a continuance of the public dialogue on abortion and supports the efforts of those who seek enactment of a constitutional amendment to restore protection of the right to life for unborn children.

Campaign statements. During the campaign, neither candidate seemed particularly anxious to turn the abortion situation into a major campaign issue.

Carter, speaking in Manchester, N.H. Aug. 3, touched on the issue of abortion. "We need to do something about teen-age pregnancies," he said. "We need a strong family planning program, better adoption procedures, better education, strong moral leadership to reduce or eliminate the need for abortions."

At a Sept. 8 news conference on the White House lawn, Ford supported the Republican Party platform plank urging constitutional protection of unborn children. It "coincides with my long-held view," he said, but he also said that "there should be a constitutional amendment that would permit the individual states to make the decision based on a vote of the people in each of the states."

Carter Sept. 9 said that abortion was a "very serious problem" for him. It was a "legitimate" issue, he said, and he understood the "deep feelings" of the anti-abortion demonstrators who were dogging his campaign trail and considered it proper for them to dramatize their view. But, he said, it would be "inappropriate" for him to "change my position to try to get their votes." Carter said he thought there would be an "adverse reaction" against any presidential candidate "who tried to take political advantage of an emotional issue like this."

Bishops review Ford abortion stand—President Ford received a favorable review of his abortion stand after a meeting Sept. 10 with a delegation from the National Conference of Catholic Bishops.

The bishops were "encouraged that the President agrees on the need for a constitutional amendment," Archbishop Joseph L. Bernardin of Cincinnati reported.

But the bishops were not "totally satisfied" with this position, Bernardin said, and the President was urged to adopt the "better approach" of supporting an outright constitutional ban. The bishops also protested to Ford about what they called an increasing number of federally financed abortions.

Neutrality in race asserted—Archbishop Bernardin called a news conference in Washington Sept. 16 to assert that his church's leadership was "absolutely neutral" in the presidential contest between President Ford and Jimmy Carter. The bishops, after a previous meeting with Carter, had expressed "disappointment" with Carter's stand on abortion.

Bernardin said the bishops had received a considerable amount of mail on their meetings with presidential candidates and much of it "expressed concern that we have endorsed one candidate over another. We have not done this."

The bishops' statements on abortion, he said, were not indicative of preference for either candidate or party and, furthermore, the hierarchy had not developed its position on abortion "in the context of what is sinful or what is not sinful."

The bishops' activity in this regard reportedly evoked widespread criticism from Catholic and non-Catholic groups and from clergy and laity among the Catholics.

TV debates—Carter and Ford held three televised debates during the campaign, and the question of abortion was touched on during an Oct. 22 exchange.

Asked whether or not it was "appropriate to the dignity of the Constitution to tack on amendments in wholesale fashion," Carter said he "would not work hard" to support any proposed amendments on gun control, school busing, balanced budgets, school prayer or abortion.

On abortion, he said:

> "I'm strongly against abortion. I think abortion's wrong. I don't think the Government ought to do anything to encourage abortion. But I don't favor a Constitutional amendment on the subject."

Carter made clear he would "honor the right" of others to seek Constitutional amendments on such issues.

Ford said he would support an amendment to outlaw abortion and favored a particular amendment to allow the states to make their own decisions by public referendum.

Carter on 'fairness.' As President, Carter told newsmen July 12, 1977 that he backed Supreme Court decisions on abortion as "adequate" and "reasonably fair." "The federal government should not be required or encouraged to finance abortions" except when the woman's life was threatened or the pregnancy was a result of rape or incest, he said. He thought the court's decision against federal funding of elective abortions "ought to be interpreted very strictly."

Carter was asked if it was fair that a woman who could afford an abortion could have one and a woman who could not afford it was "precluded from this."

"Well, as you know, there are many things in life that are not fair, that wealthy people can afford and poor people can't," he replied. "But I don't believe that the federal government should take action to try to make these opportunities exactly equal, particularly when there is a moral factor involved."

Religous & Other Developments

Bishops vs. abortions. A pastoral letter issued Feb. 13, 1973 by the National Council of Catholic Bishops warned Catholic laymen that anyone undergoing or performing an abortion "would place themselves in a state of excommunication." The message also contained unprecedented advice regarding disobediance of "any civil law that may require abortion."

According to the bishops, the Jan. 22, 1973 Supreme Court decision permitting abortions on demand was "wrong and entirely contrary to the fundamental principles of morality....The Supreme Court has certainly overstepped itself in making law rather than interpreting it." The bishops said they were "exploring all the possibilities" of overriding the court's decision.

Jesuit dismissed on abortion issue. The Rev. Eamon Taylor, provincial supervisor of New York Sept. 6, 1974 announced the dismissal of the Rev. Joseph O'Rourke, a member of the West Side Community of the Society of Jesus, who Aug. 20 had baptized the 3-month-old son of a Massachusetts woman who publicly favored a woman's right to have an abortion.

A local newspaper had reported Mrs. Carol Morreale, a member of the Immaculate Conception parish in Marlborough, favored opening a Parents Aid Society abortion clinic operated by William Baird. After the Rev. John J. Roussin, a parish priest, postponed the baby's baptism pending a review of the mother's beliefs, Mrs. Morreale's friends contacted O'Rourke, a board member of Catholics for a Free Choice, to conduct the baptism. Taylor said O'Rourke had been forbidden to perform the baptism.

In a related development, three Connecticut Roman Catholic bishops Aug. 13 warned Catholic doctors, nurses and other medical personnel that they would face excommunication if the bulk of their work involved abortions.

Catholic Conference sued. The Women's Lobby, an organization with a registered lobbyist concerned with legislation affecting women, sued the United States Catholic Conference to force it to register with Congress as a lobbying organization, or to refrain from influencing legislation, it was reported May 20, 1974.

At issue was the conference's anti-abortion activities in Congress aimed at overturning the 1973 Supreme Court decision on abortion.

The plaintiffs asserted that the "principal" activity of Msgr. James T. McHugh, director of the Conference's Family Life Division, was to secure anti-abortion legislation.

The conference said only a small portion of its $17 million budget was applied to legislation, $100,000 to the Family Life Division and $128,000 to its Office of Government Liaison.

According to Internal Revenue Service statutes, a non-profit organization could not maintain its tax exemption if registered as a lobby.

Conference takes action—The U.S. Catholic Conference announced Jan. 7, 1976 that it had formally asked the Supreme Court to reverse itself on liberalizing access to abortion. The conference also requested that the unborn's "legal personhood" be protected under the Fifth Amendment to the Constitution. In their campaign to amend the 1973 decision, the bishops contested the Court's creation of the category of "potential life."

Strong Vatican stand. A 5,000-word document issued Nov. 25, 1974 by the Congregation for the Propagation of the Faith and approved by Pope Paul VI, according to Vatican sources, said that "never, under any pretext may abortion be resorted to . . . . as a legitimate means of regulating births." Instead, the paper said, social reforms including improved adoption laws and aid for unwed mothers were appropriate.

Quakers accept abortion. A statement opposing efforts to ban abortion was adopted by the Quakers' General Committee at its annual meeting in Washington Jan. 26, 1975. The statement said:

> Members of the Religious Society of Friends (Quakers) have a long tradition and witness of opposition to killing of human beings, whether in war or capital punishment or personal violence. On the basis of this tradition, some Friends believe that abortion is always wrong.
>
> Friends also have a tradition of respect for the individual and a belief that all persons should be free to follow their own consciences and the leading of the Spirit. On this basis some Friends believe that the problem of whether or not to have an abortion at least in the early months of pregnancy is one primarily of the pregnant woman herself, and that it is an unwarranted denial of her moral freedom to forbid her to do so.
>
> We do not advocate abortion. We recognize there are those who regard abortion as immoral while others do not. Since these disagreements exist in the country in general as well as within the Society of Friends, neither view should be imposed by law on those who held the other.
>
> Recognizing that differences among Friends exist, nevertheless we find general unity in opposing the effort to amend the United States Constitution to say that abortion shall be illegal.

Baptists accept some abortions. Messengers to the 12.3 million-member Southern Baptist Convention were reported June 16, 1974 to have voted for the approval of abortion in cases of rape, incest, fetal deformity or possible damage to the health of the mother.

Methodists oppose abortion foes. The council of bishops of the United Methodist Church adopted a resolution April 4, 1975, after a meeting in Minneapolis, which upheld the "sanctity of human life" but opposed any amendment to the U.S. Constitution that would "outlaw abortion." Deleted from the resolution was a section which scored "one segment of the American religious community," a reference to Roman Catholicism, for trying to impose its values on the rest of the country. The deletion was made in order to preserve ecumenical relations between Methodists and Catholics.

Boston doctor convicted in abortion case. A Boston jury Feb. 16 found Dr. Kenneth C. Edelin guilty of manslaughter in the death of a male fetus after a legal abortion. Judge James P. McGuire sentenced him to one year's probation and immediately stayed the sentence pending the outcome of an appeal.

(The Massachusetts Supreme Judicial Court unanimously reversed Edelin's conviction Dec. 17, 1976.)

The prosecution contended the fetus was alive at the time of the abortion, some 23 weeks after the onset of the pregnancy. Its star witness, Enrique Giminez-Jimeno, a fellow hospital resident, testified Edelin held the fetus in the uterus for three minutes, suffocating it to make sure it would not live.

Dr. Edelin, who was black, said Feb. 16 that racial and religious prejudice had made a fair trial in Boston impossible. Ten of the 12 members of the jury were members of the Roman Catholic Church, which opposed abortions. Edelin said two alternate jurors had told him of instances of racial slurs made against him while the jury was sequestered, but the jury foreman denied the charge.

Members of several medical groups and women's rights advocates said the decision would make doctors fearful of performing second trimester abortions and could lead to having some aborted fetuses being kept alive by expensive medical technology. Anti-abortion advocates read the verdict as a victory in their drive to limit the effects of the 1973 Supreme Court decision that gave women and their doctors the right to terminate most pregnancies without government interference.

(In reversing the conviction Dec. 17, 1976, the state's highest court ruled that Edelin could have been guilty of manslaughter only if he had deliberately ended the life of a fetus that had been definitely alive outside the mother's body. The prosecution had accused Edelin of suffocating the fetus before it emerged from the uterus.)

Report links decrease in abortion deaths to legalization. A report made by a panel of the National Academy of Sciences showed a sharp decline in maternal deaths and injuries related to abortion since the liberalization of abortion laws. The re-report, released May 27, 1975, said that women who had had abortions since legalization had displayed no measurable increase in mental problems.

The project was lead by 11 specialists in the health and behavioral sciences who were named by the science academy's Institute of Medicine in early 1974. They were commissioned to make what members called "as objective an analysis as possible" of available abortion facts.

The impetus for the report was the 1973 Supreme Court decision that greatly liberalized states' abortion laws and the subsequent number of protests.

The report, titled "Legalized Abortion and the Public Health," noted that in 1961, when illegal abortions were common, there were 320 known abortion-related deaths. This contrasted with 47 deaths in 1973, with 16 attributed to illegal abortions.

The report noted that a healthy woman undergoing a competently performed abortion during the initial three months of pregnancy had only about six chances in a thousand of a major medical complication. During the second six months, however, the risk increased to 21 chances in a thousand.

Figures as to the number of medical complications when abortions were illegal were difficult to calculate, the committee said. But it cited a sharp drop in admissions to New York City municipal hospitals for two serious complications of abortion between 1969 and 1973. Incoming patients from septic and incomplete abortions, the report said, went from 6,524 to 3,253 in those years. Most restrictions on legal abortion in New York City were dropped in 1970.

At a news conference the day the report was released, a member of the committee said that a return to restrictive laws would probably lead to a rise in illegal abortions and the dangerous health consequences they entailed.

The committee also found that estimates of post-abortion psychoses (serious mental breakdowns) ranged from .2 to .4 per 1,000 legal abortions. This compared with the one or two associated with normal deliveries. Depression or guilt feelings reported by some women after abortions were usually described as mild and temporary.

The study panel cited figures indicating that 745,400 legal abortions were performed in the United States in 1973 and 900,000 in 1974. Of these, a third of the women were under 20, a third were between 20 and 25 and the remainder over 25. One in four was married and two-thirds were white.

The Associated Press reported May 26 that a Harris Poll survey had found that 54% of the American people supported legalized abortion, 38% opposed it and 8% were unsure.

In a related research development, Dr. William Peterson, a Washington gynecologist, reported May 20 he had developed a process that extended by a month the time in which a woman could have a suction abortion safely. He said he had performed the surgery on over 2,000 women who were beyond the third month of pregnancy.

Most doctors set three months as the outer limit for doing a suction abortion which surveys had found to have been the safest and least costly method presently in use.

Pentagon liberalizes rule. In a memorandum issued Sept. 17, 1975, the Pentagon reversed its policy restricting abortions performed in military hospitals. In 1971, President Nixon had ordered military hospitals to follow the abortion policies of the states in which they were located.

The Pentagon memo ordered base commanders in all services to heed the Supreme Court ruling.

23% of pregnancies aborted in state. About 23% of all pregnancies in Pennsylvania in 1975 were terminated by abortion, the state Health Department reported May 10, 1976. Of 43,319 abortions recorded by the department, 35% were performed on women under the age of 19. Health officials recorded 149,271 live births for the year.

There were 174 state-approved abortion facilities in Pennsylvania. They were required in 1975, for the first time, to keep records of all abortions performed.

Birth Control

Public Policy & Controversy

Birth control practices (with the exception of abortion) had gained wide acceptance in the U.S. by the 1960s despite the opposition of the Roman Catholic Church and other religious authorities to specific contraceptive methods.

'Family planning' defined. By the end of the 1960s, the term "family planning" had come into wide use in the public discussion and controversy over birth control. A "discursive" definition of the term "family planning" was prepared by the staff of the U.S. House Commerce Committee's Subcommittee on Health & the Environment. The definition:

family planning: the use of a range of methods of fertility regulation to help individuals or couples to avoid unwanted births; bring about wanted births; produce a change in the number of children born; regulate the intervals between pregnancies; and control the time at which births occur in relation to the age of parents. It may include an array of activities ranging from birth planning, the use of contraception and the management of infertility to sex education, marital counselling and even genetic counselling. Family planning has succeeded the older term, birth control, which is now felt to be too negative and restrictive in meaning. Birth control can be separately defined as the prevention of pregnancy by contraception, abortion, sterlization or abstinence from coitus.

Family planning bill passed. A bill authorizing $382 million for fiscal 1971–73 for family planning services and population research activities was approved by the House Dec. 8, 1970 and Senate Dec. 10 by voice votes. The measure sent to the President called for establishment of an Office of Population Affairs within the Health, Education and Welfare Department.

It also required development of a five-year plan for extension of family-planning services to all persons desiring them, for research programs and for training of personnel. Grants to state agencies were authorized to help provide family planning services. Low-income families were to have priority in receiving cost-free family planning services.

The original Senate version of the bill had been adopted by voice vote July 14. The bill, passed by the Senate Labor Committee July 7, was approved on the Senate floor without debate or dissent. It had been introduced by Sen. Joseph D. Tydings (D, Md.) with 30 co-sponsors.

The Nixon Administration had backed

a more limited measure with open-ended authorizations. However the committee, reporting the bill later passed by the Senate, had said that the funds authorized in the measure would make it possible to meet President Nixon's stated goal of serving the five million women in the nation estimated to be in need of family planning services.

The report of the Senate committee emphasized that the legislation included safeguards to insure that acceptance of family planning services would be on a voluntary basis and would not be a prerequisite for receiving other financial or medical aid.

A more limited House version was passed by 298–32 vote Nov. 16 before the final compromise bill was worked out.

Ford funds granted. The Ford Foundation April 4, 1970 announced grants of more than $14 million for programs designed to help curb world rates of population growth. The grants were announced in New York by McGeorge Bundy, Foundation president.

Bundy said the grants would be used to underwrite the expansion of basic research and training in reproductive biology and to develop new and better contraceptives.

Some of the institutions receiving the Ford grants were the University of Southern California Medical Center, $2.3 million; the University of Wisconsin, $1.1 million; the Worcester Foundation for Experimental Biology, $675,000; the Salk Institute of Biological Studies, $1 million; and the University of Kansas, $550,000. The World Population Council received $2 million in grants.

Expanded research sought. Roy Hertz, an associate director of the Population Council, asserted April 9, 1970 that advanced breakthroughs in contraceptive technology would require expanded research into the reproductive process. Hertz said "growing disillusionment" with present methods of contraceptives necessitated development of other techniques.

Hertz, addressing the annual seminar of the American Association of Planned Parenthood Physicians in Boston, said the reasons for the disillusionment were the known and unknown medical hazards and the difficulty in gaining widespread acceptance of the oral contraceptives and other currently available contraceptive methods among poorly motivated persons.

He said he was attempting to draw up blueprints for new birth control techniques that would circumvent the problems that had negated the overall success of the methods now in use. One approach, Hertz said, involved the vitamin folic acid, originally found in leafy vegetables. Folic acid was essential to the growth of the womb during pregnancy and to survival of the fetus. Hertz said he was seeking a substance that would interfere with the body's ability to use the folic acid. He said a substance known as prostagladin F2 Alpha was under study in England, Sweden and parts of Africa as an abortion-causing agent. Hertz suggested that should Alpha 2 prove to be safe to the woman, it could conceivably be used as a morning-after type of contraceptive.

Massachusetts law voided. The Supreme Court March 22, 1972 voided as unconstitutional a 93-year-old Massachusetts law that prohibited distribution of contraceptive devices to single persons although the same devices were legally available to those who were married.

Under Massachusetts law, persons who sold or gave birth control devices to unmarried persons were subject to prison terms.

Only Wisconsin, which had a similar restructive law, appeared to be affected by the court's decision. The court's vote in voiding the law was 4–3.

The issue came to the court in a case involving William R. Baird, a crusader for birth control. Baird was convicted in April 1967 of distributing birth control devices to a coed at Boston University and sentenced to three months in jail. State courts sustained his conviction but the 1st U.S. Circuit Court of Appeals voided the law under which he was convicted.

The opinion of the majority in the

4-3 vote was written by Justice William J. Brennan Jr., the only Roman Catholic on the bench. In his report, Brennan rejected the state's argument that the law was a proper exercise of the state's power to discourage fornication and protect people from harmful products. Brennan said this could not have been the state's real purpose because the statute applied only to unmarried persons.

Justices William Douglas, Potter Stewart and Thurgood Marshall agreed with Brennan. Chief Justice Warren Burger and Justices Harry Blackmun and Byron White dissented.

In a separate vote in the same case, the court voted 6-1 to overturn Baird's conviction. Only Burger dissented.

N.Y. curbs on contraceptives voided. **A New York State law that prohibited the distribution and sale of contraceptives to persons under 16 was ruled unconstitu-**tional July 2, 1975. The suit was seen as a test case whose results might spur other states into similar action. Among other provisions, the law had made it a crime to display or advertise contraceptives. The law also prohibited the sale of nonprescription birth-control devices—such as condoms—to minors by anyone other than physicians and limited the sale of nonprescription contraceptives to adults from licensed pharmacists. The case was *Carey v. Population Services International.*

According to the decision, arrived at by a panel of three federal judges, the law violated the constitutional rights of privacy, due process and freedom of speech. The decision overturned a section of the New York State Education Law which, in addition to prohibiting pre-16-year-olds from obtaining the contraceptives, also banned all advertising of the birth control products.

Michael N. Pollet, a lawyer for the family planning groups that challenged the law, pointed out that many other states had similar restrictions that might be contested. He said that the court decision in New York was the first "sweeping injunction on constitutional grounds" against such laws.

District Judge Lawrence W. Pierce, who wrote the decision, said that the state had asserted an interest in "promoting the morality of its young people by seeking to discourage promiscuity" by persons under 16. But he said that no evidence had been cited that showed a relationship between the restriction of contraceptives and sexual activity among young people.

Pierce further noted that the New York State Legislature already had created substantial exceptions to the prohibition on the distribution of non-prescription contraceptives to those under 16.

The ruling was upheld by a 7-2 decision of the U.S. Supreme Court June 9, 1977. Justice William J. Brennan Jr. wrote for the Supreme Court majority. On the issue of advertising, members of the majority concurred with Brennan in reiterating the court's position that certain forms of commercial expression were protected by the First Amendment.

On the other issues, the majority agreed, in various combinations, that the state had failed to prove its contention that access to contraceptives would increase sexual activities among the young; that minors, like adults, had a right to privacy in their sexual relations; that the Constitution did not support blanket prohibitions on the right of minors to obtain contraception (since it could not prevent them from obtaining abortions), and that the statutes discriminated against married New York State females aged 14-16, who were subject to the same restrictions as unmarried females in the same age group.

Chief Justice Warren E. Burger dissented without comment. Justice William H. Rehnquist also dissented, saying the decision "enshrined in the Constitution the right of commercial vendors of contraceptives to peddle them to unmarried minors through such means as window displays and vending machines located in the men's room of truck stops."

(The Supreme Court May 24, 1976 had affirmed, without hearing any arguments or issuing an opinion, a lower court ruling that voided a Utah ban on the receipt by minors of contraceptive services from federally funded welfare programs unless the minors had written parental consent. The lower court had ruled not only that the Utah ban was unconstitutional but also that it was inconsistent with the Social Security Act. The Supreme Court said that its sustaining of the lower court was confined to the judgment that the rule was inconsistent with the Social Security Act; the question of its constitutionality was not considered.)

U.S. drops condom-stamp plan. A plan for sending low-income teenagers sex information and condom stamps, first introduced in 1971 was dropped, it was reported April 28, 1975. The stamps were worth $1 for purchasing condoms. More than 43,000 boys, mostly in Philadelphia and Cleveland which were target areas for the first year's mailing, were sent the stamps, but only 254 were redeemed. The plan cost $100,000. The project director said the government's main concern was that the mailings might be construed as an invasion of privacy.

Condoms advertised on TV—Television station, KNTV, an ABC affiliate in San Jose, Calif. broadcast the first condom commercial in the U.S. July 23. It was for the Trojan brand. Following a deluge of criticism from viewers the station tentatively decided not to run it again.

But July 25 the station ran a Trojan commercial as part of its news broadcast and when it asked for viewer attitudes toward the spot it received calls that it said were 8–1 in favor of running the commercial. As a result of the response, KNTV decided to reinstate the ads.

The station was able to act independently because it did not adhere to the National Association of Broadcasters' code of ethics, which banned such commercials. Four hundred sixteen U.S. stations, about 60%, subscribed to the code and over 40% (about 3,000) of radio stations.

Family-planning service lack cited. Fewer than half of the 510,000 Pennsylvania women with low or marginal incomes who were in need of family-planning services were receiving them, according to a study released Feb. 12, 1976 by the Alan Guttmacher Institute, the research and development division of the Planned Parenthood Federation of America. The report estimated that meeting the needs of the 263,900 women in need of the services would require the expenditure of $30.6 million on family planning—$22 million more than the estimated $8.6 million spent in the state in 1974. It noted that the federal government provided 75% of the funds for the 175 clinics in the state operated by 100 agencies, with 20% coming from private sources and 5% from state and local governments.

The study, based on 1974 figures but said by an institute spokesman to be still valid, was prepared under a grant from the M. K. Kellogg Foundation as part of a nationwide series for the Guttmacher Institute.

Other items mentioned in the report included:

- Of an estimated 220,000 teenagers of all income levels in need of family counseling, approximately 150,000 remained unserved.
- Only 58 of Pennsylvania's 241 general hospitals reported the availability of family-planning services.
- Of all women between the ages of 15 and 19 served by organized programs, 56% lived in Allegheny and Philadelphia counties.
- More than 29,810 abortions were performed in the state during 1973, virtually all of them in metropolitan counties. Of the 39 hospitals reporting abortion services, 15 did not have identified family-planning programs.

Population Policy & Birth Rate

Demographer disputes 'ZPG' theory. Conrad F. Taeuber, associate director of the Census Bureau, took issue Jan. 13, 1971 with the view that zero population growth (ZPG) was necessary to conquer the nation's social and environmental problems. In a speech delivered at Mount Holyoke College (South Hadley, Mass.) and released in Washington, Taeuber said a "lower rate of growth is not an automatic solution to the problems which confront us."

Taeuber said "our population problem is one of tackling the agenda for improvement of our total environment" and that a lower rate of growth "would be only one element in the programs which need to be developed." Taeuber, who supervised the 1970 census, said three fourths of the counties in the nation were net "exporters" of people in the 1960s, suggesting that distribution of population was more important than the nationwide growth.

"Pollution, high crime rates, transportation problems and other social ills are not primarily a result of our rate of population growth," he said.

Taeuber said the nation's population increased 13% in the '60s while the total volume of goods and services grew about 60%. He said the population grew 63% between 1930 and 1968—a period during which petroleum consumption increased 300% and natural gas nearly 900%. Taeuber concluded, "changing standards and habits, in activities, technology and the style of life have much more to do with the accumulation and disposition of waste materials and pollutants than does the number of persons involved."

National population policy sought. A new coalition to support a national policy of zero population growth (ZPG) was announced in Washington Aug. 10, 1971 by Milton S. Eisenhower, interim president of Johns Hopkins University, and Joseph D. Tydings, former Democratic senator from Maryland.

The Coalition for a National Population Policy, to be chaired by Eisenhower and Tydings, included environmental and family planning organizations and such individual sponsors as United Auto Workers President Leonard Woodcock and Roy E. Wilkins, president of the National Association for the Advancement of Colored People.

The new organization backed legislation introduced in the Senate June 2 and in the House Aug. 3 to declare a U.S. policy of achieving population stabilization by voluntary means. The resolutions, sponsored by Sens. Alan Cranston (D, Calif.) and Robert Taft Jr. (R, Ohio) and Reps. Morris Udall (D, Ariz.) and Frank Horton (R, N.Y.), had the backing of 33 senators and 25 representatives.

A goal of the coalition would be a voluntary limit in family growth to an average of 2.1 children per family versus the current 2.6. Tydings said that even if the 2.1 goal were achieved immediately, there were so many young in the country that it would take 70 years to stabilize the population. At the current growth rate, he said, the population would increase from the present 208 million to 300 million by 2001.

The coalition planned to press for full funding of the $382 million authorized by the 1970 Family Planning Services & Population Research Act. Tydings said Congress had appropriated only $38 million for research and $80.9 million for services.

Tydings criticized the federal tax structure, which he said "encourages very large families and discriminates and penalizes childless couples and the unmarried."

MIT study asks end to growth. "The Limits of Growth," a study of current world production and population trends financed by the Club of Rome, predicted a catastrophic world economic and population decline in the next century, unless production and consumption habits were put under deliberate international control.

The study, conducted at the Massachusetts Institute of Technology (MIT) and set for publication in March 1972, centered on a computer model of the interrelations between such economic factors as population, natural resources, industrial and food production, and pollution.

If current trends continued, the report said, growing population and rising demand for production would deplete the dwindling supply of natural resources, including arable land. Recovery of resources would become far more expensive, leaving less capital to replace aging productive capacity, eventually causing a decline in production. This would in turn devastate the population through lack of food and adequate medical services, both of which require heavy investment of capital goods.

Various alternative sets of trends were fed into the computer, but zero population growth alone, even combined with new resource discovery, would only postpone the day of reckoning. A stable world economy with minimally adequate living standards would require "a Copernican revolution of the mind" away from growth and wastefulness.

Specifically, the report called for a halt to population and industrial growth, a reduction in pollution, an increased use of recycling, the production of lasting, repairable goods, and an emphasis on services such as recreation and education rather than consumer goods.

The study was directed by MIT professor Dennis L. Meadows, at the request of the Club of Rome, an international group of business and economic leaders.

Criticism of the study, reported Feb. 26, included charges by economists that the computer model bore little resemblance to complex reality, and that the study ignored possible new technological breakthroughs in energy and food production and in pollution control.

Fewer children born, predicted. Further indications of a long-term decline in U.S. population growth emerged with a Feb. 16, 1972 Census Bureau report on the number of children that married women expected to bear, and a report March 1 of a 6% drop in the 1971 fertility rate.

The Census Bureau report found that the average number of children expected by married women between 18 and 24, surveyed in 1971, had declined to 2.4 from 2.9 in 1967, and from 3.2 in 1955. Taking into account unmarried women, the Bureau estimated an overall expectation rate of 2.2, approaching the replacement level of 2.11, which if maintained for 70 or 80 years would result in zero population growth (exclusive of net immigration). By the year 2,000 the current finding would indicate a U.S. population total of 280 million, 25 million fewer than a 2.9 rate would produce.

The Bureau attributed the decline partly to a rise since 1960 in the average age of women at marriage, from 20.3 to 20.9, and in the proportion of women ages 20–24 who were single, from 28% to 37%. Among young married women, the two-child family was close to the norm, with 64% expecting two or fewer children in 1971, up from 44% in 1967.

The National Center for Health Statistics, it was reported March 1, said the 1971 fertility rate had declined to 82.3 births per 1,000 women ages 15–44, down from 87.6 in 1970, resulting in a 4%, or 159,000 drop in total births to 3,559,000. The fertility rate was the lowest recorded since 1940, and was nearly 50% below 1955, the peak post-World War II year.

Among the reasons for the population slowdown cited Feb. 16 by Charles F. Westoff, executive director of the U.S. Commission on Population Growth, were the use of contraceptives, liberalization of some abortion laws, "environmental ideology" and unemployment. Other experts cited the increased female role in the work force and the "marriage squeeze," or shortage of men born in the 1930's and early 1940s to marry women born in the subsequent "baby boom."

Birth rate drop continues. The National Center for Health Statistics reported March 1, 1973 that all indices of U.S. population growth had fallen in 1972 and that the crude birth rate had fallen to a record low.

The crude birth rate, the number of births per thousand population, dropped to 15.6 in 1972 from 17.3 in 1971, itself a record low. Total births dropped to 3,256,000, 9% fewer than the previous year, despite an increase of 878,000 women of child-bearing age, 15–44. It was the lowest total since 1945.

Total fertility, the average number of children born to each family, declined from 2.28 in 1971 to 2.03 in 1972, and fell further to 1.98 in the last six months of 1972.

Total U.S. population grew at a rate of .78% in 1972, the lowest rate since 1945, and less than half the rate of 1.83 in 1956, the peak post-World War II year.

A Census Bureau expert attributed the birth rate decline to the older average age of women at their first marriage, an increase in divorce, a rapid increase in the number of working women, increasing use of contraception and liberalization of abortion laws, which in itself might have accounted for about one-fourth the decline in the number of births.

Fertility rate at record low. The total fertility rate, a statistic compiled by the U.S. Census Bureau to help indicate whether the future population would decline or grow, was reported May 25, 1975 to have hit a new record low. It was the third consecutive year that the birth rate was below the replacement level.

The total fertility rate for 1974, projected onto the female population, meant that every woman would have an average of 1.86 children. The previous record low was 1.90 in 1973.

Campbell Gibson, the analyst who prepared the report, said it was still too early to tell whether the drop foreshadowed a long-term decline in the birth rate. The relatively sudden drop in the statistic suggested postponement, rather than abandonment of child-bearing, he said.

Gibson pointed out, however, that none of the recent figures reflected the full impact of the recession. Unemployment and reduced income did, traditionally, encourage lower birth rates. But Gibson noted that the number of women of child-bearing age, in relation to the general population, was larger than usual because of the post-World War II baby boom. Normally, that would mean a second baby boom when these women began their families, he pointed out.

The impact of that development had already been muted by improved methods of contraception, a tendency toward marriage and child-rearing at later ages, changes in the role of women and a general concern with environment and overpopulation, Gibson said.

But even if the current birth rate decline were sustained, Gibson noted, "we would be unlikely to hit zero population growth anytime before the year 2000."

The U.S. birth rate declined in 1975 for the fifth straight year.

The provisional natality report from the National Center for Health Statistics said the 1975 birth rate was 14.8 births for 1,000 population, down about 1 per cent from 1974's rate of 14.9.

The fertility rate was 66.7 births for 1,000 women aged 15–44 years, a decline of

U.S. Fertility Rates (1909-1971) **Births per 1,000 women aged 15–44**

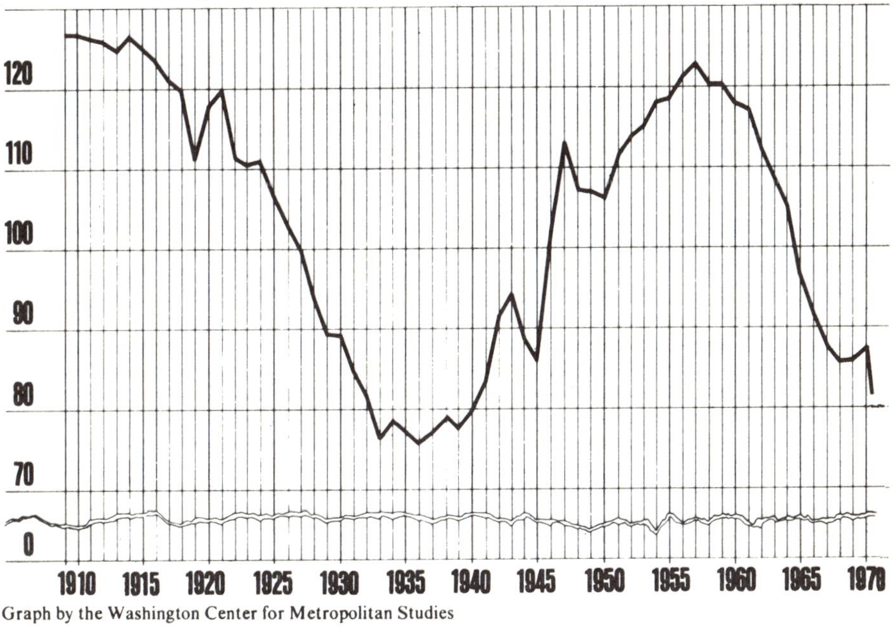

Graph by the Washington Center for Metropolitan Studies

about 2% from 1974. The fertility rate of decline had slowed from an average of 7% a year between 1970 and 1973 to about 2% between 1973 and 1975.

There were an estimated 3,149,000 live births in 1975, about 1% below 1974's 3,-159,958.

World population plan. A U.N. World Population Conference, held in Bucharest, Rumania Aug. 19–30, 1974, adopted a vaguely worded Plan of Action to slow the pace of world population growth.

The document, introduced in draft form at the beginning of the conference, was approved by acclamation after extensive revisions sought mainly by underdeveloped countries led by Communist and Latin American nations. It failed to set national or international population goals, or to focus on the possibility that overpopulation would soon overtax the world's supplies of food and other resources.

The plan subordinated population control to economic and social development, seeing the latter as the key to solving population problems. Countries which considered their birth rates "detrimental to their national purposes" were "invited to consider setting quantitative goals and implementing policies that may lead to the attainment of such goals by 1985." However, "nothing herein should interfere with the sovereignty of any government to adopt such . . . goals," the document stated.

The plan recognized that "per capita use of world resources is much higher in the more developed than in the developing countries," and urged industrial nations "to adopt appropriate policies in population, consumption and investment, bearing in mind the need for fundamental improvement in international equity."

It affirmed the basic right of couples to freely decide the number and spacing of their children, and to have the information, education and means to do so. Nations were asked to make these means and information available to their citizens, but no target date was set for compliance.

The plan also strongly recognized the right of women to contribute to economic development and to participate in all spheres of life on an equal basis with men. The improved status of women was described as essential in its own right and conducive to lower fertility.

(The plan's defense of women's rights resulted from extensive lobbying by an international group of women including anthropologist Margaret Mead of the U.S. and feminist writers Betty Friedan of the U.S. and Germaine Greer of Australia, according to press reports. There were few women among the delegates to the U.N. conference, but there were about as many women as men at the Population Tribune, a parallel, non-government conference.)

Delegates generally praised the U.N. conference and called the action plan a valuable initial step in approaching the world population problem, according to the New York Times Sept. 3. The chief U.S. delegate, Secretary of Health, Education and Welfare Caspar Weinberger, had lauded the plan Aug. 30 as a "landmark advance in international understanding and agreement on population matters." That "a population conference of 135 nations has been held at all has been a great accomplishment," he said.

However, delegates from industrial nations and many population and food experts privately expressed disappointment that the conference did not emphasize the need for urgency in finding remedies for population growth and its attending problems, the Washington Post reported Sept. 1.

"It will be said that the conference was convened on the eve of greatest famine and the the conference failed to recognize it," said Rene Dumont, a French agricultural expert who addressed the Population Tribune.

Discussions at the conference were often interrupted by political digressions, notably attacks by China against the U.S. and the Soviet Union. Chinese chief delegate Huang Shu-tse devoted the major part of his address Aug. 21 to a denunciation of the two "superpowers" as the "chief culprits" of the poverty of underdeveloped countries.

Huang said the alleged alarm of the U.S. and Soviet Union over the population explosion was "utterly groundless and . . . propagated with ulterior motives." "Each day the two superpowers talk about detente but they are continually creating tensions . . . Now they are trying to shift the blame for global problems on the Third World," he asserted. He said China opposed any outside interference in a nation's population growth.

Lev Volodsky, Soviet deputy health minister, told the conference the same day that "imperialists and colonialists" were responsible for the plight of the Third World, and that economic development was the key to resolving the population crisis.

At the Population Tribune, John D. Rockefeller 3rd, chairman of the Rockefeller Foundation and an advocate of family planning for 40 years, delivered an address Aug. 26 in which he reversed his long-standing position and proposed a birth control policy within the context of general economic and social development.

"I have changed my mind," Rockefeller said. "The evidence has been mounting, particularly in the past decade, that family planning alone is not adequate."

Rockefeller endorsed a new approach which "recognizes that rapid population growth is only one among many problems facing most countries, that it is a multiplier and intensifier of other problems rather than the cause of them. And it recognizes that motivation for family planning is best stimulated by hope that living conditions and opportunities in general will improve."

He called for a reappraisal of all work done in the population field, and a revision of "our concept of economic growth so that it could be consciously and deliberately directed toward human goals." Modern development should give greater attention to an "equitable distribution of the fruits of progress," and industrial nations should "assist in broadening the choices available to the poorer nations," Rockefeller said.

The Pill

The development of oral contraceptives—"the pill"—had been hailed by advocates of population control as a nearly ideal weapon in the campaign against unwanted births. The U.S. Food & Drug Administration (FDA) disclosed May 9, 1960 that it had issued its first approval of a birth-control pill's safety. The first accepted pill, G. D. Searle & Co.'s Enovid, had received FDA approval after a four-year test involving 1,500 women. Other birth-control pills were soon also accepted.

But disquieting reports began to surface to indicate that "the pill" wasn't always effective and wasn't always safe. By Aug. 3, 1962, the FDA had announced its intention to investigate the possible relationship between Enovid and the deaths of several women who had used Enovid or the British version of Enovid (Conviod). A number of cases of thrombophlebitis had been reported among Enovid users.

Birth-control pill caution urged. The Food & Drug Administration asked the nation's doctors Jan. 19, 1970 to familiarize themselves with the risks involved in the use of birth control pills and to explain to their patients the potential long-range side effects of the pills. The FDA sent letters to 381,000 hospital administrators and physicians, asking them to keep informed about the latest information linking birth control pills to blood clotting problems.

The letters, signed by Commissioner of Food and Drugs Charles C. Edwards, also urged the doctors to study the FDA's newly revised pill labeling system which cited the risks of thromboembolic (blood clot) problems in the use of the pills. The revised system was inaugurated in September 1969 after the FDA's Advisory Committee on Obstretics and Gynecology had conducted a full review of the pills' potential hazards.

"In most cases a full disclosure of the potential adverse effects of these products would seem advisable, thus permitting the participation of the patient in the assessment of the risk associated with the method," the letter said.

U.S. gets British data—The U.S. Department of Health, Education & Welfare received data from British medical authorities that linked the use of certain birth control pills to potential blood-clotting problems.

The British study, made public in December 1969, reported that there was a greater risk of blood clot problems in birth control pills with a relatively high content of estrogen than in those with a low estrogen level. All birth control pills contain synthetic estrogen, a female sex hormone, and progestogen, another synthetic hormone, to prevent ovulation, and if it occurs, to stop the implantation of a fertilized egg on the uterus wall.

The British study panel reported finding an abnormally high correlation between the incidence of thromboembolisms (blood clots) and the use of birth control pills composed of more than 50 micrograms of estrogen. When the British study was made public, many British women switched to pills with a lower level of estrogen. Many British companies voluntarily withdrew from the market pills that had an estrogen content of more than 50 micrograms.

Several leading U.S. physicians estimated that nearly half of the 8.5 million American women using birth control pills took pills composed of more than 50 micrograms of estrogen, either in combination or in sequence with progestogen.

'Mini-pill' testing halted—Syntex Laboratories announced Jan. 19 that it was suspending clinical tests of its "mini-pill" oral contraceptive pending further study of experiments that produced signs of breast cancer in dogs treated with the drug. The mini-pill was so dubbed because it contained only half a milligram of a progestin called chlormadinone acetate.

A spokesman for Syntex said that five dogs treated with the contraceptive developed nodules (lumps containing bacteria) in the breast tissue. One of the nodules, the spokesman said, was found to be cancerous.

The mini-pill was being taken experimentally by thousands of women in the U.S. and was marketed in France, Mexico and Great Britain. The Syntex spokesman said there had been no reports from any of the pills' users that unusual changes in breast tissue had occurred.

Senate hearings on 'the pill.' At Senate subcommittee hearings, which opened Jan. 14, 1970, prominent physicians disagreed on the potentially dangerous side effects of birth control pills. Sen. Gaylord Nelson (D, Wis.), chairman of the Monopoly Subcommittee of the Senate Select Committee on Small Business, said he had called the hearings to question whether the pills' manufacturers had deliberately under-emphasized the risks involved in using birth control pills.

Dr. Hugh J. Davis, a Johns Hopkins specialist in birth control devices, told the senators Jan. 14 that he feared that birth control pills may cause breast cancer that would remain undetected for years. Dr. Davis questioned whether it was wise to have "millions of Americans on the pill for 20 years and then [we] discover it was all a great mistake?" About 8½ million American women were reported using birth control pills.

Dr. Roy Hertz, of the Population Council and Rockefeller University, agreed with Davis. Hertz testified Jan. 15 that only two facts about birth control pills had been substantiated: the pill's high degree of effectiveness in preventing pregnancy and the pill's ability to cause blood clotting problems. Hertz said all doctors prescribing birth control pills should treat each patient as though she were part of a research program. He advocated such safety measures, he said, because too many important questions about the pill's long-range side effects remained unanswered. Hertz also cited examples of laboratory experiments in which animals treated with synthetic hormones similar to those found in the pills developed certain strains of cancer.

Dr. Robert W. Kistner, a specialist in research and treatment of illnesses related to the female reproductive system at the Harvard Medical School, disagreed with Davis and Hertz. Kistner said animals treated with birth-control hormones in laboratory experiments had produced a protective effect against cancer-producing agents. Among the patients at the Boston Hospital for Women, Kistner said, there had been no appreciable increase in the incidence of pre-cancerous conditions in the female cervix between 1964 and 1969 despite an increase in the number of women using birth control pills.

A third physician to testify Jan. 15 said the manufacturers of birth control pills had failed to inform doctors about the true risks of the pill. Dr. Edmond Kassouf said manufacturers were still distributing information that failed to say anything about current data linking such pills to blood-clotting problems. He said risks were often distorted or minimized and in some cases denied by the pills' manufacturers.

The Senate subcommittee resumed its proceedings Feb. 24 and heard a New York obstetrician link "panic" and "unwanted pregnancies" to the publicity generated by the hearings.

Dr. Elizabeth Connell, an associate professor of obstetrics and gynecology and the first woman to testify at the hearings, said "we are just beginning to see the first of the pregnancies of women who panicked in January, stopped using their pills and did not seek or use another means of birth control." Dr. Connell added that in New York some doctors were performing abortions on women who became pregnant since the subcommittee began investigating potential health hazards linked to the pill's use.

A second physician who testified Feb. 24 was Dr. Phillip Ball, who urged a five-year moratorium on the use of oral contraceptives because doctors "have been all wrong about birth control pills." Dr. Ball told the senators that he had refused to prescribe the pills for four years because of harmful side effects, including psychological changes in the users.

The director of the Planned Parenthood-World Population testified Feb. 25 that for all their supposed complications, birth control pills remained the most effective safeguard against "one of the gravest socio-medical illnesses—unwanted pregnancy." Dr. Alan Guttmacher said the potential side effects were secondary to the medical and social dangers of an unwanted pregnancy.

Dr. Guttmacher told the senators that the hearings on the safety of the pill had spread "unwarranted and dangerous alarm" throughout the world.

Pill warning. The federal government announced April 7, 1970 that it had accepted a compromise warning statement which would accompany all sales of birth control pills.

Three earlier versions of the statement cautioning women about the potential hazards of the pill had evoked strong opposition from some physicians and firms that manufactured oral contraceptives.

Secretary of Health, Education and Welfare (HEW) Robert H. Finch said the statement would be published in the April 8 edition of the Federal Register to allow comment from interested parties. (This was the initial step in making such a warning a required part of birth control pill packages.)

The new statement accepted by the government was shorter and less emphatic about the potential dangers of the pills than the others.

The warning, as revised, was inserted in the pills' packages beginning Sept. 9.

The FDA also required that physicians be provided with an 800-word brochure that reported the pills' possible side effects in detail. The pamphlet was written by the American Medical Association (AMA). It was left up to the physician to decide whether his patients received a copy.

The message said in part: "Do not take this drug without your doctor's continued supervision. Oral contraceptives are powerful and effective drugs which can cause side effects in some users and should not be used at all by some women. The most serious known side effect is abnormal blood clotting, which can be fatal."

The FDA had sought to have a 600-word warning statement carried in the pills' packages, one that FDA officials regarded as more forthright in warning women of the possible side effects of the pills, but the statement was cut after the medical profession and some pharmaceutical houses that manufactured the pills complained about the longer warning.

2 pill brands discontinued. Two large pharmaceutical houses Oct. 23, 1970 voluntarily discontinued the production of two brands of birth control pills whose chemical ingredients might have contributed to tissue changes in dogs. The action taken by Eli Lilly & Co. and the Upjohn Co. was made public by the Food and Drug Administration (FDA).

FDA Commissioner Dr. Charles C. Edwards Oct. 23 called the halt in production of the two brands of oral contraceptives "the only prudent course." At the same time Edwards said that there was no cause for alarm among women taking the pills.

The Eli Lilly product was marketed under the name C-Quens. Upjohn used the trade name Provest.

Edwards said that women using either of the two pills should continue to do so until their physicians told them otherwise.

The FDA had required continuing studies of the active chemicals in birth control pills and it was in one such study that dogs developed noncancerous nodules in their breasts when treated with large doses of two chemicals. One of those chemicals was an active ingredient in Provest. The other chemical was part of the makeup of C-Quens. The chemical in Provest was identified as medroxyprogesterone acetate, while the chemical in C-Quens was chlormadinone acetate.

'Morning-after' pill. A senior physician at the University of Michigan Health Service Oct. 25, 1971 made public findings that a "morning-after" birth control pill had safely prevented pregnancy in all 1,000 women of child-bearing age involved in a university study.

Dr. Lucile K. Kuchera described the study and her results in an article published in the Journal of the American Medical Association.

The pill used in Kuchera's experiment consisted of a synthetic estrogenic substance called diethylstilbestrol (DES), a hormone substitute used to relieve several female ailments.

In Kuchera's study, no pregnancies occurred among the 1,000 women, most of them co-eds, although almost all had had sexual intercourse without using contraception at a time when they would be most fertile. Calculations indicated that at least 20 to 40 of the women would have become pregnant if they had not used the drug.

The women in the study were given the DES-pills twice a day for five days, beginning within 72 hours of intercourse. The study was begun in 1967.

The Food & Drug Administration said Sept. 20, 1973 that it would require doctors to warn patients of possible side effects of DES when it was prescribed as a "morning-after" pill. In giving its approval to the use of DES as a contraceptive, the FDA emphasized that it did not consider the drug safe for use over the long-term. The FDA had announced Feb. 21 that it would approve the use of DES as a "morning-after" pill in emergency situations such as rape and incest.

For over 30 years DES had been approved for use in certain gynecological disorders. But it had been associated with cancer of the vagina and cervix in children of some women who were treated with it during pregnancy.

The decision to allow limited use of DES was criticized by Dr. Peter Greenwald, director of the Cancer Control Bureau in the New York State Health Department. Testifying Feb. 22 before a Senate labor and public welfare subcommittee, he said doctors would interpret the action on DES as a go-ahead and prescribe it whenever they wanted, despite the risks.

British study of pill safety. G. D. Searle & Co. May 22, 1974 released a preliminary report on a large-scale British study of the effects of using oral contraceptive pills. Financed by Searle, the study by the Royal College of General Practitioners was begun in 1968 and involved 46,000 British women.

According to the report, users of the pill faced distinct, though rare, health risks. Thrombophlebitis, blood clots in the legs, was found to be 5-6 times more prevalent among users than nonusers. Users exhibited a rate of high blood pressure twice that of nonusers. Oral contraceptives were also linked to higher than normal incidences of chicken pox and other viral infections such as stomach flu. This, the report said, suggested that the pill suppressed residual viral immunity from childhood.

On the positive side, the report indicated that oral contraceptives could reduce menstrual disorders, iron-deficiency anemia, pre-menstrual tension and benign cysts of the breast.

The report said the study had found among users a higher occurrence of lung blood clots, coronary artery disease and cervical cancer, but it said that the incidence of these conditions was too "small to justify any conclusions."

Oral contraceptive recalled. Modicon, an oral birth control pill manufactured by Ortho Pharmaceutical Corp., was being voluntarily removed from the market, it was reported Oct. 14, 1975. The company, a Johnson & Johnson subsidiary, said a routine check of pills had found reduced levels of estrogen, the active ingredient, in a small number of pills. However, the company emphasized that the move was only a precautionary one, pointing out that it was "not known if this reduction in estrogen lowers contraceptive effectiveness."

Ortho said that about 150,000 U.S. women, 1.5% of those "on the pill," took Modicon. The company advised women taking Modicon to continue taking it along with a supplemental contraceptive until their doctors could prescribe a new oral birth control pill.

A spokesman for the drug company said the problem appeared to be related to a chemical reaction between Modicon's estrogen, called ethinyl estradiol, and a red dye in the pill. Although several other companies used the same type of estrogen in some of their oral contraceptives, they were not considering recalling their pills. They discounted the Ortho findings in relation to their pills, explaining that theirs contained different dyes from those of Modicon.

Doctor changes stand on pill. Dr. Robert W. Kistner, a professor of obstetrics and gynecology at Harvard Medical School, who had spoken out against critics of oral conception and synthetic estrogens, Jan. 10, 1976 retracted his earlier statements on the subject.

Kistner acknowledged in an interview with the Washington Post that his statements regarding the safety of birth control pills and the use of estrogens in the treatment of menopause-related afflictions "cannot be substantiated." Kistner also said that he had given up research on hormonal agents seven or eight years ago and that he did not want to be known as an authority on the subject any more.

Sequentials withdrawn. At the request of the Food and Drug Administration, three major drug companies had stopped the marketing and distribution of sequential oral contraceptives, it was reported Feb. 25, 1976.

The discontinued birth control pills were Oracon, made by Mead-Johnson Company; Ortho-Novum SQ by Ortho Pharmaceuticals, and Norquen by Syntex Laboratories.

The FDA said it asked the drug companies to withdraw the pills because of new studies strongly suggesting that sequential pills posed an increased risk of cancer of the uterus.

An estimated two weeks' supply of the pill on the market was not recalled, the agency said. The sequential pills were used by 5%–10% of the 10 million American women who took oral contraceptives.

Birth control pill adds risk to smokers. The combined effect of birth control pills and cigarette smoking significantly increased the death rate among women over the age of 30, according to a report released March 30, 1977 by the Population Council, a private research group. The analysis was based on British and American studies that already had indicated that among women over 40, pill use greatly increased the risk of heart attack, stroke and death. The new findings were the first to distinguish smokers from other women.

The new data suggested that for women over 30 who smoked heavily (defined as over 15 cigarettes a day), the pill was the most dangerous contraceptive method and was more hazardous than pregnancy and childbirth.

Dr. Anrudh K. Jain, who prepared the report, called the combined effect of the pill and cigarette smoking "synergistic," meaning that the death rate among women who smoked and took the pill was higher than the combined death rates of smokers and pill users. One factor multiplied the effects of the other, a common phenomenon with certain substances such as barbituates and alcohol.

Among women aged 40 through 44 who took the pill and smoked, the death rate from heart attack was 62 per 100,000. For nonsmokers who used the pill, the heart attack death rate was 11 per 100,000; for those who smoked but did not use the pill, the rate was 16 per 100,000.

Higher mortality rates similarly applied to women in their 30s, who had a death rate of 10.2 per 100,000 among smoking pill users. Jain's findings suggested that even for women in their 20s who smoked heavily, oral contraceptives could be the most dangerous form of birth control.

Pill warning for doctors. The Food and Drug Administration said April 8, 1977 that doctors and druggists had to be told that birth control pills could cause birth defects, tumors, blood clots and, in women over 40, heart attacks. The action, directed at manufacturers of the pill, put into effect a December 1976 FDA order.

The warning would be included in "physician labeling," information for doctors and pharmacists that was included with the pill and governed advertising claims drug companies could make.

The new labeling described the pill as the "most effective method of contraception" except for sterilization. It identified potential hazards and necessary precautions for use of the pill. The FDA said it was studying a proposed requirement that women who purchased the pill receive a brochure containing the same information.

Sterilization

Rise in sterilizations. The Association for Voluntary Sterilization, a New York-based organization that kept records on the number of Americans who underwent voluntary sterilization as a method of permanent contraception, reported March 21, 1970 that the rate of requests for such operations was growing by over 100,000 each year.

The association also reported that nearly 75% of those who requested the operations were men. The male sterilization procedure was known as vasectomy. Five years previously, it was reported, almost all of the requests came from mothers with oversized families. The association reported that the number of requests it received for referral had quadrupled, from 825 in 1966 to 3,707 in 1969.

Another association reporting a significant increase in the number of callers seeking information about sterilization operations was the Margaret Sanger Research Bureau in New York. The bureau's manager March 21 said the group, which performed the operations for men, was "booked through the end of May." She said the association was planning to expand its facilities to accommodate nearly five times the number of operations it could presently handle in a week. The manager said the expansion was intended "to try to meet at least some of the demand."

Individual doctors, not associated with the Sanger Bureau or the Volunteer Association, also reported a rise in the number of requests for sterilization operations.

Sterilization program curbed. U.S. District Court Judge Gerhard A. Gesell ruled in Washington March 15, 1974 that rules proposed by the Department of Health, Education and Welfare (HEW) to cover federally-financed sterilizations of poor persons were "arbitrary and unreasonable" and failed to give sufficient protection to minors and mentally incompetent persons.

HEW had been attempting to draw up regulations because of disclosures of sterilization of retarded minors in federally-aided clinics and, as Gesell noted in his decision, evidence that welfare recipients had been threatened with loss of benefits if they refused sterilization.

The proposed rules said that legally competent adults must give "informed consent" to sterilization, and that minors and mental incompetents must give written consent approved by a third party in their behalf.

Ruling in a suit filed by the National

Welfare Rights Organization, Gesell said that neither minors nor mental incompetents could meet a standard of voluntary and truly informed consent, and that the "will of an unspecified representative" could not be imposed in a matter as serious as sterilization.

Gesell also said that the consent procedures involving competent adults must be amended to require that persons be informed that no federal benefits could be withdrawn because of a failure to accept sterilization.

Noting that in recent years 100,000–150,000 low-income persons had been sterilized annually in federal programs, Gesell said the matter was of major national significance. Government, including Congress, he said, should "move cautiously" to set regulations in "one of the most drastic methods of population control" which could irreversibly deprive unwilling or immature persons of their rights.

New sterilization technique reported. A new surgical technique for female sterilization that could be done in 15 minutes under local anesthetic was reported Feb. 10, 1975 to have been developed by Dr. InBae Yoon, assistant professor of gynecology and obstetrics at Johns Hopkins University. The operation, which was considered safer than more conventional sterilization operations, required the patient to stay in the hospital for only a few hours. It entailed a minor incision and the placement of a ring to close off the fallopian tubes. The procedure had already been performed on 1,050 patients in the U.S. and abroad.

Religion & Birth Control

San Juan clergy backs birth curb. The Most Rev. Luis Aponte Martinez, Roman Catholic archbishop of San Juan, Puerto Rico, Feb. 5, 1970 announced conditional approval by the hierarchy of a government-sponsored birth control program. Aponte clarified the clergy's position Feb. 7 by saying the church would cooperate in instructing the public on family planning and Puerto Rico's population explosion, but would oppose any massive propaganda campaign on contraceptives. The clergy's action came in response to a plea by Gov. Luis A. Ferre Jan. 14, which had called for an island-wide formal voluntary program of family planning orientation and services.

U.S. priests oppose birth edict. According to a study sponsored by the U.S. Roman Catholic hierarchy, a "substantial segment" of the priests in the U.S. believed that Pope Paul VI's 1967 encyclical against artificial birth control did not represent a "legitimate exercise" of his authority.

The New York Times reported Aug. 8, 1971 that this study of 5,000 active priests, 800 priests who had left the ministry and 250 bishops was circulated among U.S. bishops the previous week. The survey was conducted by the National Opinion Research Center under the direction of the Rev. Andrew Greeley.

The 400-page study found that 36% of diocesan priests believed that issuance of the encyclical was a "competent and appropriate use of papal teaching authority," 18% that it was within the Pope's authority but was inopportune, 33% that it was a misuse of papal authority because the Pope "failed to act with sufficient collegiality," 9% that it was beyond papal competence because the Pope "cannot impose concrete universal directives of the natural law," and 4% had no opinion.

Among the bishops surveyed, 72% regarded the encyclical as "competent and appropriate" and 25% expressed reservations. The report said 54% of the major superiors of religious orders believed the encyclical was either inappropriate or a misuse of authority; 42% gave their full approval.

Catholic rates drop. A report resulting from the 1970 National Fertility Study showed that the number of children produced and planned by Roman Catholic families in the U.S. was approaching the figures for non-Catholics, and that both were declining, it was reported May 29, 1972.

The study, funded by the National

Institutes of Health and based on a sampling of 5,600 married women of childbearing age, found that Catholic women aged 20–24 in 1970 wanted to bear an average of 2.75 children, down 20% from 3.45 in 1965. Non-Catholic women in the same age group wanted 2.35 children, down 9% from 2.57 in 1965.

Charles F. Westoff, one of the Princeton University demographers who conducted the study, said the figures indicated that "Catholics are becoming more and more like other parents in their use of the pill and other contraceptive devices."

Vatican position reaffirmed. Pope Paul VI March 29, 1974 reaffirmed the church's unequivocal opposition to birth control in a message delivered during an audience for United Nations officials. The Vatican also published the pope's prepared text, which cited his 1968 document, "Humanae Vitae."

A confidential Vatican document outlining a church campaign against governments and international agencies (widely believed to be U.N. groups) supporting birth control efforts had been made public March 11 by church sources opposed to the Vatican position.

The action, and several other unauthorized releases of internal church papers, prompted the Vatican to tighten security measures March 14. A three-page instruction book was published detailing a lengthy list of subjects given pontifical secret (or top secret) classification in an effort to prevent news leaks and limit inquiries. Punishment for violators ranged from reprimand to excommunication. According to the Vatican, the pope had personally approved the new regulations.

Birth Control Dangers

Dalkon Shield linked to death of 4. Another birth-control device was described in 1974 as possibly dangerous. A. H. Robins Co., a pharmaceutical manufacturer, informed 120,000 doctors in a letter dated May 8 that the Dalkon Shield, an intrauterine contraceptive device (IUD) made by Robbins, had been implicated in the deaths of four women, who had become pregnant while using the Dalkon Shield.

The Robbins letter stated that the company had learned of 36 septic abortions among women who became pregnant while using the IUD. Septic abortions were spontaneous abortions that sometimes caused a uterine infection called septicemia, a widespread blood infection. The four deaths cited in the Robbins letter were from septicemia.

As result of the Robbins letter, the Planned Parenthood Federation of America May 23 ordered its 700 affiliated birth control clinics to stop dispensing the Dalkon Shield and directed the clinics to inform its current users of the device of its potential dangers.

Robbins said 2.2 million women had been fitted with the Dalkon Shield since it was first marketed in 1970.

The Food & Drug Administration (FDA) June 28 ordered a ban on the manufacture and sale of the Dalkon Shield, and an FDA advisory committee recommended Aug. 22 that the ban continue until controlled trial experiments demonstrated that the shield was as safe as other IUDs. At a public hearing Aug. 21, the FDA said it had learned of 11 fatal and 209 nonfatal septic abortions among the women fitted with the shield.

But the FDA Dec. 20 ended the Moratorium on the sale of the Dalkon Shield. It said the manufacturer of the device had agreed to register all new users of the shield, as well as follow their progress. Data to be reported to the FDA by Robbins was to include the number and kind of adverse reactions, the rate at which the device was expelled by women and other details.

In October, an FDA advisory panel of medical experts had concluded that the Dalkon Shield didn't pose greater risk to women than other intrauterine contraceptives.

Dalkon IUD user wins suit, controversy grows. A jury in Wichita, Kan. awarded Connie L. Deemer $85,000 in damages against the A. H. Robins Co. in connection with her use of the Dalkon Shield, it was reported Feb. 8, 1975. She said that the device caused a perforation in her uterus and failed to prevent pregnancy. The case was the first of its kind to go to trial but was one of many similar cases pending against Robins. (Robins reported Oct. 20 that it had paid $1,548,000 to settle litigation, legal fees and other expenses from the various cases.)

The FDA advisory committee had discovered that the shield's multifilament string or "tail" could draw bacteria up into the uterus, and Robins announced Jan. 20 that it was recalling all unused domestic stocks of the shield and would not return them until a new mono-filiment tail had been developed.

The FDA, in a Senate hearing Jan. 28, pledged to control testing of the revised model in order to obtain reliable data on its safety. The promise was partly in response to complaints by the advisory panel, and the resignation of one of its members, that the agency had not done enough to control the testing of the new model. It was reported Jan. 21 that the Planned Parenthood Foundation of America and the U.S. Agency for International Development were permanently discontinuing distribution of the shield.

Robins then announced Aug. 8 that the Dalkon Shield would not be returned to the market. The manufacturer said that it believed the shield was "safe and effective" when properly used but felt that, because of unfavorable publicity, reintroduction of the device would be "difficult, if not impossible."

IUD's raise abortion death risk. The death rate from septic abortions was 50 times higher among women who continued to wear intrauterine devices (IUD's) after becoming pregnant than among those who used other methods of birth control, according to a study released by the Center for Disease Control Nov. 18, 1976.

The findings were derived from a survey of spontaneous abortion deaths in the U.S. between 1972 and 1974. The mortality rate among pregnant women who did not use the IUD was 0.28 per 100,000. In contrast, 14.8 deaths per 100,000 occurred among pregnant women who used the IUD.

FDA orders IUD labeling. Manufacturers of intrauterine birth control devices would be required, effective Nov. 7, 1977, to make brochures describing the potential risks and side effects of the IUD available to all women considering that method of contraception, the Food and Drug Administration announced May 6. The federal agency, which had originally proposed the regulations in 1975, also ordered uniform labeling for physicians that would include information on use of the IUD and dangers in prescribing it.

The FDA order required that doctors give their patients the opportunity to read the brochure before insertion of an IUD. Women could then evaluate rates of effectiveness and rates of adverse reactions.

Depo-Provera used in Tennessee. A Tennessee health official admitted Feb. 21, 1973 that his office allowed the distribution of Depo-Provera as a contraceptive for clinic patients and the mentally retarded. The Food and Drug Administration (FDA) had not approved use of Depo-Provera in the U.S. as a contraceptive because it had produced breast cancer in dogs and because scientists believed use of the drug needed more study.

The FDA had approved the drug for use in the treatment of pre-cancerous inflammation of the uterus and terminal cancer of the uterine lining. Used as a contraceptive, Depo-Provera would be injected for protection from pregnancy for up to three months.

Dr. Robert Hutcheson Jr. of the Tennessee Health Department said studies on Depo-Provera in other countries convinced state officials to use the drug in special cases where neither interuterine devices nor oral contraceptives would work. Hutcheson said Tennessee health officials had the same information as the FDA, "but they came to a different conclusion."

Hutcheson said all patients were told of possible harmful side effects. However, Anna Burgess, 21, of Cumberland County, Tenn., testified before a Senate health subcommittee hearing Feb. 21 that the State Welfare Department urged her to take Depo-Provera and at no time told her of possible bad effects or that the FDA had banned the drug as a contraceptive.

Upjohn Co., sole maker of Depo-Provera, stopped shipments of the drug to Tennessee when it found it was being used as a contraceptive, it was reported Feb. 21.

The FDA then approved limited use of Depo-Provera as a long-term contraceptive Oct. 10, but it ordered that patients be provided with detailed information of its risks.

Experimenting on People

Ethical & Legal Problems Vs. Need for Experimentation

Kennedy on benefits vs. responsibility. In a discussion in the Senate Aug. 1, 1972, Sen. Edward M. Kennedy (D, Mass.) sought to place in perspective the responsibility of society in the face of the dangers faced by human subjects of the medical experiments needed by society. This topic was part of a speech on the overall subject of bioethics. Kennedy said:

One of the most significant problems in this entire area is that of human experi-mentation. Historically the advance of modern medical science has traditionally made use of human experimentation, frequently with the scientists using themselves as experimental guinea pigs. Without some human experimentation it would not have been possible to develop the smallpox vaccine or to begin to cope with malaria. And the development of modern drugs is dependent on a certain amount of experimental drug use among special patient groups. Such drug testing has to be much more closely monitored and regulated than it has been in the past, but under the proper controlled conditions it has to occur; for human experimentation is an essential requirement for medical progress.

The thrust of my remarks today is not that human experimentation is inherently bad or that it should be banned or prohibited. Human experimentation is essential in a balanced program of medical research. But the problems posed by human experimentation—in medicine, ethics, law, and social policy—are enormous. How we resolve these issues will have a major impact on the lives of millions of Americans over the coming years.

The kind of impact human experimentation can have has been dramatically demonstrated in recent days with revelation of the tragic syphilis project at Tuskegee. The disclosure of a 40-year experiment on hundreds of poor, black men stricken with syphilis in Alabama, raises the specter of an Orwellian nightmare. Because we now have complex devices like kidney machines, and because we can now transplant a man's heart; and because we have now ended the deathly plagues of smallpox and polio—too many Americans have been lulled into a false sense of security about the powers and practices of medical science. But the news that a Federal agency—the Public Health Service—has used taxpayers' dollars to conduct a program to experiment on poor, sick, black people—without their knowing it—is an alarming revelation at best.

Many questions leap to mind with that outrageous news:

Why were not the patients treated with penicillin after that "wonder" drug had been discovered?

Why did the experiment include only men? And why were only black men included?

How many of those men are now in mental institutions, because the syphilis infection caused irreversible brain damage?

How many of those test patients fathered children who contracted congenital syphilis?

Are Federal agencies conducting any other such experiments?

And, why has the news of the Tuskegee experiment come to light right at this time?

Current Public Health Service figures show that nearly 100,000 new cases of syphilis were reported nationwide in 1971. During 1970 and 1971, the increase in reported cases rose 8 percent and 15 percent respectively. Those alarming rates definitely suggest that syphilis has reached epidemic proportions. Health authorities are particularly concerned at the fact that especially high rates are reported among our Nation's young people.

Can it be that the news about the 40-year-old Tuskegee experiment is intended to appease the national concern over the current syphilis epidemic? Since some health officials insist that treatment of the few Tuskegee survivors is useless—do they also plan to announce that treatment of today's teenagers is not required? . . .

The Tuskegee case is perhaps the most striking and heart-rending instance of human experimentation which has yet been brought to light. But many other cases exist. Some involve clearcut violations of human rights, as in Tuskegee. But many others involve complex problems of fact, of law, of medical judgment, of ethics, and social policy. The range of issues involved can be seen from the following examples:

At an institution for the mentally retarded, children were deliberately exposed to hepatitis to study the problems involved in developing immunity to the disease. The issues in this case are complex. The families of the children apparently did give their consent to the procedure, but many authorities on medical ethics question whether parents have the moral right to "volunteer" their children for experiments. And even when parents do volunteer their children in such a case, are they doing so under some subtle pressure which prevails when children are inmates of such an institution?

Another factor in this case was the fact that almost all children in this particular institution would contract hepatitis sooner or later, whether or not they were deliberately exposed. So the doctor in charge of the research asserted that deliberately exposing them under controlled conditions did not increase the danger to them. Others have argued, however, that the problem lies with the inadequate conditions at the institution. If proper sanitation were maintained, they would not contract the disease as a normal matter of course. I think this case illustrates the kind of problems we have to face in this area.

Another case involves experimenting with prisoners. In one case, prisoners who were particularly prone to serious violence have been subjected to brain surgery to try to alter their behavior characteristics and inhibit or destroy their tendency toward violence. Some medical authorities argue that this is a perfectly acceptable procedure for such cases. But others assert that it is merely a way of turning the prisoners into vegetables who will not have the capacity for violence after their operation. Even if the medical profession were to determine that this is a sound procedure in certain cases, who is to determine which individuals have a strong-enough tendency to violence that can only be treated by surgery? And what procedures are they to follow in making that decision? And even if certain individuals were singled out by such a procedure, how would they volunteer to have the operation? In their situation could they really understand all the facts involved? And can any prisoner, who is in an inherently coercive situation, really "volunteer" for anything? In this connection it is worth noting that in Great Britain the use of prisoners in human experimentation is prohibited by law, on the grounds that prisoners cannot really volunteer, in the true sense of volunteering. This problem of "what it means to volunteer" also applies to individuals in mental institutions and to patients with a terminal illness, who may be desperate to try anything.

Another case, which was the subject of a recent Washington Post editorial, involved 398 women who were mostly Mexican-Americans. In a study funded by AID, the women were divided into three groups. One group was given regular commercially marketed birth control pills. Another group was given an experimental pill which had not yet been tested out in terms of its effectiveness or its safety. The third group was given a placebo or fake pill with no effect. The startling point about this experiment, however, was that the women were not told they were participating in an experiment. Thus all the women thought they were taking birth control pills which were effective. The sad result of this experiment was that a number of the women who took the placebo or fake pill gave birth to unwanted children, with all the potential tragedy that that portends. And the experimental pill was later declared to be unsafe for human use by FDA, so that the women in that group were using a dangerous medication without knowledge that it was being administered to them.

One of the AID officials involved in dealing with the study was quoted in the press as commenting:

"The potential benefits to humanity in this kind of study outweigh the potential risks to the individual subjects."

Perhaps there is someone wise enough to make such judgments, but the essence of democracy is that we do not delegate to any officials the right to make such decisions for others. Free choice is at the basis of our Nation, and if we once allow that right to be eroded—regardless of for what purported humanitarian purposes—we have lost one of our most precious rights.

We cannot permit Government bureaucrats to make decisions which place others into experimental situations without their full knowledge and without their volunteering to participate. We must establish a national policy for human experimentation which safeguards this right and which provides Government officials with procedures to guide their actions on such matters.

Another case involving 525 members of the Air Force who had strep sore throats. It was common medical knowledge at the time of this incident that treatment with penicillin could prevent strep throat from developing into rheumatic fever; but that without penicillin some of the airmen would be likely to develop rheumatic fever. The doctors running this experiment were aware of these facts; yet they wanted to learn what the effects of withholding penicillin would be. So none of the 525 airmen received penicillin, and at least 25 of the airmen contracted rheumatic fever. According to the testimony we received at our hearing last November, none of these airmen knew they were being experimented on; they were certainly not volunteering with awareness of what was involved.

Another case of a group of 80 to 100 terminal cancer patients who were being treated with whole-body radiation at a civilian general hospital. The hospital had a contract with the Defense Department to study the effects of the whole-body radiation on the cancer patients. The results were provided to DOD for use in planning with respect to nuclear warfare; for the whole-body radiation which the patients received had some similarity to what soldiers would experience on a battlefield if they were exposed to radiation from a nuclear explosion.

There is nothing inherently wrong with such a project provided that the radiation dosage which the patients received was not affected by the requirements of the DOD contract; and that the patients knew the nature of the research they were participating in and freely volunteered to do so, after having a thorough explanation of what was involved. However, because there was considerable confusion about the facts of the case, a controversy developed with charges and countercharges being made about the project. As a result of this controversy the institution at which this treatment occurred has since suspended the project, and indicated that if it is resumed in the future it will not be with defense department funds.

I have no intent in mentioning this case to criticize the Defense Department or the institution involved. The point is that adequate policies and procedures were lacking for handling such a situation, and as a result controversy and confusion developed which were certainly not beneficial to DOD to the institution involved, or to the individual patients who participated in the research. . . .

A final illustration of the problems involved in human experimentation also involves DOD funding of a project at a civilian medical institution. This case involves patients who have cancer of the eye, and whose eyes are going to be removed in an operation. Shortly before they are due for the operation, their diseased eye is subjected to an intense beam of radiation, similar to what military personnel would receive if they witnessed a nuclear explosion in the distance. After the diseased eye is removed, the tissue is studied to help in military planning with respect to nuclear conflict. Again the case is not cited in a critical vein, but merely to indicate the existence of such projects and the need to assure that there are adequate policies and procedures to safeguard the rights of the individuals involved.

I think the foregoing examples show the range and complexity of the problems involved in human experimentation. . . .

Let me reemphasize the point that human experimentation under appropriate safeguards is an essential part of medical research. And the Defense Department has many legitimate requirements to conduct and sponsor human experimentation.

For example, when military test pilots test a new aircraft, they may have their physiological responses monitored to help in evaluating the plane and in preparing for its use in normal operations. This is a form of human experimentation, and it is of course fully justified, even though the subject's participation may involve serious risk of substantial injury or death to himself. He volunteers for such service with full knowledge of what is involved.

Similarly, testing out new undersea vehicles or deepsea diving techniques can involve substantial danger to the volunteers involved, and is a form of human experimentation, but again is fully justified. And in more conventional terms, the military has to experiment with human reactions to night combat, to undue stress and strain, and to a host of other situations which occur in military activity. . . .

Ethics panels created. The Wall Street Journal reported April 14, 1971 that there had been a large increase in the creation of medical-ethics committees at hospitals involved in research using human subjects. These committees are usually composed of doctors who are involved neither in the research nor in the treatment of the patients involved. The article, by Liz Roman Gallese, said:

Some hospitals have had ethics committees for many years. But the real impetus to establish them came in 1966, when the National Institutes of Health decided not to award research grants to hospitals or other institutions that don't have such panels. In that year there were 371 committees; today there are more than 1,900. The NIH made grants totaling $827 million in 1970, thus financing a major part of U.S. medical research

Sen. Edward Kennedy, discussing the issues raised by the article, told the Senate July 19:

One of the cardinal principles that medical-ethics committees must be guided by is the necessity to obtain the fully informed consent of every patient involved in a research project. If the patient is a minor, the consent of the parents is also required. But the Wall Street Journal article points out cases where obtaining the necessary consent presents special problems. For example, one study conducted by a Johns Hopkins University researcher involved juvenile delinquents in State institutions. One of the concerns of the American Civil Liberties Union was that proper safeguards were not being used to prevent parents from feeling coerced into giving permission.

Difficult problems arise, in many cases. Sometimes, according to Dr. John E. Plager, a member of the ethics committee at Roswell Park Memorial Institute in Buffalo:

> Real, informed consent would send patients into acute anxiety and terrify them.

New law monitors research. President Richard M. Nixon July 12, 1974 signed into law the recently approved National Research Act, which created a commission to monitor the use of human subjects in biomedical research and established a biomedical research training awards program. The bill had been passed by the Senate 72–14 June 27 and by the House 311–10 June 28.

The first U.S. legislation ever to consider the ethical questions of medical research, the act aimed at developing guidelines for research involving humans. A temporary, two-year commission appointed by the secretary of health, education and welfare (HEW)—to be succeeded July 1, 1976 by a permanent National Advisory Council for the Protection of Subjects of Biomedical and Behavioral Research—would study and make recommendations on controversial research and procedures. The temporary commission would pay close attention to research on children, prisoners, the mentally ill and live human fetuses, as well as psychosurgery, a brain operation designed to control behavior.

The commission would be without any power to enforce its recommendations and could be overruled by the HEW secretary, who would be only required to publish his reasons for rejecting the proposed guidelines. However, the permanent commission would not be obligated to publish its recommendations nor could it be overridden by the HEW secretary.

The act also required appointment of the 11-member temporary commission within 60 days of the bill's signing. Within four months of the members' appointment, the commission would recommend policies for research involving live human fetuses. Until these recommendations were presented, all fetal research using HEW funds would be prohibited, except to save the lives of infants.

Controversial Experiments

Hepatitis breakthrough. Researchers at New York University's (NYU) Medical Center in New York reported March 29, 1971 that they had apparently succeeded in immunizing a handful of children against serum hepatitis, a highly infectious and sometimes fatal liver disease.

Serum hepatitis, one of two virus diseases that involved inflammation of the liver, affected more than 150,000 Americans a year, claiming about 3,000 lives. Unlike infectious hepatitis, which was spread through contaminated food and water, serum hepatitis was generally transmitted by blood transfusions from a carrier.

The breakthrough was announced by Dr. Saul Krugman, head of the NYU research team.

In the tests described by Krugman, 14 retarded children at the Willowbrook State School were inoculated with a protective serum containing Australia antigen, a virus-like particle assoicated with serum hepatitis. Krugman said serum containing the antigen normally would transmit the disease, but that boiling apparently eliminated the infectiousness factor without affecting its ability to stimulate antibodies in the body of a patient that protect against the disease.

Ten of the 14 were inoculated with a single shot. The single injection protected five of them against a subsequent injection of infecting serum. The other four children were inoculated twice. In each case the two injections gave complete protection when an attempt was made four months later to infect them.

Willowbrook, like most other institutions for the mentally retarded, had a high rate of hepatitis and dysentery, due in part to crowded living conditions. Young children were used in the tests because hepatitis tended to be a much milder disease in children than in adults.

Krugman emphasized that his research team had obtained written consent for the tests from parents of the children involved. He said the experiments had been reviewed with government health officials before they started.

Krugman's use of retarded children for the experiments had been criticized by some legislators and physicians.

Harrison J. Goldin, a New York state senator, had called the tests "irresponsible and reprehensible" and said he considered it an outrage that mentally retarded children were used.

Another scientist, however, said Krugman had been unjustly criticized. Dr. Alfred M. Prince of the New York Blood Center said the hepatitis studies at Willowbrook and at other institutions needed to be enlarged.

Black men untreated in Tuskegee syphilis experiment. Some of the details of a U.S. syphilis study involving 600 Alabama black men that dated back to 1932 were made public July 25, 1972 in an Associated Press report.

According to AP reporter Jean Heller, the U.S. Public Health Service (PHS) conducted the study in which 400 black men with syphilis went untreated, even after a cure for the disease was known. The other 200 men, who had no syphilis, were monitored as a control group.

The study, Heller said, was organized to determine from autopsies what untreated syphilis did to the human body.

Dr. Merlin K. DuVal, assistant secretary of health, education and welfare for health and scientific affairs, said July 25 he would begin an investigation at once. Other federal health officials said they were giving whatever medical services they could to the project's survivors while they continued to chart the disease's course.

The experiment, known as the Tuskegee Study, was begun by the PHS in 1932 with 600 black men from Tuskegee, Ala. At that time, Tuskegee had the highest syphilis rate in the nation. The men were induced to join the program with promises of free lunches, free transportation, free medicine for any disease other than syphilis and free burial after autopsies were performed. Four hundred of the group had syphilis and never received deliberate treatment for it. The other 200 had no syphilis and received no specific therapy.

The study was begun 10 years before scientists found penicillin to be a cure for syphilis. But even after penicillin's healing qualities were known, the group of 400 with syphilis were not treated with it.

According to the AP report, a 1969 study by the PHS's Center for Disease Control in Atlanta found that seven men of the original syphilitic group of 400 had died of the disease. Another 154 died of heart failure that U.S. health officials said was not specifically related to syphilis.

A Health, Education & Welfare Department (HEW) advisory panel said in a report made public June 13, 1973 that the syphilis study had been "ethically unjustified." The panel recommended that a permanent governmental authority be established to regulate all federally supported research involving human subjects.

CIA subject of LSD experiment committed suicide in 1953. The widow and the children of a Central Intelligence Agency (CIA) employe who killed himself in 1953 after unknowingly taking LSD in a job-related experiment learned the circumstances of his death only after reading the Rockefeller Commission report on CIA activities, published in June 1975, according to July 10 news accounts.

The family of Frank R. Olson—his wife, Alice, his sons Nils and Eric and his married daughter Lisa Hayward—decided after weeks of discussion to contact reporters "to get the story out, so our father's friends and colleagues—and also our friends—could know what the CIA has done," the New York Times July 10 quoted Eric Olson as saying. The Times also said that David W. Belin, director of the Rockefeller panel, had confirmed Olson's death. Belin added: "The staff didn't feel it was necessary to talk to the family. They didn't know what it would add—once we found out what had happened."

In a statement given to reporters at the family home in Frederick, Md., Mrs. Olson said her husband had been a researcher for the CIA in biological warfare at nearby Fort Detrick, Md., and that two weeks before his death he had attended several days of meetings and been given LSD "without his knowledge or consent." He returned home and "was very quiet, he was an entirely different person," Mrs. Olson said. "I didn't know what had happened. I just knew that something was terribly wrong. The entire weekend he was very melancholy and talked about a mistake he had made. He said he was going to leave his job." During the following week, Olson was taken to New York City to consult Dr. Harold A. Abramson, a psychiatrist, and several days later his family was told he had committed suicide by jumping from the 10th floor of the Statler Hotel in Manhattan. Mrs. Olson declared that a CIA employe, her husband's escort, had told of waking up at 1:30 a.m. and seeing Olson run across the room and jump through both a closed window and a drawn shade.

The New York Times July 11 cited a 1953 police report by Detective James W. Ward which gave another version of Olson's visit to New York. It said he had arrived with Col. Vincent Ruwet, also attached to Fort Detrick, and had returned to Washington after two consultations with Dr. Abramson. When Olson came back to New York later that day, according to Ward's report, he was accompanied by a man who called himself Robert Lashbrook. "They again visited the doctor and as a result of this visit Olson was advised to enter a sanitarium as he was suffering from severe psychosis and delusions," Ward said. That night, Lashbrook told Ward, he woke up at about 3:20 a.m. to a "crash of glass," telephoned the hotel operator and, "at this time, learned that Olson had jumped out of the window."

The New York Times July 12 said the Olson family believed Lashbrook and a man they identified as Sidney Gottlieb had given the drug to Frank Olson, but the CIA refused to say whether either Lashbrook or Gottlieb had ever been employed by the agency.

The Washington Post July 13 reported a telephone interview the previous day with James Roethe, the attorney in charge of the Rockefeller Commission's study, who said the document did not contain all the panel had learned about CIA drug experiments. Roethe said: "I really don't feel that I'm going to be in a position to make a comment unless something so outrageous comes out that I feel I have to, and at this point I haven't seen anything." The Post printed a list of names, furnished by the Olson family, of those present at the 1953 meeting in which Frank Olson and others were given the LSD.

Lashbrook says Olson agreed—Robert V. Lashbrook, a former CIA employe who was with Frank Olson at the time of his suicide in 1953, said July 17 that Olson had agreed in principle beforehand to be the subject of an LSD experiment.

In a telephone interview with the New York Times, Lashbrook, now a high school science teacher in Ojai, Cal., declared: "It was my understanding that actually everyone there had agreed in advance that such a test would be conducted, that they were willing to be one of the subjects. The only thing was that the time was not specified." He said it would be "misconstruing things quite a lot to say that any individual or group of individuals were the subject of anyone doing them in." In its account of the interview with Lashbrook, the New York Times July 18 quoted a section of the Rockefeller Commission report that said: "Prior to receiving the LSD, the subject [Olson] had participated in discussions where the testing of such substances on unsuspecting subjects was agreed to in principle. However, this individual was not aware that he had been given LSD until about 20 minutes after it had been administered."

Lashbrook said he himself had been a "guinea pig" several times in LSD tests and "didn't like it." He noted, however, that any "direct relationship" between the drug and Olson's death "would be a little hard to justify" because Olson's body would have eliminated all elements of the drug long before his death, which took place more than a week after the experiment. "Possibly LSD had brought up something in his past that was bothering him," Lashbrook ventured.

The Washington Post July 18 reported that when asked who had decided to administer the drug to Olson and when, Lashbrook replied he was "not too sure" and that "in any case, I don't really want to name them."

Gottlieb destroyed LSD data—The New York Times July 18 reported that Dr. Sidney Gottlieb, a biochemist and former head of the CIA's program of testing LSD, had destroyed the program's records in 1973, ten years after the experiments were believed to have been halted.

The Times, alluding to sources on the staff of the Rockefeller Commission, said Gottlieb had thrown out a total of 152 separate files and that Richard Helms, then director of the agency, had also destroyed records.

Olson files released—Alice Olson, Frank Olson's widow, made public Jan. 10, 1976 the CIA documents that dealt with her husband's death. She had received the documents after President Ford ordered the CIA to turn them over to her.

The attorneys for the Olson family said that the documents, although containing "inaccuracies and self-serving statements," nevertheless "make it quite clear that Frank Olson was unknowingly given LSD by CIA officials as a result of which he died on Nov. 28, 1953, and that an intentional cover-up followed his death."

The cover-up charge rested on the decision of the CIA to give police investigating the death as little information as possible, so that it would be taken for a routine suicide. Also, a cover identity, as an Army consultant, was provided for the CIA agent with Olson at the time of his death.

The documents did not give firm answers to certain questions relating to Olson's death, or to the policy of the agency regarding the LSD experiments. It was not clear whether the CIA employes responsible for giving LSD to Olson had been reprimanded. A CIA official, Luis de Florez, had argued shortly after the death that "in the interest of maintaining the spirit of initiative and enthusiasm so necessary to our work," no reprimand should be issued. Documents dated Feb. 1954 seemed to indicate that Florez' view was adopted. However, documents apparently prepared in early 1975 stated that two employes had been reprimanded.

The documents also raised doubts whether there had been a review board for experiments "in which human lives could possibly be jeopardized." Allen W. Dulles, then director of the CIA, ordered one established after Olson's death, but there was no record in the documents of its establishment or functioning.

The documents described orders issued six months before Olson's death by two senior CIA officials, Richard Helms and Frank Wisner, requiring their permission for experiments involving LSD. Records showed, however, that neither official was notified before the experiment involving Olson.

The papers furnished to Mrs. Olson were only a small proportion of those which had originally existed on the case.

Army also tested LSD. News sources reported July 18, 1975 that the Department of the Army had conducted LSD experiments with some 1,500 persons in the 1950s and the 1960s, some of them at the Edgewood Arsenal in Maryland, the Army's chemical warfare research counterpart to Ft. Detrick, where Frank Olson was a CIA employe at the time of his death.

A total of 585 persons, most of them soldiers, were said to have participated in experiments at the Edgewood Arsenal, at Fort Bragg in North Carolina, Fort McClellan in Alabama, Dugway Proving Ground in Utah and Fort Benning in Georgia.

An additional 900 civilians were tested in Army-sponsored experiments at the University of Maryland Psychiatric Institute, the New York Psychiatric Institute, the University of Wisconsin, the University of Washington Medical School and the Tulane University Department of Neurology and Psychiatry.

The tests were reported to have been conducted between 1956 and 1967.

Army suspends drug test program—The Army said July 28 it was suspending drug and chemical experiments on human subjects in order to "determine all the facts connected with the test programs." The announcement said that the Army planned to find all those on whom it had tested LSD so that it could give them physical and mental exams to find out whether they had suffered any ill effects.

The New York Times reported July 29, however, that suspension of the testing had occurred partly because of questions raised about the background of the head of the research program, Dr. Van M. Sim, as well as queries from the press, members of Congress and former test subjects.

Sim, at a Pentagon press conference July 23, had defended the test program, which involved 900 civilian and 6,983 military volunteers over a 20-year period. The Army had ended its testing of LSD on humans in 1967, but continued experiments on soldiers with other drugs that produced hallucinations similar to those caused by LSD, said Sim, civilian medical research director at the Army's Edgewood Arsenal in northeastern Maryland.

Sim said none of 585 Army volunteers given LSD was told the name of the drug or that it sometimes produced side effects. To have identified the drug and its possible effects would have prejudiced the experiment, he said. (Sim added that follow-up studies had been done on 10% of the men, but he retracted this statement Aug. 2, saying he had made a mistake and that the Army had done a follow-up on only two test subjects.)

He said he considered the experiments "very important" to national security and did not consider them hazardous because the subjects were carefully supervised. He knew of no deaths or prolonged hospitalizations resulting from the LSD experiments, Sim said. Seven men subsequently showed side effects, but the doctors treating them were sent "full explanations" of the experiments, Sim said.

Sim, who said other test subjects in the Army's program were given drugs ranging from alcohol to barbiturates, claimed he was unfamiliar with the LSD experiments involving 900 civilians. These tests were conducted by universities and private institutions under Army contracts, he said.

Following Sim's news conference, the Army disclosed that 2,940 of the program's military volunteers had been tested with BZ (3-quinuclidinyl benzilate), a hallucinogenic drug more powerful than LSD. BZ, whose effects of disorientation and hallucinations lasted up to 80 hours, was developed for use in situations such as civilian riots, protection of military combat areas and military rescue missions, the Army stated. (No follow-up examinations on volunteers who took BZ were performed, the Army said Aug. 14.)

The Washington Post reported Aug. 3 that the Army had manufactured BZ in 1963–64 and was still stockpiling the drug at its Pine Bluff Arsenal in Arkansas. The Post said that the international protocols banning biological and toxic chemical weapons signed by President Ford Jan. 22 excluded several riot control agents, including BZ.

Nerve gas tests admitted—Dr. Sim Aug. 8 confirmed a report by Rep. Thomas J. Downey (D, N.Y.) that the Army had tested lethal nerve gas on soldiers at the Edgewood Arsenal without telling them exactly what the substance was. Downey said more than 1,000 human subjects had been exposed.

Sim described the nerve gas as similar to agricultural pesticides and claimed it was administered in small doses, with no resulting serious illness. The purpose of the tests, he said, was to develop antidotes for nerve gas. He added that information from the experiments, conducted between 1955 and 1967, had been widely utilized in the treatment of farmers and crop dusters exposed to lethal pesticides.

1953 fatality linked to drug test—The Army disclosed Aug. 12 that a patient in a New York City mental hospital had died in 1953 during an Army-sponsored experiment with a hallucinogenic drug. The patient, Harold Blauer, 42, died shortly after being injected with a derivative of mescaline, said the Army, which had not previously admitted sponsoring the experiment.

According to the Army, Blauer had been given the drug in a series of five tests at the New York State Psychiatric Institute by civilian physicians working under an Army contract with the institute. The first four tests, the Army said, produced mild or no effects. However, Blauer apparently suffered an allergic reaction on the fifth test and his cardiovascular system collapsed.

Army officials indicated they could not say whether Blauer, a tennis pro, had consented to the experiment. One of his daughters, Elizabeth Barrett, 35, said she remembered being told that the drugs were administered on his doctor's orders.

Blauer's widow, who was never told of the Army's involvement, sued the New York State Department of Mental Hygiene and the institute but later settled out of court for $13,000.

The daughter, who said she was only 13 years old at the time of her father's death, recalled being told by her mother (who died in 1974) that her father had received LSD. In addition, she said her mother had said that her father had been given experimental drugs twice before his death and had reacted badly both times. She said her father "absolutely" had not volunteered for the experiment.

Project Sanguine report. Sen. Gaylord Nelson (D, Wis.) Dec. 10, 1975 made public the results of a 1973 scientific inquiry into the effects of the Navy's Project Sanguine on the human body. Project Sanguine, also known as Project Seafarer, was a proposed system by which the Navy would use low-frequency radio waves to communicate with its submarines. The proposal had come under strong attack from environmentalists.

The Navy had commissioned a seven-member panel of scientists in 1973 to assess the biological consequences of the project at its Wisconsin test site. The panel found that low-frequency radiation raised the level of triglycerides in the blood of six of eight people working near the site. Triglycerides, a blood fat related to cholesterol, had been linked to heart disease.

Nelson charged the Navy with suppressing the panel's findings. "For at least the last two years," he said, "I have asked admirals who have visited my office about Sanguine, whether there was anything to indicate that the system had adverse environmental impact and was told there was nothing."

The Sanguine project head, Navy Capt. W. C. Cobb, denied any coverup. He added that "we do not think that harmful, adverse effects" from Sanguine-type emissions "have been validated."

Plutonium tested in humans in 1940s. The Energy Research and Development Administration (ERDA) had confirmed that the government injected plutonium into human subjects from 1945 to 1947 to determine what the poisonous, radioactive substance would do to workers manufacturing the atom bomb. The Washington Post reported Feb. 22, 1976.

The injections were administered in varying quantities to eighteen persons (13 males and 5 females) ranging in age from four to 68. All were believed suffering from terminal illnesses.

Officials of the ERDA said records on the experiment were so unclear that it was not known how the subjects were selected or who ordered the tests. The ERDA could only be certain that one person had consented to the injection.

According to a fact sheet prepared by the ERDA, the purpose of the experiment was to gather information that would permit scientists to determine the amount of plutonium to which humans could safely be exposed.

The fact sheet said that seven persons who received injections lived less than one year afterward; three lived between one and three years; two between 14 and 20 years; and one 28 years. The fate of two was unknown, and three were still living.

A-tests on prisoners—ERDA confirmed Feb. 28 that its predecessor, the Atomic Energy Commission, had used 131 prisoners in radiation experiments in the 1960s.

According to the ERDA, the AEC beamed x-rays into the testicles of 131 prisoners in Oregon and Washington to see if heavy radiation could cause sterility. A spokesman for the ERDA said that the prisoners had given written consent to the experiment and later undergone vasectomies to avoid fathering deformed children due to the damage caused by the test on their reproductive systems.

It is not known whether the radiation produced cancer in any of the subjects because no comprehensive follow-up studies had been made.

HEW lifts fetal research ban. Acting on a recommendation from a national review board that conducted hearings on the subject, Caspar W. Weinberger, secretary of health, education and welfare, July 29, 1975 ended a 13-month ban on federally funded research with human fetuses.

The moratorium had begun in 1973 when the National Institutes of Health said

April 17 that it had banned research by NIH-supported scientists on all live, aborted fetuses. The NIH had been studying guidelines, suggested in 1971 by an independent group of doctors, under which research would be permitted if the aborted fetus were no older than 20 weeks, were no larger than 500 grams (1.1 lbs.), and no longer than 25 cm. (9.8 in.). The presumption was that such fetuses were incapable of surviving.

The 1975 rules allowed experimentation with fetuses both inside the mother's womb and, in many cases, on aborted fetuses temporarily alive. Research was still prohibited on live fetuses if it would kill them, or keep them alive artificially.

If the fetus was still in the womb, the research had to be either necessary for keeping it alive, or to seek important facts which could not be learned otherwise. The regulations added that the experimentation must pose only "minimal" risk beyond any the fetus already faced.

The recommendations, which were first made by the National Commission on Protection of Human Subjects of Biomedical and Behavioral Research, were approved by Weinberger without major changes.

The rules required the mother's consent in all cases. They required the father's consent except where his identity could not be learned or if pregnancy resulted from rape.

Because risks to the fetus could be assessed differently in different cases HEW was charged by the commission to establish a set of national ethical review boards to review questionable research. The new rules applied officially only to HEW projects, but almost all fetal research was federally funded. Also, hospitals' ethical review committees generally applied the same rules to all research as was applied to federal projects.

Opposition to the renewal of such research came, in large part, from anti-abortion groups, including the U.S. Catholic Conference, which maintained that no fetal research was ethical. The anti-abortion groups argued that a fetus was unable to give consent and that a woman planning an abortion had given up her right to decide what was done to the fetus.

However, an introduction to the new rules said a woman "may not be presumed to lack interest in her fetus" even if she had decided to opt for an abortion. Therefore, she could be "validly asked to consent for research."

The study commission heard a number of research reports on the usefulness of fetal research. One such report, made by the Battelle Institute of Columbus, Ohio, said that certain fetal research had saved the lives of hundreds of thousands of babies.

The report focused on four medical advances that resulted from such research. Included was a treatment of Rh hemolytic disease of the newborn. The disease resulted from an incompatibility of blood types between the mother and the fetus. Advances through fetal research eventually led to a vaccine that saved 450,000 fetuses between 1930 and 1975, the Battelle report said.

Also touched on in the report were the development, through fetal research, of a vaccine to fight rubella, a viral infection, and its resultant birth defects; research on a respiratory distress syndrome of newborns; and the development of amniocentesis, a technique for sampling fetus cells from the fluid surrounding the fetus of the womb. The director of the Battelle project said that none of the research could have been done on animals.

One member of the commission hearing the report said the study, submitted March 14, was the "most striking evidence we've heard yet on the potential future importance of fetal research."

Dr. Maurice J. Mahoney, a Yale scientist who was heading another research project for the commission, said there had been a "quantum jump" in fetal research in recent years. In the report, first submitted to the Commission for the Protection of Human Subjects Feb. 15, Mahoney cited over 1,000 studies worldwide. He attributed the rapid growth to advancing medical science and the legalizing of abortions that made fetuses more available.

"By far the smallest" number of studies Mahoney said, was in one of the most controversial areas of research involving the early fetus outside of the womb. Mahoney said he could only cite three studies in which fetuses were purposely kept artificially alive for a time. They were all part of attempts to develop a new type of fetal incubator for "test-tube births," where the mother could not herself carry the baby.

Another report made by a team of scientists headed by Dr. Richard Behrman, head of pediatrics at Columbia University, and presented to the commission March 15, said more prematurely born fetuses survived than was expected. The survey indicated that annually, several hundred babies might be surviving birth before the end of the first two-thirds of pregnancy in the U.S.

The report also said that research done on fetuses younger than 24 weeks still in the womb, and studies after birth on a fetus younger than 25 weeks, were biologically safe. No fetuses that young had been known to live more than minutes without artificial assistance, and none survived to leave the hospital, the report said.

Opposition to fetal experimentation continued, however. In its platform for 1976, the Republican Party said:

> While we support valid medical and biological research efforts which can produce life-saving results, we oppose any research on live fetuses. We are also opposed to any legislation which sanctions ending the life of any patient.

Massachusetts curbs fetal research—Gov. Francis Sargent of Massachusetts June 26, 1974 signed a bill prohibiting doctors from testing vaccines on developing fetuses.

Rep. William Delahunt, principal sponsor of the bill, said June 27 that the law would not interfere with most fetal research. He added that researchers should be grateful that the law was not as restrictive as a recently enacted Illinois statute barring research on living or dead human fetal tissue.

Dr. Michael N. Oxman, a Boston microbiologist, was critical of the new legislation. Vaccine studies, he contended June 28, "can only be done by administering the vaccine to women already planning abortions and then testing the fetal tissues to see if the vaccine reached the fetus."

Amniocentesis safe—Amniocentesis, a medical procedure which determined certain defects in babies developing in the womb, was found to have been safe and accurate, according to a federal research project. The conclusions were released Oct. 20, 1975 by the National Institute of Child Health & Human Development, the sponsor of the study.

The research involved 1,040 women who had the procedure performed and 992 who did not. In amniocentesis, a small amount of fluid surrounding the fetus was removed for analysis by means of a hollow needle. The researchers found that the rate of fetal loss—spontaneous abortion and still birth—was 3.5% in those who had the test performed as opposed to 3.2% in the control group. The difference was not considered statistically significant.

Since 1968, when it was first found to have been effective in detecting Down's syndrome (mongolism), a major genetic problem, the procedure had been done on 3,000 patients annually. The test was most useful for pregnant women who were 35 or over. The chance of their fetus having Down's syndrome or another chromosome abnormality was one in 100 as opposed to one in 2,000–3,000 for women under 25.

'Genetic Engineering'

Research and experimentation in genetics has produced both scientific knowledge and profound uneasiness. Many scientists warn about the accidental creation of dire diseases or human monsters. Some scholars and religious thinkers, while understanding the desire to overcome genetic defects, express concern over the moral implications of such questions as: What genetic traits are to be judged undesirable? Who is to make these judgments? What action should be taken on the basis of such judgments? And when?

Complete gene synthesized. Scientists at the University of Wisconsin June 3, 1970 announced the first complete synthesis of a gene, the basic unit of heredity. Although other scientists had used a natural gene to form a new one, the Wisconsin group was the first to piece together a molecule link by link.

The synthesis was achieved by piecing together 77 links of a large yeast molecule. It was accomplished by Dr. H. Gobind Khorana, who won a Nobel Prize in 1968 for work in genetics, and his colleagues after experimenting for nearly five years. Although some scientists said the feat came earlier than expected, others predicted that it would be a long and arduous task to tie the work to manipulation of the hereditary material in plants, animals and man.

A human cell was estimated to have six billion such links as compared to the yeast molecule's 77.

(The gene, the basic unit of heredity, comprises an helexical double strand of deoxyribonucleic acid [DNA]. In any one gene, the sequence of the DNA's chemical sub-units determines genetic instructions for a living cell. The sum of coded chemical messages in all the genes of a cell gives it complete instructions, determining what the cell can do and what it can become.)

Gene signal decoded and synthesized—Scientists at the Massachusetts Institute of Technology reported Sept. 10, 1974 that they had synthesized and deciphered the chemical structure governing the turning-on of heredity instructions in a gene.

The MIT team of researchers, headed by Nobel Prize laureate Har Gobind Khorana, reported to the American Chemical Society that it deciphered what it believed to be most or all of the "on" signal for a gene they had succeeded in synthesizing in 1973. Khorana said the team also had learned a significant amount about the "off" signal. The synthesized gene was found naturally in the common human intestinal bacterium Escherichia coli.

Bacterial gene made & implanted—Scientists at the Massachusetts Institute of Technology said Aug. 28, 1976 that they had successfully constructed a bacterial gene, complete with regulatory mechanisms, and had implanted it in a living cell where it functioned normally. The gene synthesis, which would allow scientists to study how genes were controlled, was considered a major step toward understanding the influence of the basic unit of heredity upon the health or illness of the organism.

A tyrosine transfer RNA gene from the bacterium Escherichia coli was produced by assembling from scratch the sequence of its 199 pairs of nucleotides (the four fundamental chemicals of the genetic code). These nucleotides had the chemical names adenine, thymine, guanine and cytosine and were abbreviated A, T, G and C. The synthetic gene was assembled entirely from commercially available A, T, G and C.

The first 52 nucleotide pairs, called the "promoter," started the formation of the gene's product. The next 126 pairs specified instructions for the gene to produce tyrosine transfer RNA, a molecule that transported the amino acid tyrosine to ribosomes (granules containing ribonucleic acid) within the cell. There the tyrosine would combine with other amino acids to make protein molecules. The last 21 pairs, the "terminator," halted the formation of a new molecule. This method of synthesis made it possible to alter specific segments of the nucleotide sequence and thus modify the gene's instructions and function.

The breakthrough technique in genetic engineering, developed by Dr. Har Gobind Khorana, was limited to one species and to modifications in only one gene of that species. It was not considered to hold hazards similar to recombinant DNA experimentation, which involved the transplanting of natural genes from one organism to another.

Dr. Khorana's method also differed significantly from that of a Harvard University group which had synthesized a mammalian gene by chemically reversing the gene-to-product sequence and had derived the gene from the product.

Human cell particle produced in lab. Two New York University scientists disclosed June 1, 1970 that they had produced the first man-made part of a human cell, the lysosome, in a laboratory. The two scientists, Dr. Grazia Sessa and Dr. Gerald Weissmann of NYU's School of Medicine, reported their achievement at a meeting of the International Inflammation Club in Kalamazoo, Mich.

Scientists and research biologists said the feat could open the way to a more detailed study of the body's response to disease and to the inflammatory process that led to arthritis and rheumatism. Other biologists called the achievement "a good thing" and "interesting," but emphasized that it represented only a small step in efforts to reproduce the human cell in the laboratory.

Weissmann said the man-made lysosome had been produced from fatty substances called lipids. These tended to form thin layers, and the process of forming the layers in such a way as to make the lysosome behave in a test tube environment exactly as did its natural counterpart took Weissmann and Sessa five years.

Mammal gene constructed. Four Harvard University scientists had developed the first artificial animal gene, the New York Times reported Dec. 6, 1975.

The scientists, Drs. Argiris Efstratiadis, Fotis Kafatos, Allen Maxam and Thomas Maniatis, achieved the synthesis through a combination of methods for making, in a test tube, complete double-stranded sequences of the chemical DNA of rabbit hemoglobin, a blood component.

One of the techniques used by the Harvard team, reverse transcriptases, was developed by two of three 1975 Nobel Prize winners in medicine, Drs. David Baltimore and Howard Temin.

The synthesis of the rabbit hemoglobin was seen as a major advance in the study of genetics, hereditary diseases and the human genetic evolution.

Scientists urge halt to genetic tests. A committee of scientists endorsed by the National Academy of Sciences urged colleagues throughout the world to observe a temporary ban on certain types of experiments involving genetic manipulation of bacteria (reported July 18, 1974). Such a moratorium should be declared, the ad hoc panel said, because gene-transplantation experiments might accidently increase the resistance of some microorganisms to drugs or lead to the spread of some types of cancer-causing virus. The panel was made up of researchers in the forefront of developing techniques to isolate particular genes and insert them into living cells.

The group asked that two types of experiments be avoided—the insertion into bacteria of bacterial genes determining resistance to antibiotics and toxin formation, and genes from cancer-causing or other kinds of virus. The committee also suggested that experiments involving insertion of animal genes into bacteria should "not be undertaken lightly," given that many types of animal cells contained genes common to certain tumor viruses. Conceding that its recommendations would "entail postponement or possibly abandonment of certain types of scientifically worthwhile experiments," committee members requested that their colleagues observe the ban until a conference could be convened in 1975 to assess potential hazards.

The panel especially urged caution in experiments with the bacterium Escherichia Coli (E. Coli), which was commonly found in the human digestive tract. A genetically hybrid E. Coli, the committee warned, "might possibly become widely disseminated among human bacterial, plant and animal populations with unpredictable effects."

In some experiments, new types of plasmids resistant to antibiotics might be created, the panel said. A plasmid is a self-replicating DNA element resistant to antibiotics. As an example of an experiment to be avoided, one of the panel members, Dr. Stanley H. Cohen of Stanford University, cited the introduction of a penicillin-resistant gene into the bacteria pneumococci, which was sensitive to penicillin.

The committee was chaired by Dr. Paul Berg of Stanford, and had among its members Dr. James Watson of the Cold Spring Harbor (N.Y.) Laboratory, who along with English geneticist Francis Crick deciphered the structure of DNA.

Research guidelines set. A conference of 139 molecular biologists from 17 nations, held Feb. 24–27, 1975, approved a set of guidelines to reduce the risks in gene-grafting research.

The conference, held at the Asilomar Conference Center in Pacific Grove, Calif., had been called by a committee of U.S. scientists, who feared such experiments might accidently produce drug-resistant or cancer-causing organisms.

As a result of the conference, gene-transplant research was expected to resume. At the urging of the conference's conveners—an ad hoc National Academy of Sciences committee chaired by Stanford University biochemist Paul Berg—U.S. biologists previously had voluntarily agreed to observe a moratorium on some research until safeguards could be drawn up. The ban had become part of the regulations of the Medical Research Council in Great Britain and was generally followed throughout the world.

Essentially, the scientists were concerned with laboratory techniques by which genes of one organism were grafted to the DNA of another organism. Transplanted genes became a permanent part of the recipient organism and its descendants.

The research background of the Asilomar conference was this:

Stanford biologists had discovered a peculiarity of the relatively simple, single-celled bacterium. While most of the DNA in a bacterium was found in their chromosomes, they also had plasmids that often lay outside the chromosomes. The biologists learned to extract a strand of plasmid DNA, cut out a segment and insert in its place a segment of foreign DNA. Moreover, the technique, which also could be used with certain viruses infecting bacteria, was refined so that almost any kind of cell could be grafted to bacteria.

Researchers investigating gene recombination argued that the potential benefits of such grafting were incalculable, but they conceded that there were potential dangers. If it were true that certain bacterial plasmids were resistant to antibiotics, a strain of recombinant streptococcus (the cause of rheumatic fever and other diseases) could be rendered resistant to penicillin, some scientists suggested. Of equal concern were experiments in early 1974 in which DNAs of viruses infecting animals were recombined in test tubes. In one experiment, genes from a virus infecting humans were combined with genes thought to cause cancer in hamsters. The hybrid strand of viral DNA was then inserted into bacterial plasmid DNA. The scientists stopped short of grafting the virus genes to bacteria, however.

Against this background, the National Research Council of the National Academy of Sciences asked Berg to chair a committee to look into the dangers of gene recombination.

As the scientists were basically worried about recombinant organisms that might escape the laboratory, the guidelines drafted at the Asilomar conference concerned "containment." The suggested containment procedures ranged from those in use in hospital-type bacteriology laboratories to high-security measures involving use of protective clothing and air locks. In addition, the guidelines urged scientists to determine necessary containment procedures before beginning experiments.

NIH panel urges use of guidelines—An advisory committee to the National Institutes of Health (NIH), meeting in San Francisco Feb. 28, recommended that federal grants for research in genetic engineering be conditioned on the recipients' agreeing to follow the guidelines adopted by Asilomar conference.

Dr. A. A. Bayev, the leader of the Soviet Union's delegation to the Asilomar conference, said Feb. 27 that the guidelines were "reasonable and acceptable." (The Soviets attended but did not participate in the conference.)

Genetic research curbed. Guidelines that banned certain forms of genetic experimentation and strongly regulated others were issued June 23, 1976 by the National Institutes of Health.

The new rules barred experiments involving highly poisonous substances, the transfer of drug-resistant properties to dangerous bacteria and the deliberate release of synthetic genetic material into the environment.

Safety precautions included providing ventilation and sewage facilities designed to filter outgoing air and wastes, the transfer of supplies through airlocks and confinement of high-security laboratories to isolated areas.

The guidelines directly applied to the 25,000 NIH grantees and contractors, which included most of the nation's universities. The NIH was the government's main agency for the conduct and support of biomedical research.

The issuance of the guidelines ended the two-year voluntary national moratorium on recombinant DNA research.

Cambridge (Mass.) ban. The Cambridge (Mass.) City Council voted July 7, 1976 for a three-month moratorium on recombinant DNA research at Harvard University, where officials recently had approved plans to construct a genetics research laboratory. The nine-member council also voted to organize a review board of scientists and citizens to investigate further potential hazards.

Scientists urge wider DNA guidelines. Recombinant DNA research guidelines should apply to all federal, academic and industrial groups engaged in such experimentation, scientists testified Sept. 22, 1976 before the Senate Labor & Public Welfare Committee's subcommittee on health. To date, National Institutes of Health (NIH) guidelines to assure that genetically modified bacteria did not escape from laboratories and create health hazards applied only to recipients of NIH funds.

NIH director Donald S. Frederickson said that nearly all federal agencies, except the Agriculture Department and the Central Intelligence Agency, had agreed to comply voluntarily with the NIH restrictions. Senators Edward M. Kennedy (D, Mass.) and Jacob K. Javits (R, N.Y.) made public a letter they had written July 19 to President Ford urging him to take steps to require adherence to the NIH guidelines "in all sectors of the research community."

Sen. Kennedy, chairman of the subcommittee, said that his concern over industry's compliance with the guidelines was raised when the General Electric Co. refused to send a spokesman to the hearings. General Electric was currently working on developing a bacterial species capable of eating up oil spills.

New York Attorney General Louis J. Lefkowitz convened a public hearing Oct. 21 to discuss whether legal restrictions should be placed on potentially dangerous genetic engineering experiments in the state. The public hearings focused on the questionable stringency of the federal guidelines, which did not apply to industrial research and were not backed by legal sanctions.

Patent order lifted. The Commerce Department Feb. 24, 1977 suspended an order issued Jan. 10 which had accelerated the granting of patents to companies involved in recombinant DNA research. The order had bypassed a major guideline laid down by the National Institutes of Health (NIH), by allowing private industries to withhold data and protect trade secrets which would otherwise have been reviewed by a safety board. The NIH guidelines, which applied only to federally funded research projects, required advance disclosure of bacterial or other genetic material to be used in experimentation.

The regulation was rescinded after Health, Education and Welfare Secretary Joseph A. Califano Jr. and two California State Assembly committees protested the ruling. In a letter Feb. 7 Califano asked that the Commerce Department await the recommendations of a federal interagency committee currently considering how to regulate firms involved in genetic research.

Major U.S. pharmaceutical companies currently conducting recombinant DNA experiments included Hoffmann-La Roche, Upjohn and Eli Lilly. Abbott Laboratories in North Chicago, Ill. issued a statement Mar. 9 that although they were preparing staff, facilities and techniques for such research, they were "not at present actually recombining DNA molecular pieces."

NAS forum on DNA research. The National Academy of Science sponsored a public forum on recombinant DNA research Mar. 7-9 in Washington, D.C., where opposing viewpoints were heard on whether such work ultimately would help cure diseases or unleash new ones. Those who voiced concern about disrupting the natural genetic heritage of life were countered by a majority of biologists who felt the work would lead to the discovery of life-saving drugs.

Hours before the conference opened, a group called the Coalition for Responsible Genetic Research announced its formation and called for "an immediate international moratorium on all research that would produce novel genetic combinations between distant organisms which have not been demonstrated to exchange genes in nature."

The new group, claiming 400 sponsors from the U.S. and abroad, included Harvard University biologist and Nobel Prize winner Dr. George Wald, who described recombinant DNA research as perhaps the biggest issue in the history of science.

NIH builds gene research facility. The National Institutes of Health was preparing the nation's first certified P4 level laboratory, where the most hazardous genetic experiments could be conducted, in Ft. Detrick, Md., the Washington Post reported March 8. The $3-million facility would be housed in a remodeled building previously used to develop the Army's germ warfare projects.

The P4 classification, the most stringent physical containment level outlined in the NIH recombinant DNA guidelines, required airlocks, use of protective clothing and sterilization of all wastes. P4-level experiments involved any work with the DNA of primates (monkeys or man) or with an animal tumor virus.

Administration urges U.S. DNA control. Federal legislation to regulate biological experimentation with recombinant DNA was proposed by the Carter Administration April 6, 1977. The proposals were based on the recommendations made March 16 by a federal interagency panel that had been assigned to study the controversial field of genetic research.

The committee, representing all 16 federal agencies concerned with the research, had advised that the Department of Health, Education and Welfare (HEW) assume primary responsibility for recombinant DNA regulation and that federal law supersede state and local laws on the same subject. Exceptions to the federal supremacy rule would be allowed in cities or states that set standards "as stringent as, or more stringent than," the federal regulations, as in the case of Cambridge, Mass.

HEW Secretary Joseph A. Califano told the health and scientific research subcommittee of the Senate Human Resources Committee that "legislation in this area constitutes unusual government involvement in the workings of basic science." He said, however, that the potential hazards of the revolutionary gene-splicing technique "justify such a measure at this time."

Scientists reproduce insulin gene. Drs. Howard M. Goodman and William J. Rutter of the University of California at San Francisco reported May 23, 1977 that they had mass-produced the gene for insulin. They used the recombinant-DNA technique and spliced the genetic material that produces insulin in rats into colonies of the bacteria Escherichia Coli (E. Coli). Bacteria normally did not make insulin and had no natural genetic instructions for doing so.

The bacteria duplicated the transplanted genetic material, thus marking a major step toward providing limitless supplies of insulin, a vital hormone needed by diabetics, whose own bodies could not produce it.

The possibility of developing new drug resources had been a major goal of advocates of recombinant DNA technology.

Diabetics currently obtained insulin from the pancreas glands of pigs and cattle.

The Mind

Behavior Modification

"Drugs, electrical stimulation of the nervous systems and operant conditioning have become powerful tools in a behavioral technology aimed toward significantly changing people's behavior. Many feel that the issues of personal and social values are irrelevant to the use of these tools and that problems over the direction of change will be worked out within the current social and political context, with no professional involvement necessary. Others feel that, in the application of such technologies, there are major value issues which must be considered. . . . Dr. Holland examines some issues in behavioral control that have wide ethical consequences." (From "Current Ethical Issues in Mental Health," National Institute of Mental Health, 1973; brief introduction to paper presented by Dr. James G. Holland in March 1970. Excerpts from Holland's paper follow.)

Ethics & behavior modification. Ethical problems posed in behavior modification were explored by Associate Prof. James G. Holland of the University of Pittsburgh at a workshop held at an annual meeting of the American Orthopsychiatric Association in San Francisco in March 1970. Among Holland's remarks:

"Behavior modification shares with other therapies all of the usual ethical problems of informed consent, privileged communication, etc. But behavior modification procedures add new problems. The new ethical considerations arise from the very strength of the technique. . . .

"The basic research in the experimental analysis of behavior has provided the means for the development of effective procedures for changing behavior in a variety of settings. . . . [T]here has been extensive use of programed instruction and contingency management in classrooms, manipulation of behavior of mental patients on the ward as well as in individual therapy, and a host of other applications. When a behavior modification procedure is developed, all aspects are empirically defined and hence replicable. . . . With a little training anyone able to arrange the necessary reinforcers or aversive stimuli can carry out the procedures, and training workshops are common for teachers, parents, psychiatric nurses, prison personnel, and others to prepare them to use behavior modification. . . .

". . . The science is at the service of those who command the means to use it.

". . . For example, when it was discovered that in past wars less than 25% of the men in combat actually fired their weapons, [a Human Resources Research Organization psychologist] . . . prepared training procedures to increase the soldier's willingness to fire more frequently and effectively. . . .

"... A survey among experts in weapons systems conducted by Rand Corp. projects the behavioral control of mass populations as a major weapons system. Most of the experts expect it to be reality by 1980—American know-how beating by four years the English masters of *1984*....

"... Philip Sperling, in his address as president of the APA Division of Military Psychology, promotes 'political psychology' as the newest and most critical aspect of military psychology. 'Political psychology,' Sperling (1968) says, '... deals with problems of control of the behavior of groups.'...

"... The behavioral psychologist is preparing procedures which ... facts indicate will be used by those in positions of power for their ends rather than for the objectives of the individual whose behavior is being manipulated...."

Pupils get behavior drugs. The Washington Post reported June 28, 1970 that 3,000 to 6,000 primary-school pupils in Omaha, Neb. had been getting "behavior modification" drugs prescribed by local physicians to improve their in-class conduct and their capacity for learning. The program was introduced in the Omaha public school system, which had a total enrollment of 62,000 students, in the spring of 1969.

Dr. Byron B. Oberset, an Omaha pediatrician, was credited with starting the "behavior modification" drug program with pupils who had been identified by their teachers as "hyperactive" and unmanageable to the point of disrupting normal classroom activity. Oberst said five drugs were most often used in the program. He said that Ritalin, a brand name for methylphenidate hydrochloride, a stimulant, was the drug principally used. The others used were Dexedrene, Deaner, Aventyl and Tofranil.

Oberst said Ritalin "increased the ability to concentrate." He said that although "nobody knows the mechanisms of how they [the drugs] function . . . we know these children become more successful."

The program was not without its critics. One physician said Ritalin had been developed "in an effort to find a substance with the 'mood elevating' effects of amphetamine minus its drawbacks." But Ritalin, the physician said, had been a disappointment because it appeared that the drug "might not achieve a full separation of amphetamine's desirable and undesirable effects. . ."

The U.S. Food & Drug Administration (FDA) disclosed Sept. 29 that it had warned Dr. Oberst against the further use of two drugs in the program. The disclosure that he had been advised to stop using the amphetamine-type drugs was made by FDA officials who appeared before a House Government Operations Committee hearing on the right to privacy. One of the congressmen on the committee, Rep. Cornelius Gallagher (D, N.J.), said "we should suspend the use of these drugs for this purpose until more is known."

The two drugs cited by the FDA in its Aug. 6 letter to Dr. Oberst were Tofranil and Aventyl. FDA officials told the House committee that neither Tofranil nor Aventyl should be used by children and that the agency "now specifically warns against such use."

A Nixon Administration official said Oct. 11 that the government would convene a panel of scientists and pediatricians to draw up a warning statement about the use of amphetamine drugs to improve the in-class conduct of overactive school children.

Dr. Edward F. Zigler, director of the Office of Child Development, said he was concerned about the use of amphetamine drugs on children who did not require them. Zigler's office was also charged with responsibility for the Head Start plan for needy pre-school children.

Peace drugs proposal stirs dispute. Dr. Kenneth B. Clark, president of the American Psychological Association, touched off a dispute within America's scientific and medical community when he proposed Sept. 4, 1971 the creation of mind-affecting drugs that could be given to the world's political leaders to subdue and curb their aggressive and hostile tendencies.

Clark's view was challenged Sept. 6 by a wide range of prominent psychologists who said they doubted that the drugs envisioned by Clark could be developed. They added that even if the mind-affecting drugs could be developed there would be enormous social and political problems over the control of their use.

Clark had advanced his plan in an address at the APA's annual meeting in Washington. He said conventional means of trying to prevent inhumane acts and the threat of a nuclear holocaust were too slow to insure the survival of man. He said it was time to develop new mind-affecting drugs or agents that world leaders could routinely be given to subdue their propensity for violence.

Clark described his plan as a form of psychological disarmament. He said that such a form of disarmament might be negotiated among nations as military disarmament was now discussed.

Behavior modification reviewed. The National Institute of Mental Health (NIMH) July 9, 1975 released the first federal policy statement on the controversial topic of behavior modification. According to the NIMH, 60,000 Americans were undergoing behavior modification treatment by doctors.

According to the new study, behavior modification had been a "marked success" for the treatment of such problems as phobias, compulsive behavior and sexual dysfunction. However, it was noted that the use of the treatment for depression and schizophrenia had been far less successful "and may not be as good as existing forms of treatment."

Scientifically, behavior modification was the process of trying to change a person's way of reacting by applying "positive" or "negative" reinforcement. In practice, this generally amounted to giving rewards like food treats or punishments like electric shocks or loss of privileges.

The institute's conclusions were published in a report, intended as a guide to therapists, titled "Behavior Modification: Perspective on a Current Issue." The report noted that persons considering such treatment should carefully review its overall benefits and drawbacks.

"One of the main problems" of the treatment, according to an NIMH spokesman, was the lack of "quality control." He said that at least a third of the sex therapists using the method were "outright quacks." Aside from private patients, the technique was being used at hospitals, prisons and schools.

The Institute was financing $2 million in research into the method in 1975, and another $1 million in research was being done by federal alcohol and drug abuse agencies. The Law Enforcement Assistance Administration and the Bureau of Prisons, after a rash of public criticism of the uses of the method, ended most such programs in federal prisons in 1975.

However, in a report released by the General Accounting Office (GAO) Aug. 6, it was revealed tht the Bureau of Prisons still applied such techniques to some prisoners in solitary confinement. Rep. Ralph Metcalfe (D, Ill.) who had asked for the report said the programs were "inhuman" and should be discontinued.

According to press reports Aug. 6, Metcalfe said the treatment as administered was "nothing short of long-term punishment under the guise of what is in fact pseudo-scientific experimentation."

The GAO report on the programs, which were begun in 1972, was somewhat less critical of the program than Metcalfe. It said "the effort has not been well managed," but added that it had stressed rewards and minimized punishments and included "counseling, work, education, recreation and other activities."

Soviet political psychiatric abuses charged. The U.S. concern over possible misuse of behavior-modification methods was aired in an atmosphere made more tense for international psychology and psychiatry by continued charges that the Soviet Union was abusing psychiatric techniques to repress political dissidence.

Drugging of prisoners charged—In a letter written March 13, 1971 and published five days later, two political prisoners charged Soviet prison hospital attendants with drugging psychiatric patients in order to change their views. Andrei D. Sakharov, the human rights activist, supported the prisoners' claim in a telegram March 18 to Interior Minister Col. Gen. Nikolai A. Shchelokov.

The authors of the letter were Viktor

Fainberg, who had been involved in a protest against the 1968 Soviet invasion of Czechoslovakia, and Vladimir Borisov, accused of distributing anti-Soviet leaflets in 1969. Fainberg and Borisov, inmates of a Leningrad psychiatric hospital, said authorities administered mind-altering drugs to political prisoners, threatened them with electric-shock therapy and placed dissidents in the company of mental patients with homicidal tendencies. They added: "Medicine, one of the most humane of professions, is thus being turned into a servile handmaiden of the regime's correction agencies in their hangman functions."

The men also charged that prisoners were being held in mental hospitals for as long as 15 years, contrary to a law which limited forced psychiatric treatment to two years.

In a related development, a female poet in the Turkmen Republic was reported Sept. 27 to have been confined to a mental hospital after sending to the Communist party Central Committee in Moscow a document citing unfavorable living conditions in her home area. Annasoltan Kekilova was said to have had her poems withdrawn from publication after complaining of "substantial faults in our republic," according to a petition mailed to the Central Committee by her mother, Ogulsakhat Seidova. After losing her job and deciding to renounce Soviet citizenship and leave the country, Mrs. Seidova said, Miss Kekilova was taken to a psychiatric hospital.

West publishes Medvedev text—Western sources reported Sept. 16, 1971, that Zhores A. Medvedev, Soviet biologist and dissident who had been arrested and given a forced psychiatric exam, had written an account of the incident and that it had been published in London that week.

The volume, entitled "A Question of Madness" and published by Macmillan, told of Medvedev's arrest May 29, 1970 and his examination two days later at the hands of a group led by Boris V. Shostakovich of the Serbsky Institute of Forensic Psychiatry and Dr. Alexander Y. Lifshits of the Kaluga Psychiatric Hospital.

A chapter written by the biologist's brother, Roy A. Medvedev, described a summons he received to the office of the secret police (KGB) and an interview in which it was agreed to "close the case" of Zhores Medvedev if the government destroyed "the false medical record" accusing the scientist of "incipient schizophrenia" and "paranoid delusions of reforming society."

In an introduction to the text written in September 1970, Zhores Medvedev declared: "Now, three months after the main events of the story, it has become clear that the other side has not kept its part of the bargain, and this unties my hands." He said he had written the account "to call attention to the dangerous tendency of using psychiatry for political purposes, the exploitation of medicine in an alien role as a means of intimidation and punishment—a new and illegal way of isolating people for their views and convictions."

Hospitalization denied—The government newspaper Izvestia denied Oct. 23 that healthy persons were put in mental hospitals. Izvestia said: "The malignant critics are concerned about only one thing, to portray insane persons as 'fighters for ideas'." The paper maintained the only people in mental hospitals were those "who committed socially dangerous acts while not responsible for their actions or became ill during a pretrial investigation, during actual court proceedings or after the passing of sentence."

Psychiatrists bar condemnation—The World Psychiatric Association Congress, at its meeting in Mexico City, rejected Dec. 1, 1971 an appeal by the Soviet dissident Human Rights Committee that it condemn the use of psychiatry for political purposes. Delegates argued that the organization's constitution provided no mechanism for such a statement.

The Soviet dissidents' letter, published Oct. 23, said: "Especially serious is the problem of the rights of people forcibly held in psychiatric hospitals by court order or on any other basis. The lack of firm guarantees to insure the rights of people ruled mentally ill, or subjected to in-patient psychiatric examinations, facilitates abuses in this area."

The letter also warned against "the application of procedures and means of treatment which result in irreversible clinical changes. It should not be forgotten that such abuses can be practiced as a method of political persecution." Signing the letter were the committee's four full members—Andrei D. Sakharov, Andrei N. Tverdokhlebov, Valery N. Chalidze and Igor Shafarevich, a mathematician at Moscow University.

Bukovsky sentenced—A member of the dissident movement in the U.S.S.R. who had worked to focus foreign attention on conditions in Soviet prisons was sentenced Jan. 5, 1972 to seven years imprisonment and five years of exile. Vladimir Bukovsky was convicted of giving Western newsmen information about the alleged Soviet policy of sending dissidents to psychiatric hospitals.

Bukovsky was convicted of trying to bring a printing press into the country, of "disseminating slanderous lies about the social and government system of the U.S.S.R.," and of trying to persuade two Red Army officers to help send information abroad.

The London Times said Jan. 3, 1972 that three unidentified former inmates of the "special psychiatric hospital" in Leningrad had volunteered to give evidence in Bukovsky's defense.

U.S. doctor checks detentions—Dr. Alfred M. Freedman, president of the American Psychiatric Association, said Nov. 2, 1973 that after talks with Soviet psychiatrists and a visit to a Soviet psychiatric hospital he had the "impression that differences of opinion, criticisms and opposition were considered as bizarre behavior and important manifestations of illness." He expressed his belief that six Soviet dissidents interned in psychiatric hospitals, whose dossiers were provided by Soviet psychiatrists, had been unnecessarily detained.

Freedman and 12 other Western psychiatrists had been allowed to visit one building at the Serbsky Institute in Moscow Oct. 15, while two others were allowed to visit dissident Gen. Pyotr Grigorenko at a hospital near Moscow that day. Freedman said Grigorenko's refusal to accept the services of an official Soviet interpreter during the visit had been cited by a Soviet psychiatrist as a sign of paranoia.

The psychiatrists had been in the Soviet Union to attend scientific conferences.

Twenty-one members of the presidium of the Soviet All-Union Society of Neuropathologists and Psychiatrists wrote in a letter published Oct. 2 that no one had been detained for his opinions or been given psychiatric drugs with harmful effects. But the writers said "violations of public order" and "spreading of slander" could be symptoms of disorder requiring confinement.

Plyushch freed, reports in West on hospital treatment—Soviet mathematician Leonid Plyushch was released Jan. 9, 1976 from a psychiatric hospital in the Ukraine in which he had been interned since 1973 after being charged with anti-Soviet acts.

The 36-year-old Plyushch, with his wife and two sons, arrived in Vienna Jan. 11 where he was examined by psychiatrists who reported him free of mental disorders. One doctor noted, however, that, during his internment, the mathematician had been "forced to take drugs like insulin and haloperidol that were harmful to his health. It cannot be excluded that his health will remain permanently affected by the large doses."

In its statement reporting Plyushch's release from the Dnepropetrovsk psychiatric hospital, the official Soviet news agency Tass said Jan. 8 that the mathematician had been found ill by a team of psychiatrists at the time of his 1972 trial and that "his health had so much improved after treatment [in the hospital] that the court had found it possible to grant his wife's request that she be allowed to look after him."

Upon his arrival in Vienna, Plyushch, described as looking frail and trembling, said that 60 other "political patients" were being held in the Dnepropetrovsk mental hospital. Officials of the London-based human rights organization Amnesty International stated that that figure would represent a "shattering" increase in their estimate of the number of individuals accused of political crimes who were being held in Soviet mental hospitals. The Amnesty officials said they had compiled dossiers on 120 such cases over the past five years and noted that the Dnepropetrovsk institution was but one of at least six Soviet psychiatric hospitals.

At a press conference in Paris Feb. 3, Plyushch termed himself a "neo-Marxist" and said Soviet authorities had tried to destroy his political beliefs in the hospital. He said political prisoners were mixed with the criminally insane in the "horror of the madhouse" where patients were regularly abused by attendants who were actually criminals serving out sentences. Plyushch said he was given a treatment known as "neuroleptics," a Soviet term for drug treatment that changed neural functions, and described regular injections of sulfur and the depressants haloperidol and triftazine, as well as insulin therapy.

Plyushch named some of the 60 political prisoners he said remained interned in the Dnepropetrovsk mental hospital and appealed for their release and the release of several other imprisoned political dissidents. Of his own background, the mathematician noted that he had been dismissed from his position at the Institute of Cybernetics of the Academy of Sciences of the Ukraine in 1968 after having sent a letter of protest to a Soviet newspaper regarding two writers who were being tried for anti-Soviet activities. He was arrested in 1972 after several years of publishing articles in clandestine publications and he was interned in the Dnepropetrovsk institution from July 1972 until January 1975.

Moscow denies psychiatric abuses—In an article published Feb. 4 in the Soviet daily Literaturnaya Gazeta, the U.S.S.R. denied that persons were sent to psychiatric hospitals because of political beliefs and asserted that it was in the West that recourse was made to psychiatry to "control political opponents."

The article characterized a number of emigre dissidents who had been placed in Soviet mental institutions as mental cripples, many of whom were similarly interned upon arriving in the nations to which they had emigrated. The article cited the cases of Alexis Tummerman and Anatoly Yakovson, who, it said, were hospitalized in Israel; Lev Kostantinov, who had been hospitalized in Vienna; and Viktor Fainberg, interned in Great Britain.

(According to the French newspaper Le Monde Feb. 6, Fainberg had never been interned, while the others, having undergone some hospitalization, were presently living "normally and at liberty.")

Behavior-heart attack link confirmed. Researchers at the Boston University School of Medicine reported in the June 6, 1974 issue of the New England Journal of Medicine that men who exhibited high degrees of so-called Type A behavior were twice as likely to have heart attacks as men who did not.

The scientists selected 2,750 men free of heart disease and had them fill out computer-scored questionnaires for Type A personalities, which were found among those who strived to achieve and were perfectionist, tense, unable to relax, active and energetic. After four years, the Boston University doctors found, those scoring high on Type A behavior had twice as many heart attacks as those who scored low.

Behavior modification of aid in physical treatment. The report of the President's Biomedical Research Panel, published by the Department of Health, Education & Welfare April 30, 1976, suggested that behavior-modification techniques could be of value in treating physical ills. The report said:

"In the area of physical health, the strongest case for a strictly behavioral activity of relevance is for programs designed to change behaviors associated with risk. The potential importance of such efforts can be made clear for the specific example of cardiac disorder. It has been estimated that the elimination of Type A behavior alone could reduce the incidence of cardiac disorder by 31%. The elimination of other behavior contributing to vulnerability to coronary disease (smoking, overeating) would reduce the incidence further. For many programs that reduce vulnerability, the methods of behavior modification and the related biofeedback procedures show considerable promise. They may very well be capable of teaching an individual to bring dangerous behavior (Type A activity) and even internal processes (blood pressure) under a degree of control. . . ."

The report said that "obstacles to progress in the behavioral sciences" include "the effects of laws on privacy, confidentiality, and full disclosure. Although we recognize the essentiality of such laws for the protection of human dignity, it is already clear that their indiscriminate application is standing in the way of scientific progress. For example: (1) Investigators in educational research have been denied access to student populations (and even the names of students and their parents) because of fear on the part of the school administrators that such information would violate the students' rights of privacy. This happens even in cases where the studies involve nothing in the way of sensitive information. (2) In some clinics, permanent records are being systematically impoverished in order to minimize the amount of information that can be disclosed. Research in the future (for example, the historical demography of family structure) is sure to suffer from this. (3) Many researchers have interpreted informed consent regulations to require disclosures that make some types of laboratory research impossible because the participant's naivete is essential to the investigation. Such scientists are moving to 'safer' lines of investigation that may be less productive."

Psychosurgery

Psychosurgery has always been a controversial topic. As Peter McL. Black wrote in the Humanist (July-August 1977), "it carries with it the stigmata of political coercion and mass manipulation." The controversy ranges from the question of whether psychosurgery should ever be performed to the issue of what constitutes adequate consent for such procedure, especially in view of the fact that candidates for psychosurgery may not be completely rational.

Definition & controversy. A "discursive" definition of the term "psychosurgery" was prepared by the staff of the U.S. House Commerce Committee's Subcommittee on Health & the Environment. The definition: ***psychosurgery***—surgery which is done for the purpose of changing the patient's personality, thought, emotions or behavior, rather than for the treatment of a physical disease. The term is used irregularly: for instance, sometimes referring to all surgery done on the human brain for whatever purpose.

Peter McL. Black, resident in neurosurgery at Massachusetts General Hospital and former fellow in medicine, law and ethics at the Center for Bioethics, Kennedy Institute, Georgetown University, noted in his article (actually part of a debate) in the Humanist that definitions of psychosurgery proposed by authorities "have in common a destruction, removal or disconnection of brain tissue explicitly aimed at changing behavior. . . ."

Thomas S. Szasz, professor of psychiatry at Upstate Medical Center in Syracuse, N.Y., conceding that he was "often identified . . . as a leading opponent of psychosurgery," wrote in the Humanist debate that while a person should be free to seek psychosurgery, no persons, even if "dangerous to himself or others," should be *required* to undergo such operation. He quoted from his book Heresies (Doubleday Anchor, 1976):

"When surgeons operate on the brain of a person with brain disease, they call what they do 'neurosurgery'; when they operate on the brain of a person without brain disease, they call it 'psychosurgery.' It's a nice arrangement for neurosurgeons: it allows them to operate regardless of whether their patient has or has not a disease of the brain; and, because the persons without brain diseases but destined for such surgical interventions are often declared to be legally incompetent on account of 'mental illness,' it also allows them to operate regardless of whether their ostensible patient requests or rejects the operation. . . ."

In a resolution introduced in the Senate in 1973, Sen. J. Glenn Beall Jr. (R, Md.) proposed the following definition:

> The term "psychosurgery" means brain surgery on (A) normal brain tissue of an individual, who does not suffer from any pathological disease, for the purpose of changing or controlling the behavior or emotions of such individual, or (B) on diseased brain tissue of an individual, if the sole object of the performance of such surgery is to control, change, or affect any behavioral or emotional disturbance of such individual. Such term does not include brain surgery designed to cure, or ameliorate the effects of epilepsy; nor shall such term be construed to include electric shock treatments.

Court bars psychosurgery. A Wayne (Mich.) County court ruled July 10, 1973 that state funds could not be used for experimental psychosurgery on persons confined against their will in state institutions, even when the patient's consent was formally obtained.

The court declared unanimously that even if an involuntarily detained patient were to agree to the surgery, the procedure would violate his First Amendment rights of free speech by damaging his ability to generate ideas. The decision, however, left open the possible use of psychosurgery when the procedure had advanced to the level where its benefits outweighed its risks. The court said that not enough was presently known about how the brain functions to permit the experimental surgery.

Beall for caution. Sen. J. Glenn Beall Jr. proposed a two-year moratorium on the use of federal funds and facilities for psychosurgery "or psychiatric surgery." He told the Senate March 29, 1973 that testimony heard by the Health Subcommittee of the Senate Labor & Public Welfare Committee gave him reason for urging caution. Beall said:

During the 20 years between 1935 and 1955, a surgical technique known as lobotomy was widely practiced in this country and throughout the world. It is estimated that approximately 50,000 Americans underwent this radical surgical technique which produced extreme changes in personality, emotional disturbances, impairment of judgment, and a frequent lack of control of basic impulses. During his testimony before the Health Subcommittee, Dr. Bertram S. Brown, the Director of the National Institute of Mental Health, stated:

Unequivocally, that no responsible scientist today would condone a classical lobotomy operation.

Mr. President, I do not wish to simplistically equate the more sophisticated psychosurgical techniques with the classical lobotomy, but I do believe that we should take reasonable and responsible steps designed to protect our citizens from these new and essentially experimental surgical procedures. The classical lobotomy, which permanently disabled tens of thousands of our fellow citizens, fell into disuse only after the American public became aware of its dire consequences. The Congress, the American Medical Association, and the American Psychiatric Association all failed to take decisive action to bring this practice to an end.

In the context of the current situation, it is estimated that between 500 and 700 psychosurgical operations are performed each year in this country. Many psychosurgeons, including Dr. O. J. Andy, who testified before our Health Subcommittee, no longer consider this technique to be experimental. Thus, the potential exists for rapid expansion in the number of operations taking place each year, and I believe that the time has come for the Federal Government to assert itself in such a way as to insure that our citizens are not once again victimized by the specious promise of a quick and lasting surgical cure for mental illness. . . .

In response to a question, Dr. Brown stated that we know much more about the functioning of the human brain today than we did 30 years ago—"but we know very little of what we need to know." I believe that this observation succintly sums up the reasons for suspending Federal support to psychosurgical projects until such time as we have, at our disposal, the type of comprehensive information needed to make a valid policy decision. Dr. Brown reinforced this point when he stated:

We have no reliable data on the extent of the practice or psychosurgery in this country, the types of patients subjected to this technique, or the after effects on patient behavior. The most systematic attempt (in this country) to assess the effects of psychosurgery on patient behavior and intellectual capacities was the Columbia-Greystone project which was conducted in 1954. Since then, many changes in psychiatric and medical practice have taken place: chemotherapy has dramatically changed the nature of the patient population in mental hospitals, and new surgical procedures have been introduced which are quite different from those studied by the Columbia-Greystone project. In order to make any specific recommendations for overseeing or controlling the clinical practice of psychosurgery a systematic survey of the field must be conducted—perhaps by one of the many professional societies and private foundations that have recently begun to focus on ethical issues in life sciences. We need to gather existing data available from patient histories and other sources which never come to our attention because they are not federally funded. In order to answer the "hard" questions, we must first find out what's going on.

Stokes for psychosurgery ban. Rep. Louis Stokes (D, Ohio) told the National Commission for the Protection of Human Subjects of Biomedical & Behavioral Research June 11, 1976 that psychosurgery should be banned in all federally connected health care centers. He said that "psychosurgery has no therapeutic value," that "it is impossible to give informed consent to psychosurgery" and that "psychosurgery has awesome potential as a tool for the social and political repression of minority groups, political dissenters and the poor." Stokes noted that Dr. Bertram S. Brown, director of the National Institute of Mental Health, had said "psychosurgery should be regarded as an experimental therapy...." Stokes continued:

... Indeed, psychosurgery is a highly experimental surgical procedure. Unlike other surgical procedures it has no inherent validity for there is no apparent disease present in the brain tissue. In other words, this procedures is performed even though the brain is healthy and free from disease. Because psychosurgery involves delving and digging deeply in to the human brain, healthy tissues are destroyed in the process.

Tragically, since brain cells do not regenerate, the function which they govern is also obliterated forever. Consequently, the risks involved in this procedure are high. According to the record in *Kaimowitz* v. *Department of Mental Health* (Cir. Ct. Wayne Co., Mich., July 10, 1973), "Psychosurgery ... poses a substantial danger to research subjects, and carries unknown risks". Moreover, "psychosurgery flattens emotional responses, leads to lack of abstract reasoning ability, leads to a loss of capacity for new learning and causes general sedation and apathy. It can lead to impairment of memory, and in some instances unexpected response to psychosurgery are observed. It has been found, for example, that heightened rage reaction can follow surgical intervention on the amygdala, just as placidity can."

In short there are no "successful" psychosurgery operations. However, there are examples of failures. There is the 1968 case of the California prison system's operation on three (3) prisoners. These prisoners were severely damaged by the operations. And there is the case of the thirteen mental patients confined in state institutions in Michigan who were lobotomized. The federally funded State Department of Mental Health financed these experiments sometime between 1968 and 1972. Though the fate of ten of the patients remains under investigation, three of these persons operated on remain at Northville State Hospital as examples of the failure of the experiments.

There is also the example of Morris N. Kallen, Jr., who underwent psychosurgery in Philadelphia's Hahnemann Hospital in 1971. Kallen had undergone psychosurgery under the assumption that he would overcome his heroin addiction. The surgery was a failure and he died a year later.

These examples of the failures of psychosurgery lend credence to the growing belief that the reports on the successes of this procedure are fallacious. According to Dr. Peter Breggin, psychosurgery is no more "... a medical procedure than mutilation of an arm as punishment of a crime is a medical procedure." Thus, it should follow that informed consent cannot be given to the intrusive and permanently damaging experimental procedure now known as "psychosurgery."

In the *Kaimowitz* case, the court addressed the question of institutionalized patients giving consent to psychosurgery. The Court held that the inherently coercive atmosphere of a lengthy institutionalization so greatly diminishes an individual's capacity to give informed consent reasonably and voluntarily that it was *legally impossible* to give consent to psychosurgery. Although this lower court decision had no binding precedential effect in Michigan or any other state, it was the first judicial pronouncement on psychosurgery. Because of the importance of this case, the court's rationale deserves further discussion. The ruling raised very significant constitutional issues. It made the major point that institutionalization *per se* erodes the ability of an involuntarily confined person to render informed consent. Moreover, the pressure upon a patient to conform, to cooperate and to consent in order to placate his supervisors or the parole board, vitiates the possibility of ever obtaining truly voluntary consent.

An excerpt from a January 17, 1973 letter written by the persons chosen as subjects of the experiment in *Kaimowitz* illustrates the coercive impact of institutionalization. The inmates wrote the following letter to Attorney Gabe Kaimowitz:

"We the remaining C.S.P.'s, all undersigned, are very much interested in the job you've undertaken in the case of Louis Smith.

"We've been following the Free Press coverage on the case quite closely since it concerns us all.

"We are all, very possibly, being held unlawfully and have been since 1968. In some cases, there may be other additional grounds for legal action. There are among us a couple of other guinea pigs, those asked to take the medicine mentioned in the newapaper article as the way out. The rest of us are potential guinea pigs if the Department of Mental Health is allowed to get away with such things as they are trying.

"We all want out, and want to stay out, to be cured or at least to be able to control our acts. Becoming guinea pigs is a lot to ask though. We don't want to be vegetables, or incapable of reproducing in the future, or dead. Most of us are young men and have a long life ahead of us. Our freedom is important to us, [out] we want to be free men, young men not too old to enjoy, and not "an it" that can't enjoy."

This letter appeared as an exhibit in the *Kaimowitz* case and is a good example of why physician controlled consent standards should be viewed skeptically. As a lawyer who has argued before the Supreme Court in support of constitutional rights my belief is that the reasoning of the *Kaimowitz* opinion, though commendable, should be taken a step further. I agree with the opinion that an individual can *never* give truly informed consent to psychosurgery because of the unpredictableness of the procedure. Thus, it is impossible for an individual to possess the competency, knowledge and voluntariness necessary to waive his or her constitutional right of consent. Moreover, because of the potential psychosurgery has to docilize its victims, it violates the patient's right to freedom of speech. . . .

As a result, all suits are brought on an aggrieved party's behalf. The result is that the victims of psychosurgery are relegated to the status of subcitizens.

In sum, my position is that no one can give informed consent to psychosurgery. This includes not only involuntarily but voluntarily confined mental patients, as well as, children and persons incarcerated in penal institutions.

The number of psychosurgery operations performed today does not compare in epidemic proportion to the 40,000 lobotomies performed between 1940 and 1955, yet the 500 to 600 operations performed each year are no less dangerous. While it appears that the majority of recent psychosurgery operations have been performed on middle-class women, there today remains a politically inspired move to employ psychosurgery to "rehabilitate" prisoners, "cure" sexual deviants, detoxify drug addicts, quiet unruly children and generally silence political dissenters.

In 1967, two very disturbing letters were published in the journal of the American Medical Association which dealt with the correlation between urban "rioters" and possible brain "dysfunction". The letters were written by three (3) Boston physicians, Dr. Vernon Mark, Director of Neurosurgery at Boston City Hospital, Dr. William Sweet, Chief of Neurosurgery at Massachusetts General Hospital, and Dr. Fran Ervin, a Psychiatrist at Harvard Medical School.

The Physicians wrote:

"That poverty, unemployment, slum housing and inadequate education underlie the nation's urban riots is well known, but the obviousness of these causes may have blinded us to the more subtle role of other possible factors, including brain dysfunction in the rioters who engaged in arson, sniping, and physical assault.

"The real lesson of the urban rioting is that, besides the need to study the social fabric that creates the riot atmosphere, we need intensive research and clinical studies of the individuals committing the violence. The goal of such studies would be to pinpoint, diagnose, and treat those people with low violence thresholds before they contribute to further tragedies."

Mark, Sweet, and Ervin were awarded grants totalling more than $600,000 from the National Institute of Mental Health and the Law Enforcement Assistance Administration to continue their studies on violence control.

Unfortunately, the award of these grants gave financial and moral encouragement to the medical community to use psychosurgery. The most flagrant examples of abuse occured in settings in which those least able to object to the psychosurgical procedures were housed. For example, in 1972, the California Prison system was formulating an elaborate program of psychosurgery on prisoners. Correspondence between prison officials and a local hospital discussed the funding of the first dozen operations, planned at San Francisco's Langley Porter Neuropsychiatric Institute, following the initial workup at the Vacaville Prison. Fortunately, public opinion and media opposition terminated these projects.

As previously mentioned, there were the unwitting participants in the *Kaimowitz* case. In that case, Louis Smith alias "John Doe" and twenty-three (23) patients in Michigan public institutions were to have undergone psychosurgery in a state funded study on "uncontrollable aggression". The purpose of the study was to make a comparison between a drug that would check the flow of male hormones and psychosurgical operation on the amygdaloid portion of the limbic system of the brain. Luckily, the Circuit Court for Wayne County, Michigan freed Smith from the threat of psychosurgery.

Neither the black man operated on at Michigan's Northville State Hospital nor Morris N. Kallen, Jr., who was operated on at Hahnemann's Hospital in Philadelphia, were so fortunate. According to officials, psychosurgery was performed on the black man to "cure" him of injuries which resulted from beatings sustained after his arrest by police during the Detroit riots of 1967. He now sits at Northville State Hospital like a vegetable: Kallen's "cure" for heroin addiction failed and he died a year later.

In the March 14, 1972 issue of the "Philadelphia Daily News", Dr. M. Hunter Brown of Santa Monica, California voiced approval of the operations done at Hahnemann. In fact, Dr. Brown conceded that he had ". . . performed the operation 267 times . . .".

Dr. Brown is joined by his colleague from Mississippi Dr. Orlando Andy in support of psychosurgery. Both advocate that violence can be controlled through surgery and that psychosurgery should be used on selected incarcerated criminals. Dr. Brown has even volunteered his services to the prison sys-

tem, while Dr. Andy has suggested operating on "violent" and "disturbed" children. In fact, Dr. Andy has operated on 13 or 14 children ranging in age from six to nineteen. Interestingly these physicians are presently seeking to minimize the political designs of psychosurgery, and yet it is clear that psychosurgery has received considerable encouragement from reactionary politicians.

In 1973, California Governor Ronald Reagan, who is currently campaigning to become the President of the United States, announced the formation of a new Biomedical Center at UCLA's Brain Research Institute and Department of Psychiatry called the Center for the Reduction of Life-Threatening Behavior. The purpose of the center was to explore the causes of "life threatening behavior" which may or may not exist within the brain. Two of the target groups were to be youths and rioters.

The Center was scheduled to receive almost one million dollars in state funds and federal LEAA allocations. However, due to a variety of reasons, including the collapse of the Nixon Administration, the LEAA made the decision not to fund the research center.

If psychosurgery is not banned, blacks, the poor, the young, and the social and political activists are likely to be its victims. The only reasons why these groups have been relatively spared from psychosurgery in recent years is because of pressure from reform groups; the *Kaimowitz* decision; the cut-off of federal funds; the moral importance of the establishment of this Commission, and my proposed legislation. Collectively, they have dissuaded psychosurgery's widespread use. However, psychosurgery remains a threat because a few physicians have encouraged patients in private institutions to "consent" to this procedure. Moreover, existing federal regulation does not effectively control the practice of psychosurgery. I submit that the practice of psychosurgery is not amenable to effective regulation by either the public or private sector, and thus it must be totally banned.

Federal panel backs operation. Psychosurgery "should not be categorically prohibited," according to a report approved Sept. 10, 1976 by the 11-member National Commission for the Protection of Human Subjects of Biomedical and Behavioral Research.

The group recommended that psychosurgery should continue to be permitted but only under strict government supervision. Safeguards would include:

- Certification of both a surgeon's competence and a patient's suitability for psychosurgery by institutional review boards that met Department of Health, Education and Welfare (HEW) standards.
- A requirement that operations on minors be permitted only after a court hearing where the patient had legal representation.
- A requirement that an operation be requested by a confined patient or prisoner or that person's legal guardian, not by the confining institution.

The commission recommended that HEW establish some means of assessing psychosurgery results to determine "the extent to which specific procedures may relieve various psychiatric [symptoms and] disorders." In 1973, the head of the National Institute of Mental Health (NIMH) had opposed psychosurgery on the basis that doctors did not know enough about the brain.

Other Developments Involving Mental Problems & the Law

Better Alabama mental care ordered. U.S. District Court Judge Frank M. Johnson Jr. ordered Alabama April 13, 1972 to meet detailed guidelines for psychiatric treatment and custodial care in its institutions for the mentally ill and retarded. It was considered a landmark case.

Johnson, ruling on a suit brought by patients and staff members, called conditions at two mental hospitals "grossly deficient," and those at a school for the retarded "grossly substandard." If the legislature did not provide funds for remedial action, or if the Alabama Mental Health Board failed to abide by the specific standards enumerated in the order within six months, the court pledged to appoint a master to oversee operations.

Minimum professional and nonprofessional staff-patient ratios were set, as well as minimum educational time and class size limits for the school. An "individual treatment plan" for each patient would be required, and federal minimum wages would be paid for any work performed, which could not in any case by compulsory.

Seven-member "human rights committees," with a patient on each, were named for each facility, to review all programs and aid patients who claimed rights abuses.

Alabama sanity laws voided—A three-judge federal court panel ruled 2–1, Dec. 14, 1974 that Alabama's state laws on the involuntary commitment of persons to mental institutions were unconstitutional. The panel found that current commitment procedures violated constitutional standards of due process.

The decision stipulated procedures to be followed in subsequent civil commitments. They included a prompt hearing, preferably before a jury, the right to legal counsel, the right to call witnesses, and the right to an "independent expert examination." While it sanctioned emergency commitments, the court added the requirement that a hearing be held within seven days.

The court also ordered the state to begin releasing or give new hearings to the 3,000 persons confined under the voided commitment statutes.

Mental hospitals probed. A Stanford University psychologist reported in the January 1973 issue of Science that he and seven other persons had successfully been admitted to 12 different mental hospitals, where they stayed up to 52 days without detection. Dr. David L. Rosenhan ran the experiment over a three-year period to determine whether mental hospitals could tell the sane from the insane. His conclusion was they could not, the New York Times reported Jan. 20.

The pseudo-patients resumed normal behavior after being admitted because they heard strange voices. Once admitted, anything they did was seen as an "aspect of pathological behavior," even pacing of the halls out of boredom and waiting outside the dining room before meals—the high point of the day for some of the patients. One nurse ascribed copious note-taking by one of the fakers to a crazy compulsion.

When each patient was finally discharged, it was with the diagnosis of "schizophrenia in remission," never a clean bill of health or a suggestion of misdiagnosis.

Benefits to bias victim ordered. A Michigan state hearing referee ruled that Chrysler Corp. had to pay workmen's compensation benefits, including psychiatric care expenses, to a black employee whose nondisabling psychotic tendencies had been aggravated by plant racism and unfair work conditions, causing him to kill three supervisors after he was fired in 1970, it was reported March 7, 1973.

James Johnson had been found legally insane at his trial and placed in a state mental hospital. In the latest ruling, a state examiner said Johnson had developed paranoic feelings toward whites during his childhood on a Mississippi plantation. He had then been unfairly assigned to undesirable jobs at the plant, denied advancement opportunities, called "nigger" and "boy" by a foreman, denied medical benefits, suspended unfairly and fired after refusing what he considered a dangerous job.

U.S. suit seeks rights for retarded. A Department of Justice suit filed in U.S. district court in Baltimore Feb. 21, 1974 charged that the State of Maryland had deprived residents of the state's largest institution for the mentally retarded of their constitutional rights to proper care, treatment, education and safekeeping.

The suit, the first of its kind filed by the Justice Department, was an attempt to force the courts to establish minimal standards of care and treatment for 200,000 persons in mental institutions in the U.S.

Filed on behalf of the 2,400 residents of the Rosewood State Hospital at Owings Mills, the suit named as defendants Dr. Neil Solomon, Maryland secretary of health and mental hygiene; Bert W. Schmickel, director of the state's mental retardation administration; and Rosewood superintendent Dr. Marvin M. Malcotti.

J. Stanley Pottinger, an assistant attorney general, said: "In all too many cases, when one who is mentally retarded is institutionalized, little or no treatment or habilitation is provided. Under these circumstances, commitment can become a 'life sentence' with no trial by jury or other due process protections—safeguards that are routinely accorded to those . . . convicted of the most heinous crimes."

According to the suit, the defendants failed or refused to hire a professional staff large enough to insure minimum treatment and habilitation; provide appropriate programs for residents, including physical therapy, nursing and health care and academic instruction; and provide a humane psychological and physical environment in which training and habilitation could take place.

The suit also alleged that the defendants had failed to hire sufficient personnel to supervise the residents and prevent them from harming themselves and others.

In some cases, the suit charged, residents were employed without pay in nontherapeutic work and were kept in the institution solely because of their willingness or ability to do a job.

The Justice Department cited as the suit's legal basis the 8th Amendment prohibition against cruel and unusual punishments, the 13th Amendment ban on involuntary servitude and the 14th Amendment guarantee of equal protection under the law.

Acknowledging that about half of Rosewood's inmates were classified as severely or profoundly retarded (below 35 IQ), the suit said all or nearly all inmates were capable of benefitting from care intended to enable them to cope with personal needs and to improve physical, mental and social efficiency.

Homosexuality no mental disorder. In 1974 U.S. psychiatrists agreed formally that homosexuality per se should no longer be classified as a mental disorder.

The American Psychiatric Association reported April 8 that its membership had approved the December 1973 action by trustees revising the organization's list of mental disorders. According to the new definition, homosexuality would be considered a "sexual orientation disturbance" only if a person was disturbed by the condition and desired treatment for it. The trustees had said the diagnostic category would be distinguished from homosexuality, "which, by itself, does not necessarily constitute a psychiatric disorder."

I.Q. tests curbed. A federal judge ruled in San Francisco Nov. 27, 1974 that intelligence quotient (I.Q.) tests must not be given to black children in California if the tests did not reflect the children's cultural background.

U.S. District Court Judge Robert F. Peckham made the ruling in a suit brought by the NAACP Legal Defense and Educational Fund Inc. and other groups. He had ruled two years earlier that San Francisco schools could not use I.Q. tests to determine whether black children should be placed in classes for the educable mentally retarded.

Three black psychiatrists held a press conference after the ruling Nov. 27 and estimated that 75% of the black children in classes for the mentally retarded did not belong there. I.Q. tests were based on "white middle class standards," said Dr. William Pierce.

Curb on confining mentally ill. The Supreme Court June 26, 1975 unanimously ruled that mental patients could not be confined in institutions against their will if they were not dangerous to others and could live on the outside on their own.

"May the state fence in the harmless mentally ill solely to save its citizens from exposure to those whose ways are different?" asked Justice Potter Stewart, author of the court's opinion. "One might as well ask if the state, to avoid public unease, could incarcerate all who are physically unattractive or socially eccentric. Mere public intolerance or animosity cannot constitutionally justify the deprivation of a person's physical liberty."

The decision in the case (O'Connor v. Donaldson) concerned a damage suit by Kenneth Donaldson, 67, who had spent 15 years in a Florida mental hospital before his release in 1971. Donaldson, who had sued two supervising doctors at the institution for allegedly depriving him of his constitutional rights and failing to provide treatment to him, had been committed to the state facility in 1957 by his father, who said his son was suffering from delusions. In its ruling, the high court ordered the case returned to federal district court for determination of whether one of the supervising doctors had been entitled to instruct the original state trial jury—which awarded Donaldson $38,000—that he could not have reasonably known that the Florida law supporting custodial care was invalid.

In a concurring opinion, Chief Justice Warren E. Burger said he did not feel that all legally confined persons had the right to treatment, or that providing treatment might justify the confinement of an otherwise functional person.

N.J. ruling upholds commitment—A three-judge federal court panel April 15, 1976 upheld the New Jersey regulations concerning the involuntary commitment of individuals to mental institutions. The decision, which affirmed the constitutionality of regulations on involuntary commitment adopted in September 1975, rejected the contention of a former mental patient that he should have been accorded the same rights of due process given criminal defendants. Under current regulations, a person could be confined without a hearing for a period as long as 20 days after an adult and two psychiatrists had stated that the individual's continued freedom would pose a danger to himself or herself or to society.

A report by the New Jersey Mental Health Planning Committee, made public June 28, said the state's mental health program placed too much emphasis on hospital-based care and not enough on community-based, out-patient mental health centers. The 18-member task force, appointed in 1974 by state Health Commissioner Dr. Joanne Finley and Institutions and Agencies Commissioner Ann Klein, called for the integration of the state's psychiatric hospitals and community-based programs and ultimately the creation of a state Department of Mental Health.

Mental illness linked to economy. The economic recession and accompanying inflation were responsible for a marked increase in admissions to mental health facilities, according to two psychiatrists writing in the Journal of the American Medical Association Jan. 26.

Drs. Louis E. Kopolow and Frank M. Ochberg of the National Institute of Mental Health said, "the present economic recession and concomitant inflation are taking their toll on the mental and physical health of the nation."

These conclusions were based on information obtained through telephone surveys made of community mental health centers and state and private mental health facilities in areas of high unemployment.

The surveys showed an increase in the treatment for mental illness, particularly among men 45–60 years of age. The occupational group most affected was the semiskilled production worker on assembly lines.

According to the psychiatrists, the same stresses that brought about mental illness also contributed to the development of such ailments as coronary artery disease and peptic ulcers.

One-family housing for retarded upheld. The Appellate Division of the New York State Supreme Court May 3, 1976 upheld the right of a private organization to establish a group home for retarded children in a neighborhood zoned for one-family housing.

The court's ruling opened the way for eight retarded children—ranging in age from five to 10—to move into a home in the Little Neck section of Queens, under the supervision of a married couple. The home had been purchased in 1975 for $108,000 by the Working Organization for Retarded Children.

Some people in the neighborhood opposed the agency's plan to open a group home on the basis that the area was zoned for one-family houses.

In handing down its decision, the court stated that "a group home which is organized pursuant to the social services law is specifically designed to emulate in appearance a reasonably sized biological unitary family."

The court also dismissed the contention that such a home would alter the local quality of life or disrupt the neighborhood.

Care standards ordered. Patients at the Camden County (N.J.) Psychiatric Hospital in Lakeland were "entitled as a matter of constitutional right to adequate treatment in the least restrictive environment," according to a ruling handed down July 19, 1976 by state Superior Court Judge Michael P. King.

A class-action suit, filed May 8, 1975 on behalf of the hospital's patients (currently 414), had charged that living conditions there were poor, staff training was inadequate, patients' records were not being reviewed periodically, administrators were refusing to release patients from locked wards after court-ordered releases, patients' constitutional rights were being violated and patients were receiving poor care and treatment because of inadequate staffing.

King's 29-page decision did not generally address accusations of mistreatment or neglect, however. It said the hospital's staff and administrators had been "struggling uphill and against the tide" and ordered the county's board of chosen freeholders to provide funds for the hiring of more staff.

King also called for better recreational facilities, longer visiting hours, more security for patients' belongings and continuation of a $4.6-million county program to upgrade the physical plant of the 50-year-old institution.

"This court sees its duty in this case as one setting forth standards which should be met by the board [of freeholders] in the operation of the institution to ensure that patients, about 90% of whom are involuntarily committed, will receive the constitutionally mandated treatment in a humane environment," King said.

In a somewhat similar situation, Judge Harold M. Nitto of the Passaic County (N.J.) Juvenile & Domestic Relations Court ruled Oct. 20 that persons involuntarily committed to mental institutions had the right to quality care.

In so deciding, Judge Nitto ordered the state Department of Institutions and Agencies (I&A) to provide individual psychiatric care, a "meaningful program of social development" and an educational program for Robert George Williamson, 19, of Wayne, who had been committed to Greystone Park Psychiatric Hospital in 1974 after being found mentally incompetent to stand trial for the murder of a neighbor in 1973.

Nitto, who declared Williamson to be "perniciously mentally ill," said the criminally insane had a right to treatment, not simple incarceration, since the latter amounted to imprisonment.

The judge issued an order requiring I&A to "expend such funds as are necessary" within the next 30 days to insure quality treatment for Williamson at a suitable place, "whether public or private, whether within the State of New Jersey or elsewhere."

Judge Nitto said in his 28-page opinion that he had heard expert testimony that "equated Greystone to a warehouse for the mentally ill." Unless Williamson received "one-to-one" psychotherapy, Nitto said, his "condition would likely harden and become exceedingly difficult to treat in the near future. . . ."

New Jersey had 20,000 persons in its mental institutions. Of that number, 7,000 had been committed involuntarily and 165 had been adjudged criminally insane.

U.S. study of situation at Farview—In an additional situation involving the legal rights of mental hospital patients, officials of the National Institute of Mental Health, a subdivision of the U.S. Department of Health, Education and Welfare, had concluded that Farview State Hospital in Waymart, Wayne County, was unable to provide even minimal treatment for patients and that the task of bringing Farview into compliance with acceptable standards would likely be "near impossible," the Philadelphia Inquirer reported Oct. 10, 1976.

The NIMH report, based on a survey made July 20–22 at the request of the U.S. Social Security Administration (SSA), had prompted the federal government to cut off Medicare payments to the hospital, the Inquirer reported. Farview, the only state institution devoted exclusively to the criminally insane, had received some $500,000 annually under the program.

An SSA spokesman said Farview had not been in compliance with federal regulations since 1974. He noted that prior to that year his agency had relied on the word of state health inspectors that the hospital met federal standards.

In its report, the NIMH team questioned "whether or not any institution of this kind can or should exist." Citing a severe lack of adequately trained professional personnel at Farview, it wrote of a "pretense of providing psychiatric treatment" and said the institution served merely to provide "relief for the rest of the community" by isolating "the most difficult persons living in Pennsylvania—those who are poor, criminal and psychotic."

The team also criticized shortcomings in the physical plant, the poor training of staff, shoddy record-keeping, an unsanitary kitchen and a poor water supply.

In a series of articles beginning June 27, the Philadelphia Inquirer had alleged there were patterns of brutality, mysterious deaths, neglect, inadequate treatment and other abuses and substandard conditions at Farview. The series had prompted the formation June 29 of a special investigating committee of the state Senate. Committee members had toured the institution July 8 and opened public hearings on it July 28. Following the July 8 inspection tour, Sen. Henry J. Cianfrani (D, Philadelphia) had said, "This in no way resembles a hospital. This is nothing but a prison."

Independently of the Senate probe, Wayne County Coroner Robert Jennings was conducting an inquest into alleged "suspicious" deaths at Farview. The bodies of several former patients had been exhumed during the course of the inquest.

The NIMH team said they had found "no evidence of brutality" and that a review of three cases of "sudden and unexpected deaths had revealed no exceptional difficulties in clinical management" beyond the general lack of professional supervision, guidance and treatment.

Following are excerpts from the National Institute of Mental Health's report on Farview State Hospital:

The hospital is a large prison-like institution that presents itself both internally and externally as stark, cold, uninviting. The hospital has a basic philosophy of security first and other considerations second. . . .

STAFF

There is absolutely no way in which the Farview State Hospital meets even minimum requirements for staffing which is necessary to provide for active psychiatric treatment.

Of the three professions, psychiatry, psychiatric nursing and psychology, there can only be said to be one fully trained person, the chief of psychology, in those three professions who presently works at the hospital.

This is a rather stark and dramatic indication of the failure of the governing body to provide the appropriate resources to provide adequate psychiatric treatment. . . .

Farview State Hospital has received the most difficult psychiatric and behavioral problems of the state and has been staffed almost exactly the opposite of the way it should be to treat these people.

At the time of the previous surveys there were just four nurses available. That number has presently risen to 30, however, of these 30 nurses none is a fully trained psychiatric nurse and only two or three actually have bachelor degrees. This means that those persons on the wards, for the most part, are unable to exert the professional leadership needed to change the pattern of activities from custodial and security to therapeutic. . . .

SUMMARY

Farview State Hospital today is the result of a complex number of factors which include societal, management and clinical areas. The hospital has been set up and has functioned as the last stop for the most difficult persons living in Pennsylvania—those who are poor, criminal, and psychotic.

The hospital has been used by the Department [Bureau] of Corrections, Department of Justice and by the rest of the mental health system as a way of punishing patients or as a way of relieving these other institutions of difficult management problems.

On the other hand, the hospital has been managed by essentially untrained, unqualified persons for dealing with these severe behavioral disorders and has been run under the philosophy of security as the primary and ultimately over the years the only reason for the hospital. It is no wonder that the present allegations made toward the hospital concerning patient brutality come up if one realizes that the setting is such that if brutality does not come up it would be rather surprising. However, we must point out in our survey we saw no evidence of brutality; charts reviewed of three of the patients who are being presently investigated for sudden and unexpected deaths revealed no exceptional difficulties in clinical management or no failure in clinical management beyond those manifested for every other patient in the overall sense that there is simply not enough professional supervision, guidance, and treatment provided.

The largest single group in the hospital, the psychiatric security aides, have a long history of . . . efforts . . . directed toward security, maintaining it and . . . have in a sense been responsible for the hospital.

The above mentioned factors therefore clearly point not to individual malfeasance within the hospital nor even individual apathy in the hospital but rather to an overall failure of the governing process—a failure to provide adequate resources, adequate administrative and managerial support, adequate monitoring and ultimately having failed to be accountable for the institution called Farview State Hospital.

ISSUES

The issues at Farview are not those that are being played up in allegations of brutality; the issue at Farview is whether or not any institution of this kind can or should exist and if it does, how to monitor it, manage it, and staff it so that there is adequate treatment provided to those patients who are in it.

Internally it seems that the management of Farview could be and should be more aggressive in defining itself more clearly in attacking those practices which leave it as a dumping ground and which keep its population at a level which makes active treatment for anyone highly unlikely. This really refers to the need for Farview and its governing body insofar as the Department of [Public] Welfare is considered to be the governing body to address issues with the corrections department as well as to address the issue of other state hospitals learning to manage their own difficulties.

But even beyond this there is clearly a need for the governor and the legislature not to investigate Farview, not to castigate it but rather to address themselves and the people of the state as to whether or not the people of the state wish to continue to treat criminal, poor, and psychotic persons in this manner or whether they wish to address their mental health needs in a different way.

Certainly by these findings not being in compliance it is clear that medicare recertification is not possible and there is a good chance obviously that the governing body will decide that there is no other way, nothing else they can do and therefore at least the pretense of providing psychiatric treatment can be dropped and the state can face the fact that what they are providing is relief for the rest of the community.

The present hospital administration at the top is realistic, idealistic, aware and forward looking; however, immediately below the top there is an enormous paucity of clinical management persons and above the top there is little indication from our stay that there is any activity constructively aimed towards either changing Farview or addressing the needs of these persons who are incarcerated there in a different way. Therefore, it seems likely that this administration will be left with a near impossible task.

Problems of Death

When Does Death Occur?

Medical advances have brought into question the very fact of death. When has a person died? When the heart has ceased beating? If so, does the transplant surgeon commit murder when he removes the still pulsating heart of an accident victim whose brain shows no sign of life? The legal and moral implications of these and similar questions about death are still not completely settled.

The difficulty of definition. A "discursive" definition of the term "death" was prepared by the staff of the U.S. House Commerce Committee's Subcommittee on Health and the environment. The definition: ***death***—a permanent cessation of all vital functions; the end of life (often called mortality). A simple concept whose actual occurrence medicine has made very difficult to define and measure. A concensus appears to be forming that death occurs when all measurable or identifiable brain functioning (electrical or any other kind) is absent for over 24 hours.

The problem of definition had been discussed by Dr. Eliot Corday in the May 7, 1970 issue of the Hospital Tribune. "Already, in view of the known resuscitative methods and life-support systems that may revive a patient from apparent death," he wrote, "the public has begun to question the criteria by which a live heart is removed from a dead donor."

Corday warned that the medical profession appeared "to be moving toward a double standard. One standard would be to accomodate the transplanters—certifying that death has occurred when there are no reflexes and the EEG trace is linear—in other words, cerebral death. The other standard for the everyday practice of medicine would be to continue to accept the age-old definition of death as the irreversible cessation of perceptible heart beat and respiration. And today this may have to imply that cardiac resuscitation, assuming it was available, had been attempted and failed—a question that has come up in at least one court case."

Corday recalled that a Harvard ad hoc committee had drafted a definition of irreversible coma. The criteria would include: maintenance of respiration only by artificial means and inability to maintain spontaneous respiration when artificial means are withdrawn; no awareness of externally applied stimuli; no spontaneous muscle movement or reflexes; a flat EEG. These criteria had been generally accepted as justifying a diagnosis of cerebral death and thereby permitting the removal of organs, but Corday noted that "some transplant surgeons, however, have declared cerebral death while spontaneous respiration was still present."

Similar criteria were adopted in 1968 by 24 surgeons, immunologists, neurologists and heart specialists who met in Geneva on the call of the Council for International Organizations of Medical Science, under the aegis of the World Health Organization and UNESCO. These conferees insisted on two further criteria, Corday recalled: "(1) the donor's heart must be in perfect condition at the time of removal; (2) an immunological examination should be made before the operation to determine the compatibility of donor and receiver." The addition of these two requirements could indicate that some question remained in the minds of conferees as to the adequacy of the criteria they were accepting and that they were proposing to balance the desirability of saving another's life against the uncertainty over whether the potential donor had actually died. Corday noted that the scientists had added still another requirement—that "two independent teams should be deployed in heart transplant operations, one to establish the donor's hopeless condition, the other to perform the operation."

Corday held that there was still "need to determine whether there is adequate evidence that the moment of death may now be advanced to coincide with brain death, though cardio-respiratory activity is spontaneous."

4 MDs cleared in transplant case. Four doctors—three transplant specialists and a state medical examiner—were acquitted May 25, 1972 by a jury in Richmond, Va. of wrong-doing in removing the Va. of wrong-doing in removing the heart of a 56-year-old man for a transplant operation although under the legal definition of death he was still alive.

The jury set a precedent in allowing the medical definition of death to take precedence over the legal definition. Most medical authorities regarded a person as no longer alive if the brain was dead even if other life systems could be kept going by mechanical means.

At issue in the trial was whether Drs. David Hume, Richard Lower and David Sewell, members of a transplant team, ended the life of Bruce O. Tucker May 25, 1968 so they could use his heart in a transplant operation. The fourth doctor named in the suit was Dr. Abdullah Fatteh, the state medical examiner, who released Tucker's body for the transplant team's use.

Legal definition of death at issue. An Oakland, Calif. superior court jury convicted Andrew Lyons of involuntary manslaughter May 24, 1974 despite his contention that his victim, whose brain-wave activity had stopped, had not died until surgeons removed his still-beating heart for transplant into another person.

Dr. Norman Shumway, one of the surgeons involved in the case and a heart-transplant specialist at Stanford University in Palo Alto, Calif., testified at the trial May 19 that irreversible cessation of brain activity, rather than an end to heartbeat, was the best way to legally determine death. (The recipient of the manslaughter victim's heart died a month after receiving it.)

AMA for postponing definition law. In an action Dec. 3, 1974, the House of Delegates of the American Medical Association adopted a resolution calling on state medical societies to ask legislatures to postpone enactment of statutes defining death. Calling statutory definition "neither desirable nor necessary," the delegates said death should "be determined by the clinical judgment of the physician." The "permanent and irreversible cessation of function of the brain" was suggested as a possible clinical criterion for death.

Definition complicates slaying. Walter Burton Carey 3rd, a 27-year-old ex-convict, pleaded innocent Dec. 7, 1976 to charges of second-degree murder, murder in the commission and furtherance of a felony and first-degree robbery in the slaying of an Islip, N.Y. high school student.

Carey was accused of killing Karen Ann Pomroy, 17, in a Nov. 29 robbery. Pomroy had been found unconscious, her skull partially crushed, that afternoon on the grounds of Islip High School. She was operated on that evening at Southside Hospital in Bay Shore by Dr. William H. Bloom, a neurosurgeon and the president of the county medical society.

According to Bloom, Pomroy had gone into an irreversible coma on Tuesday, Nov. 30, "with a total absence of reflexes." Bloom said tests revealed blood was not reaching her brain. She was placed on a respirator early Wednesday morning, Dec. 1, and electroencephalograms were administered to measure brain activity. These scans, said Bloom, had shown no brain activity was present. Pomroy was removed from the respirator Thursday, Dec. 2, after her corneas and her kidneys had been removed for transplant with her parents' consent.

(Carey was arrested for assault Dec. 1 and charged with murder Dec. 3. According to papers submitted to the court Dec. 3, he had told a detective, "I grabbed her. I grabbed her pocketbook. She started screaming, and I kept hitting her with a [iron railroad] spike.")

Suffolk Assistant District Attorney Gerald Sullivan Dec. 7 indicated he believed Carey's attorneys would challenge the murder charges on the ground the actual cause of death had been her removal from the respirator, not the blows Carey had allegedly struck. Bloom Dec. 3 said, in his opinion, "brain death" had occurred at approximately midnight on Nov. 30. Pomroy had not been pronounced dead until 3:45 PM, Dec. 2.

Sullivan said the Carey trial would be the first of its kind, since New York State had no legal definition of death. Bills proposing legal definitions had failed to pass in the state legislature.

'Death With Dignity': The Senate Hearings

Ethical, medical & legal problems. Hearings were held by the Senate Special Committee on Aging Aug. 7–8, 1972 on what the committee chairman, Sen. Frank Church (D, Ida.), said in his opening statement was a subject "sometimes called 'Death With Dignity,' or 'The Right to Die,' or ... other titles which question the right to prolong life by extraordinary means when all hope for recovery—or in some cases, even for consciousness or lucidity—has vanished."

Church indicated that the advances of medical science had caused the ethical, medical and legal problems being explored by the committee. He said: "At least 80% of the population of this nation now dies in institutions—hospitals, nursing homes, and other facilities of one kind or another. Yet, not very long ago, the largest percentage of Americans died in their own homes.... Lingering illnesses, of course, occurred with some frequency, but more often than not there was no practical way of keeping persons alive after they had lost conscious relationship to the world around them. Today, the very institutions and medical talent that have triumphed over many illnesses are also coming under criticism because of the way in which they deal with the terminally ill, or apparently terminally ill, patient."

Dr. Arthur E. Morgan, former president of Antioch College, testified March 7. He said:

"In many cases, continued living is an unalloyed liability, giving none of the values of life to the person involved. However, the decision to cease living should have legal consideration before action. Even the decision of the person himself may have been induced against his own judgment, simply by acquiescence. Should it not be social custom in matters of life and death that a legal verdict be required? Quite commonly the issues will be so clear that legal determination will be little more than a form. Furthermore, in cases where the person chiefly involved may be largely without self-determination, a legal and social judgment would seem to be sound public policy.

"...[T]he real burdens sometimes placed upon others by the necessity of caring for persons for whom life has lost all meaning, or for the hopelessly aged or infirm, must also be considered. There are diseases and disabilities characterized by disorganization of the brain ... which lead to permanent and irrecoverable and complete loss of intelligence and awareness which lasts through life, sometimes 20 or 30 years or more. In many instances the care of such cases through the years monopolizes family activities and attention with no relaxation and the certain prospect of no recovery. The necessary continuance of life in such cases often represents unrelieved tragedy for the responsible individuals or families, or the waste of institutional facilities. Experienced and representative physicians hold that this class of totally incurable disability has called long and loudly for relief which up to the present has been denied. . . ."

Dr. Laurance F. Foye Jr., education service director of the Veterans Administration, offering a dissenting opinion, said:

"A number of complex problems are encompassed by the popular but obscure phrase 'death with dignity.' These include: the hopeless case, prolongation of suffering, active and passive euthanasia, the 'right to die,' and the 'living will.' Essentially, these are all medical problems relating directly to the responsibilities and decisions of the physician in his relationship with his patient. Rational consideration of these questions is unfortunately and customarily confused by opinions based upon misconceptions and emotion.

"A recent newspaper article on this problem clearly demonstrated and contributed to the confusion by quoting priests, rabbis, theologians, the pope, a state governor, a poet and several physicians. It is a disturbing observation that, to my knowledge, every religious spokesman on this subject has come out in favor of passive and occasionally active euthanasia in hopeless cases. . . .

". . . [W]e must not equate incurability with hopelessness. Diabetes, emphysema, practically all heart disease, baldness and flat feet are incurable but rarely hopeless. While approximately one-third of cancer patients can be cured of their disease, the remaining two-thirds are today incurable. The incurable cancer patient may live three months . . . or 30 years with his disease, possibly earning a living, raising a family, and enjoying life during this period. He may or may not require treatment along the way, and he may or may not die of this incurable disease. These statements are generally true of all incurable diseases. . . .

"Every physician can . . . describe a number of patients for whom he predicted a rapidly fatal outcome—saying, 'I knew they were going to die'—and was wrong. The patient who was told by his doctor that he had six months to live but is alive years later is legendary. Thus, since the practice of any form of euthanasia, active or passive, can only be justified by certainty of outcome, and we can't be certain for any specific patient, we dare not authorize or practice euthanasia. If a physician withholds maximum effort from patients he considers hopelessly ill, he will unavoidably withhold maximum effort from an occasional patient who could have been saved. Patients will die because of the physician's decision not to treat actively. This approach and concern cannot be fostered or condoned, legally or otherwise.

"Typically, at this point in the discussion, the proponent of euthanasia then describes in detail a patient being kept alive 'uselessly' with tubes and machines and urges that the machines be turned off and the tubes removed 'so the patient can die peacefully and with dignity.' Neither I nor anyone else knows how to decide when being alive becomes 'useless'; I can only point out that 'tubes and machines' are used because they save lives, relieve symptoms and permit many patients to survive critical stages of an illness. Since it is usually a serious life-threatening problem that calls for these measures, they don't always work, and . . . some patients will die. One cannot then say, because such a patient dies, that these measures were a waste of time . . . since when they are initiated it is not known in which patient they will be successful.

"The statement made by noted clerics that the physician is not obligated to use 'heroic or extraordinary' means in a 'hopeless' case now becomes meaningless, since we can't be certain the case is hopeless, and it is precisely in such critical cases that 'extraordinary' measures must be considered and may be effective. . . .

"The 'living will,' a document in which the patient permits and instructs his physician to let him die if his condition is hopeless, really solves nothing but does create problems of its own. The danger is that relatives, deciding for any number of reasons that active treatment should be stopped, will attempt, with or without legal support, to prevent the doctor from continuing his life-saving efforts, or that the doctor will find that the existence of such a document will be one 'reason' to terminate his active treatment. . . .

"The 'right to die' concept implies that, if our death is certain and immediate we have the 'right' to make it even more immediate. The now obvious fallacy is that the patient or the doctor can know when death is certain. . . . We must never forget that on occasion patients, their families, and their physicians will conclude that a disease has reached the hopeless stage and death is imminent—and be wrong. If they can stop treatment on the basis of their hopelessness, the prophecy becomes self-fulfilling. Whether the patient was going to die or not, their action ensures his death and the physician's confidence is his ability to predict death is dangerously enhanced. . . .

"Finally, what many laymen fear is that the doctor, in a pointless attempt to postpone death, will keep them in agony for long periods of time—the prolongation of suffering problem. A number of studies have shown, and this corresponds to my experience, that the majority of critically or terminally ill patients do not have pain and that those who do can be controlled by the judicious use of pain-killing medicines. . . ."

Dr. Walter W. Sackett, a member of the Florida House of Representatives, told the committee Aug. 7 that he considered "euthanasia . . . more closely akin to death with dignity than it is to mercy killing." "Euthanasia means happy death," he continued. "[T]his philosophy is almost unanimously accepted by the general population. I have asked for a referendum on it. I have asked for a constitutional amendment. . . ." Sackett also said:

". . . I have been accused by a few rattlebrains, I think, of . . . trying to act like God. Now, when I keep a person such as we have been describing alive, I feel then I am acting like God, and I am being very inhumane to that person by continuing his suffering. . . .

"You talk about there are no diseases that are actually incurable. . . . There are. When the central nervous system is injured, that is permanent. That is forever. When the brain tissue, spinal cord tissue, is injured, that is it. It will never get any better. That is final. There is no return from it. . . ."

Church asked: ". . . Dr. Sackett, . . . you have said that in your practice of medicine you have let patients die?" Sackett replied, "Hundreds of them." He estimated that "75% of the doctors" do likewise.

Dr. Henry K. Beecher of Harvard Medical School told the committee Aug. 8 that "death occurs at several levels: There is cellular death. Human cells can be maintained alive in tissue cultures for years; so we cannot define death as the loss of all vital functions. There is 'physiological' death when the vital activities have ceased; that is, death occurs when integrated tissue and organ functions cease. There is intellectual death, spiritual death and social death. . . . Or to approach the problem with more generality: There is subcellular and cellular life, life of organs, life of the individual and beyond this, life of the individual as a member of the community. However, it is phrased, our basic concern is with the presence or absence of physiological life, especially neurological life. The lack of an accepted definition of death handicaps many of the activities within the hospital, the cadaver transplant problem. This is a medicolegal problem; it is also a sociolegal problem. . . ."

Beecher recalled Pope Pius XII's speech on "The Prolongation of Life" before the International Congress of Anesthesiologists Nov. 24, 1957. The pope said that the physician had a duty to use all reasonable ordinary means to restore vital functions and consciousness and to employ such extraordinary measures as are available to him. "But," the pope said, "normally one is held to use only ordinary means—according to circumstances of persons, places, times, and culture—that is to say, means that do not involve any grave burden for oneself or another. A more strict obligation would be too burdensome for most men and would render the attainment of the higher, more important good too difficult. Life, health, all temporal activities are in fact subordinated to spiritual ends. On the other hand, one is not forbidden to take more than the strictly necessary steps to preserve life and health, as long as he does not fail in some more more serious duty."

Alexander Morgan Capron of the University of Pennsylvania School of Law discussed the legal aspects of the subject. He said:

"... The crux of the problem ... is whether dignified death is inconsistent with good medical care. There is a pressing need to make clear that these are consistent and indeed that good medical care is a means to achieving a dignified death as well as a dignified life.

"If there is an inconsistency between what medicine ought to be doing and present practices, at least part of the blame can be laid at the door of the law. So far as I know there are no clear and certain answers to such questions as: (1) When can a dying patient choose to cease being treated? (2) Who else can exercise that authority on the patient's behalf? (3) What interests do physicians and the state have in prolonging treatment and what weight do these interests carry compared with others? (4) What action could be taken against a physician who—on his own initiative or at the request of a patient or his relatives—ceased treatment?

"The law's initial answers to these questions are contained in a group of cases that arose from refusals by Jehovah's Witnesses to accept blood transfusions which physicians believed were necessary to save the patients' lives. American courts are divided in their response.

"In one leading case, *In re Brooks Estate* ... (1965), the Illinois Supreme Court held that a competent adult who steadfastly opposed blood transfusions for her chronic peptic ulcer should not have been compelled to receive blood under a court order. Unfortunately, the appellate court's reasoning is not particularly useful for this discussion because it was grounded in the patient's First Amendment right to free exercise of her religion.

"A number of courts have reached an opposite conclusion. For example, in *application of President and Directors of Georgetown College,* 331 F.2d 1000 (D.C. Cir.), *cert. denied,* 377 U.S. 978 (1964), Judge J. Skelly Wright, sitting alone on an emergency appeal, ruled that a hospital was entitled to an order permitting it to administer blood over the patient's objections. While I disagree with the action taken by Judge Wright, this case is still useful for the issues it raises which, aside from the religious factor, seem very similar to those raised in the death with dignity situation....

"...The creation of an explicit legal right for patients to decline potentially lifesaving treatment presents a second issue discussed in the *Georgetown* case: the court's analogizing of the refusal to be treated with 'self-homicide.'

"Accepting, *arguendo,* that the state has a legitimate interest in prohibiting suicide, I do not believe that this interest or its rationale should be extended to preclude the choice of a dignified death. Suicide concerns the state because it devalues life as much as any form of murder and because the attempts at suicide so often imperil the lives of other people. The same cannot be said of a dying patient, for he is not rejecting life but only declining further treatment with the recognition that death is inevitable.

"In another case, *John F. Kennedy Hospital* v. *Heston,* 58 N.J. 576, 279 A. 2d 670 (1971), in upholding the appointment of a guardian to consent to blood transfusions for a Jehovah's Witness who needed an operation for a ruptured spleen, the New Jersey Supreme Court equated refusal to receive blood with suicide and declared that 'there is no constitutional right to choose to die.' Chief Justice Weintraub wrote that, 'If the state may interrupt one mode of self-destruction, it may with equal authority interfere with the other.' He then continued with *obiter dictum* which is highly relevant to this discussion: 'It is arguably different when an individual, overtaken by illness, decides to let it run a fatal course. But unless the medical option itself is laden with the risk of death or of serious infirmity, the state's interest in sustaining life in such circumstances is hardly distinguishable from it interests in the case of suicide." ... "

The 'Right to Die' & Mercy Killing

California gets right-to-die law. California Gov. Edmund G. Brown Jr. Sept.

30, 1976 signed into law a bill allowing adult patients to make a "living will" authorizing their doctors to turn off life-sustaining equipment if, in the judgment of the doctors, the patient was unquestionably dying and the equipment was only serving to stave off the moment of death.

The legislation—the first such to be enacted by any state in the U.S.—required that the "living will" be witnessed by two persons who were not doctors and were not relatives of the patient. A doctor who acted under the authority conveyed by such a will could not be held liable for a patient's death that resulted from the disconnecting of life-support equipment. The law—which then went into effect Jan. 1, 1977—also provided that such deaths could not be classed as suicides for the purpose of denying life-insurance benefits.

The bill had cleared the California legislature Aug. 30.

Courts orders Karen Quinlan be allowed to die. The New Jersey Supreme Court ruled unanimously March 31, 1976 that the mechanical respirator that had kept Karen Anne Quinlan alive for more than 11 months could be disconnected if attending physicians and a committee of hospital officials concluded she would never recover.

"If . . . there is no reasonable possibility of Karen's ever emerging from her present comatose condition to a cognitive, sapient state, the present life-support system may be withdrawn . . . without any civil or criminal liability . . . on the part of any participant, whether guardian, physician, hospital or others," the court said in its 59-page opinion written by Chief Justice Richard J. Hughes.

In so ruling, the court agreed to appoint Joseph Quinlan, Miss Quinlan's adoptive father, as her legal guardian. He was to have "full power with regard to the identity of treating physicians," the court said.

While rejecting arguments by Paul W. Armstrong, attorney for parents Joseph and Julia Quinlan, that the right to seek removal of the respirator was grounded in the constitutional guarantees of freedom of religion and against cruel and inhuman punishment, the court asserted that Miss Quinlan had a "right to privacy" that would allow her to make life-sustaining medical decisions. Moreover, the court held Miss Quinlan had the right to make such a fatal decision "in much the same way" as a woman who decided to terminate a pregnancy under certain conditions.

"We have no doubt," the court said, ". . .that if Karen were herself miraculously lucid for an interval . . . and perceptive of her irreversible condition, she could effectively decide upon discontinuance of the life-support apparatus, even if it meant the prospect of natural death."

However, since she was legally incompetent to make this decision, her father, acting as guardian, should do so, the court ruled.

"If a putative decision by Karen to permit this noncognitive, vegetative existence to terminate by natural forces is regarded as a valuable incident of her right to privacy, as we believe it to be, then it should not be discarded solely on the basis that her condition prevents her conscious exercise of the choice," the court added. (It had been brought out in testimony in the Superior Court trial in 1975 on the Quinlans' request to turn off the respirator that Miss Quinlan had at one time said she would not want extraordinary means used to keep her alive if she were beyond hope of recovery.)

Under the court's ruling, Joseph Quinlan would have to discuss his daughter's condition with her doctors. If they agreed the respirator should be disconnected, his request would have to be submitted to the hospital's "ethics committee or like body" for a ruling on her prognosis. If the committee agreed she had no hope of ever becoming conscious again, the respirator could then be turned off.

The court said, however, that if the attending physicians or the hospital balked at shutting off the respirator, Joseph Quinlan should seek out doctors or a hospital willing to so act.

The court's ruling also noted arguments by Morris County Prosecutor Donald G. Collester Jr. and others that disconnecting the respirator would be criminal homicide. "There is a real and in this case determinative distinction between the unlawful taking of the life of another and the ending of artificial life-support systems as a matter of self-determination," the court concluded.

Excerpts from the New Jersey Supreme Court's ruling March 31 in the case of Karen Anne Quinlan:

The matter is of transcendent importance, involving questions related to the definition and existence of death, the prolongation of life through artificial means developed by medical technology undreamed of in past generations of the practice of the healing arts; the impact of such durationally indeterminate and artificial life prolongation on the rights of the incompetent, her family and society in general; the bearing of constitutional right and the scope of judicial responsibility, as to the extraordinary prayer for relief of the plaintiff. Involved as well is the right of the plaintiff, Joseph Quinlan, to guardianship of the person of his daughter. . . .

Because Karen's neurological condition affects her respiratory ability (the respiratory system being a brain stem function) she requires a respirator to assist her breathing. Attempts to "wean" her from the respirator were unsuccessful and have been abandoned.

The experts believe that Karen cannot now survive without the assistance of the respirator; that exactly how long she would live without it is unknown; that the strong likelihood is that death would follow soon after its removal, and that removal would also risk further brain damage and would curtail the assistance the respirator presently provides in warding off infection. . . .

From all this evidence, and including the whole testimonial record, several basic findings in the physical area are mandated. Severe brain and associate damage, albeit of uncertain etiology, has left Karen in a chronic and persistent vegetative state. No form of treatment which can cure or improve that condition is known or available. As nearly as may be determined, considering the guarded area of remote uncertainties characteristic of most medical science predictions, she can *never* be restored to cognitive or sapient life. Even with regard to the vegetative level and improvement therein (if such it may be called) the prognosis is extremely poor and the extent unknown if it should in fact occur. . . .

The character and general suitability of Joseph Quinlan as guardian for his daughter, in ordinary circumstances, could not be doubted. The record bespeaks the high degree of familial love which pervaded the home of Joseph Quinlan and reached out fully to embrace Karen, although she was living elsewhere at the time of her collapse. The proofs showed him to be deeply religious, imbued with a morality so sensitive that months of tortured indecision preceded his belated conclusion (despite earlier moral judgements reached by the other family members, but unexpressed to him in order not to influence him) to seek the termination of life-supportive measures sustaining Karen. A communicant of the Roman Catholic Church, as were other family members, he first sought solace in private prayer looking with confidence, as he says, to the Creator, first for the recovery of Karen and then, if that were not possible, for guidance with respect to the awesome decision confronting him.

To confirm the moral rightness of the decision he was about to make he consulted with his parish priest and later with the Catholic chaplain of St. Clare's Hospital. He would not, he testified, have sought termination if that act were to be morally wrong or in conflict with the tenets of the religion he so profoundly respects. He was disabused of doubt, however, when the position of the Roman Catholic Church was made known to him as it is reflected in the record in this case. . . .

We have no doubt, in these unhappy circumstances, that if Karen were herself miraculously lucid for an interval (not altering the existing prognosis of the condition to which she would soon return) and perceptive of her irreversible condition, she could effectively decide upon discontinuance of the life-support apparatus, even if it meant the prospect of natural death. . . .

We have no hesitancy in deciding . . . that no external compelling interest of the state could compel Karen to endure the unendurable, only to vegetate a few measurable months with no realistic possibility of returning to any semblance of cognitive or sapient life. . . .

Although the Constitution does not explicitly mention a right of privacy, [U.S.] Supreme Court decisions have recognized that a right of personal privacy exists and that certain areas of privacy are guaranteed under the Constitution. The court has interdicted judicial intrusion into many aspects of personal decision, sometimes basing this restraint upon the conception of a limitation of judicial interest and responsibility, such as with regard to contraception and its relation to family life and decision.

The court in Griswald [v Connecticut] found the unwritten constitutional right of privacy to exist in the penumbra of specific guarantees of the Bill of Rights "formed by emanations from those guarantees that help give them life and substance." Presumably this right is broad enough to encompass a patient's decision to decline medical treatment under certain circumstances, in much the same way as it is broad enough to encompass a woman's decision to terminate pregnancy under certain conditions. . . .

The claimed interests of the state in this case are essentially the preservation and sanctity of human life and defense of the right of the physician to administer medical treatment according to his best judgment. In this case the doctors say that removing Karen from the respirator will conflict with their professional judgment. The plaintiff answers that Karen's present treatment serves only a maintenance function; that the respirator cannot cure or improve her condition but at best can only prolong her inevitable slow deterioration and death; and that the interests of the patient, as seen by her surrogate, the guardian, must be evaluated by the court as predominant, even in the face of an opinion *contra* by the present attending physicians. Plaintiff's distinction is significant. The nature of Karen's care and the realistic chances of her recovery are quite unlike those of the patients discussed in many of the cases where treatments were ordered. In many of those cases the medical procedure required (usually a transfusion) constituted a minimal bodily invasion and the chances of recovery and return to functioning life were very good. We think that the state's interest *contra* weakens and the individual's right to privacy grows as the degree of bodily invasion increases and the prognosis dims. Ultimately there comes a point at which the individual's rights overcome the state interest. It is for that reason that we believe Karen's choice, if she were competent to make it, would be vindicated by the law. Her prognosis is extremely poor,—she will never resume cognitive life. And the bodily invasion is very great,—she requires 24-hour intensive nursing care, antibiotics, the assistance of a respirator, a catheter and feeding tube.

Our affirmation of Karen's independent right of choice, however, would ordinarily be based upon her competency to assert it. The sad truth, however, is that she is grossly incompetent and we cannot discern her supposed choice based on the testimony of her previous conversations with friends, where such testimony is without sufficient probative weight. Nevertheless we have concluded that Karen's right of privacy may be asserted on her behalf by her guardian under the peculiar circumstances here present.

If a putative decision by Karen to permit this non-cognitive, vegetative existence to terminate by natural forces is regarded as a valuable incident of her right of privacy, as we believe it to be, then it should not be discarded solely on the basis that her condition prevents her conscious exercise of the choice. The only practical way to prevent destruction of the right is to permit the guardian and family of Karen to render their best judgment, subject to the qualifications hereinafter stated, as to whether she would exercise it in these circumstances. . . .

The wide debate thus reflected contrasts with the relative paucity of legislative and judicial guides and standards in the same field. The medical profession has sought to devise guidelines such as the "brain death" concept of the Harvard Ad Hoc Committee mentioned above. But it is perfectly apparent from the testimony we have quoted . . . and indeed so clear as almost to be judicially noticeable, that humane decisions against resuscitative or maintenance therapy are frequently a recognized *de facto* response in the medical world to the irreversible, terminal, pain-ridden patient, especially with familial consent. And these cases, of course, are far short of "brain death."

We glean from the record here that physicians distinguish between curing the ill and comforting and easing the dying; that they refuse to treat the curable as if they were dying or ought to die, and that they have sometimes refused to treat the hopeless and dying as if they were curable. In this sense . . . many of them have refused to inflict an undesired prolongation of the process of dying on a patient in irreversible condition when it is clear that such "therapy" offers neither human nor humane benefit. We think these attitudes represent a balanced implementation of a profoundly realistic perspective on the meaning of life and death and that they respect the whole Judeo-Christian tradition of regard for human life. No less would they seem consistent with the moral matrix of medicine, "to heal," very much in the sense of the endless mission of the law, "to do justice. . . ."

We would hesitate, in this imperfect world, to propose as to physicians that type of immunity which from the early common law has surrounded judges and grand jurors, so that they might without fear of personal retaliation perform their judicial duties with independent objectivity.

Nevertheless, there must be a way to free physicians, in the pursuit of their healing vocation, from possible contamination by self-interest or self-protection concerns which would inhibit their independent medical judgments for the well-being of their dying patients. We would hope that this opinion might be serviceable to some degree in ameliorating the professional problems under discussion. . . .

The evidence in this case convinces us that the focal point of decision should be the prognosis as to the reasonable possibility of return to cognitive and sapient life, as distinguished from the forced continuance of that biological vegetative existence to which Karen seems to be doomed. . . .

We conclude that there would be no criminal homicide in the circumstances of this case. We believe, first, that the ensuing death would not be homicide but rather expiration from existing natural causes. Secondly, even if it were to be regarded as homicide, it would not be unlawful. . . . There is a real and in this case determinative distinction between the unlawful taking of the life of another and the ending of artificial life-support systems as a matter of self-determination. . . .

The trial court was apparently convinced of the high character of Joseph Quinlan and his general suitability as guardian under other circumstances, describing him as "very sincere, moral, ethical and religious." The court felt, however, that the obligation to concur in the medical care and treatment of his daughter would be a source of anguish to him and would distort his "decision-making processes." We disagree, for we sense from the whole record before us that while Mr. Quinlan feels a natural grief, and understandably sorrows because of the tragedy which has befallen his daughter, his strength of purpose and character far outweighs these sentiments and qualifies him eminently for guardianship of the person as well as the property of his daughter. Hence we discern no valid reason to overrule the statutory intendment of preference to the next of kin.

We thus arrive at the formulation of the declaratory relief which we have concluded is appropriate to this case. Some time has passed since Karen's physical and mental condition was described to the Court. At that time her continuing deterioration was plainly projected. Since the record has not been expanded we assume that she is now even more fragile and nearer to death than she was then. Since her present treating physicians may give reconsideration to her present posture in the light of this opinion, and since we are transferring to the plaintiff as guardian the choice of the attending physician and therefore other physicians may be in charge of the case who may take a different view from that of the present attending physicians, we herewith declare the following affirmative relief on behalf of the plaintiff. Upon the concurrence of the guardian and family of Karen, should the responsible attending physicians conclude that there is no reasonable possibility of Karen's ever emerging from her present comatose condition to a cognitive, sapient state and that the life-support apparatus now being administered to Karen should be discontinued, they shall consult with the hospital "Ethics Committee" or like body of the institution in which Karen is then hospitalized. If that consultative body agrees that there is no reasonable possibility of Karen's ever emerging from her present comatose condition to a cognitive, sapient state, the present life-support system may be withdrawn and said action shall be without any civil or criminal liability therefor on the part of any participant, whether guardian, physician, hospital or others. . . .

By the above ruling we do not intend to be understood as implying that a proceeding for judicial declaratory relief is necessarily required for the implementation of comparable decisions in the field of medical practice.

The U.S. Supreme Court Nov. 1 refused to review the decision.

Lower-court ruling reversed—The decision to authorize the disconnection of the respirator reversed a Nov. 10, 1975 decision of a state Superior Court judge.

In refusing her parents' request, Judge Robert Muir Jr. had cited the fact that, although Miss Quinlin had lost all ability to think or function as a normal person, she was still legally and medically alive and as such retained the right to live.

The legal dispute had begun in September 1975, when the Quinlan parents, sure their daughter had no chance of recovery, petitioned the court to have her returned to "her natural state" and "leave her to the Lord" by having the respirator removed. The Quinlins, Roman Catholics, were upheld in their views by their parish priest. The parents had made their decision after Miss Quinlin had been in a coma for seven months and had fallen into an irreversible "persistent vegetative state," according to doctors.

The Quinlins went to court after a request to attending physicians to disconnect the respirator was turned down. Muir left the final decision on use of the respirator with the doctors. He authorized Daniel R. Coburn, a Morristown lawyer who acted as Miss Quinlin's guardian for the court hearings, to continue as the guardian of "her person." Coburn would not be authorized to initiate any new medical procedures but would be available for consultation with the attending physician.

Respirator removed—Miss Quinlan's respirator was removed May 22, 1976, and she continued to breathe without it. Her doctors described her June 3 as being in stable condition.

In their first public statement since the court ruling, Quinlan's doctors—Robert Morse and Arshad Javed—and officials of St. Clare's Hospital in Denville said that Quinlan's treatment was in keeping with "prevailing medical practice and moral constraints" and would be guided "in addition" by "an irreversible tenet to protect life." The doctors had opposed removing the respirator. The statement said that Quinlan would continue to receive "appropriate nutrients and antibiotics to fight infection, along with other procedures indicated by her condition."

Dr. Joseph F. Fennelly of Madison, N.J. was reported May 30 to be spokesman for a group of seven doctors who had agreed to look after Quinlan as a "chronic care patient." She was moved June 9 from St. Clare's Hospital to the Morris View Nursing Home in Morris Township, N.J.

According to published reports, Quinlan was not connected to a respirator or any other mechanical life-supporting device. Attendant physicians at St. Clare's had over a three-week period weaned her from the mechanical respirator that had been thought needed to keep her breathing. Since May 19, she was reported to have been breathing unaided.

According to a report in the June 2 Morristown Daily Record, the parents of Miss Quinlan, Joseph and Julia Quinlan, had begun searching for a facility other than St. Clare's after they and their attorneys had reached an impasse May 18 with hospital officials over future treatment of the comatose woman. The hospital and its doctors, the Daily Record said, had apparently refused to change their position expressed at the 1975 trial on Joseph Quinlan's petition to disconnect the mechanical respirator then thought to be keeping their daughter alive. The doctors and the hospital opposed withdrawal of high calorie nutrients and antibiotics, the Daily Record reported.

Following the meeting, the Quinlans attempted to find a local nursing care facility willing to accept their daughter but were apparently turned down a number of times because of the notoriety that would accompany acceptance.

The decision by Morris View, a 375-bed facility operated by Morris County for indigent patients, was presaged in guidelines for admission of comatose patients adopted by the county's welfare board June 3. The guidelines required that a patient be in a coma for at least six months if the condition were the result of trauma or unknown causes and three months from other causes. The guidelines further stipulated that treating physicians and family agree recovery was unlikely and that "aggressive treatment of any acute problem . . . or readmission to a hospital" was inappropriate.

Quinlan's treating physicians at St. Clare's had stated they would have used blood transfusions, and if need be, reconnected the mechanical respirator to fight infections or other problems affecting her.

On June 10, the day after Quinlan's admission to Morris View, a newly formed ethics committee at the county nursing home ruled the 22-year-old woman was in an irreversible coma with no reasonable possibility of recovery to a "cognitive, sapient state." In so finding, the committee set the stage for the withholding of extraordinary means to rescue Quinlan from any medical crisis that might arise. The committee also agreed, however, that "normal" levels of food and antibiotics should be continued.

In a related development, state Atorney General William Hyland said June 10 he believed the state Supreme Court's ruling in the Quinlan case would allow doctors to withhold food and medicine from terminally ill patients to let them die. But Hyland told a news conference this did not mean he thought feeding of Quinlan should be stopped.

Quinlan 'alive' a year off respirator—Karen Anne Quinlan was breathing normally March 31, 1977, a year after the state Supreme Court had ruled that the machine could be turned off. Joseph and Julia Quinlan, who had felt the respirator was preventing their daughter from dying "with decency and dignity," continued to make daily visits to the nursing home where Karen Anne was being fed a high-calorie food formula and receiving antibiotics to guard against infection.

Quinlan, now 23 and weighing about 70 pounds, had gone into a coma on April 14, 1975 after accidentally mixing barbituates and alcohol. Her doctor said her current blood oxygen level was adequate for her body's limited needs, meaning she could continue to breathe unassisted. He said, however, that in the event of a respiratory collapse, Quinlan would not be placed back on a respirator.

The Quinlan case continued to generate interest in "right to die" legislation that allowed individuals to fill out "living wills" limiting the amount of medical treatment they would receive in the event that they became hopelessly terminally ill. Right-to-die bills had been introduced in the legislatures of 38 states in 1977, but to date only two had been passed and signed into law, in California and Idaho.

AMA & mercy killing. Dr. Malcolm C. Todd, elected by the House of Delegates of the American Medical Association June 28, 1973 as the organized physicians' next president, said that day that mercy killings "have their place" in certain "uncorrectable" fatal illnesses. Todd added, however, that doctors should not be forced to make the euthanasia decisions by themselves.

Six months later the House of Delegates Dec. 4 adopted a report reiterating opposition to mercy killing. However, the delegates agreed that a doctor should respect the wishes of a dying patient concerning the amount of medical care he wanted. "The cessation of the employment of extraordinary means of prolonging the life of the body when there is irrefutable evidence that biological death is imminent is the decision of the patient and/or his immediate family," the report said.

Mercy killer freed. In practice, juries have often been reluctant to convict and punish people accused of hastening the death of loved ones who were termially ill and in great pain. For example, in Freehold, N.J. Nov. 5, 1973, a jury accepted a plea of temporary insanity as it decided that Lester Zygmaniak was not guilty of the mercy killing of his brother, George Zygmaniak, who had been severely crippled by a motorcycle accident.

The jury acted in the knowledge that Zygmaniak, 23, admitted putting his brother to death. Zygmaniak had told police that George, 26, paralyzed from the neck down, had pleaded with him to end his suffering.

A Louis Harris survey made public April 23 indicated that those polled believed by 62%-38% margin that "a patient with a terminal disease ought to be able to tell his doctor to let him die rather than to extend his life when no cure is in sight."

However, the same sample group opposed by 53%-37% euthanasia, under which a terminally ill patient could tell his doctor to put him to death.

Euthanasia rejected. The Church of England, after a four-year study, said euthanasia—mercy killing—should not be legalized, the Washington Post reported March 18, 1975.

Regulation

Government Policy

The sale of medicines has almost always been a lucrative business. It has made many people wealthy regardless of whether or not their products actually help. In many cases, it is charged, some alleged medicines actually do harm rather than good—sometimes because the potion itself is harmful, other times because a useless medicine, even if basically harmless, might keep the user from seeking effective treatment. A variety of federal and state laws and agencies have, therefore, been created to regulate this business.

Investigational drugs & the FDA. The main federal agency charged with regulating the trade in medicines is the Food & Drug Administration (FDA). Sen. Abraham A. Ribicoff (D, Conn.), chairman of the Senate Subcommittee on Executive Reorganization & Government Research, charged in the Senate Sept. 19, 1973 that the FDA had been lax in its regulation of "investigational new drugs—drugs approved for testing but not for public sale." These were drugs, he said, that "had been administered in clinical experiments to human subjects." Ribicoff made his charge on the basis of an investigation conducted on his orders by the Government Accounting Office (GAO). Ribicoff said in a statement published in the Congressional Record:

The GAO study discusses only 10 of the more than 6,000 drugs currently classified as investigational new drugs. But the results of the GAO study and the subcommittee staff findings strongly suggest that FDA regulation of investigational new drugs has been lax and has not adequately protected the patients who take these drugs. They also show a failure to adopt safe testing procedures by certain drug companies, as well as resistance to FDA regulation. The FDA and the companies involved have shown a disregard for public safety which is incompatible with their responsibility to protect and promote public health.

Specifically, the report found that in eight cases, FDA failed to halt human tests after receiving indications that the drugs were not safe. As a result, over 2,000 people were exposed to the hazard of unsafe drugs. GAO further found that the drug companies unnecessarily delayed reporting adverse drug effects to FDA and that once this data was received, FDA did not require necessary patient followup in six cases to protect the health of the people who had been given suspect or unsafe drugs.

Since the passage of the Kefauver-Harris amendments of 1962, the law has required the FDA to regulate the use of all drugs shipped in interstate commerce for investigational use on human beings. Under FDA procedures established pursuant to this statute, FDA has required the sponsor—usually a drug company, but in some cases an institution, such as NIH—to submit an investigational new drug application before such shipment could take place. Prior to August 14, 1970, a sponsor could begin clinical experiments on human subjects immediately upon submission of its application—that is, prior to any FDA review of its data. Since August 14, 1970, however, FDA has required sponsors to wait 30 days after submission of an IND application before initiating human testing. No positive FDA approval is required once 30 days have passed, and sponsors may initiate such testing unless FDA has affirmatively directed them not to do so.

FDA's procedures for the testing of investigational new drugs are divided into three phases:

Phase I covers the first trials in human subjects. This trial is normally limited to a group of 20 to 50 healthy people. If the results are satisfactory, testing proceeds to phase II.

Phase II involves testing the drug on 100–200 patients with the disease the drug is expected to treat. If phase II results are satisfactory, testing may proceed to phase III.

Phase III involves expanded trials on a much larger group of patients. It is not uncommon for phase III testing to include several thousand patients.

Before an experimental drug may be administered to human beings, it must first be given to animals. Prior animal testing is required because there is often some correlation between the ability of a drug to produce adverse effects in animals and its ability to produce such effects in human beings. While the precise relationship between animal results and human results is often indeterminate, it is clear that a drug that has been shown to produce cancerous tumors in animals presents a greater potential risk to human beings than a drug that has shown no adverse health effects in animals.

Current FDA regulations require both substantial animal testing and substantial human testing before a drug is approved for general public sale, rather than investigational use. Under current FDA practice, a drug may be administered to human beings in phase I studies for up to 2 weeks after only 2 weeks of animal studies and prior to full evaluation of those animal studies. Human subjects in phase I and phase II experiments may be given the drug for up to 3 months after only 1 month of animal studies, and may be given a drug for an unlimited period after only 3 months of animal studies. Phase III subjects may be given the drug for an unlimited period after only 6 months of animal studies.

The GAO study contains a comprehensive discussion of each of the drugs it reviewed. . . .

The GAO survey showed a consistent pattern for FDA delay in reviewing the data submitted with the IND application. For Practolol, the delay was 3 months. For Triflocin, it was 8 months. In both cases, animals given the drugs developed cancerous conditions. For the other drugs reviewed, the delay ranged from 4 months to a full year. During this time, the drug companies routinely began human testing. . . .

The most dramatic example of FDA's failure to halt human testing after notice of evidence of cancer in animal tests is the drug Practolol, sponsored by Ayerst Labs. When the test data was reviewed, the medical officer concluded that "this study is indefensible and unacceptable." On March 11, 1970, FDA recommended to the sponsor than human testing be discontinued. Testing continued. On April 8, FDA again advised the sponsor to discontinue testing, but the sponsor refused. At that time, the sponsor submitted to FDA the results of a study showing that cancerous tumors had been found in mice. (Ayerst had notice and substantial documentation of the results of this study on August 14, 1969, but had failed to provide it to FDA until nearly 8 months later. By contrast, the Canadian Food and Drug authorities had had possession of the study since August 27, 1969.) Still, FDA took no effective action to terminate testing on human subjects.

In January 1971, FDA tried for a third time to persuade the sponsor to discontinue tests on human beings. Ayerst not only refused to discontinue the tests, but also refused even to make the finding of the mouse study—indicating cancerous tumors—available to the doctors who were conducting the experiments. Those doctors thus had no way of evaluating the risks to which their patients were being subject. Finally, on August 27, 1971, fully 17 months after FDA had first advised the Ayerst to discontinue testing, and after a fourth request from FDA to discontinue, the tests were stopped.

This case is not unique. Another similar case history is that of Oxprenalol Hydrochloride, sponsored by Merrell-National Labs. In this case, it took the FDA 6 months and two requests to stop human testing after tumors had been found in mice. . . .

The GAO found that the time lag between discovery of the effects of human and animal tests and reporting them to FDA ranged from 40 days to 19 months. The case of Triflocin, sponsored by Lederle Labs, was typical. There, the sponsor took 7 months to analyze the results of a study which eventually showed bladder cancer in rats. Meanwhile, human testing was in progress. FDA concluded that the delay was "not unjustified because such delays were apparently standard operating procedure for this company. FDA stated that it "did not consider the delay unusual." The fact that the delay was not unusual, rather than supporting a finding that it was justified, seems to point to the very opposite conclusion.

With respect to Practolol, sponsored by Ayerst Labs, the sponsor failed for 8 months to supply FDA with the results of a study showing cancerous tumors in mice.

In the case of MK–665, an oral contraceptive sponsored by Merck, Sharp and Dome Research, the sponsor waited over a month before notifying FDA that cancer had been found in dogs treated with the drug. The Justice Department declined to bring a criminal prosecution in this matter. . . .

Ribicoff insisted that the FDA "should more closely monitor all human testing" and require test sponsors to perform follow-up checks on FDA orders. Companies that failed to perform proper follow-up tests should be disqualified as IND (investigational new drug) sponsors, Ribicoff declared. He said:

Several of the cases reported by GAO illustrate the need for these steps. One of them was MK–665, sponsored by Merck, Sharp and Dome, which was shown to cause breast cancer in dogs. Only about one-third of the patients who received the drug in clinical tests have been examined.

Another is Hexobendine. When dogs, which were given the drug developed cataracts, human testing was halted in September 1971. The sponsor, Merrell-National Labs, resisted an FDA request to do a followup on all patients who received the drug. As of December 22, 1972, 48 percent of the patients who had received followup eye examinations showed evidence of cataract development. While it cannot be said with certainty that this cataract development was drug related, as of March 1973, only 48 percent of the persons who had received Hexobendine had received eye examinations. The FDA regarded this followup as inadequate. (One problem the FDA encountered with respect to Hexobendine was that no one—neither FDA nor the sponsor—seemed to know precisely how many people had taken the drug, how long they had taken it, and when it had been administered.)

One of the most flagrant cases of a drug company's resistance to FDA with respect to followup is that of Cinanserin, sponsored by E. R. Squibb & Sons. Human testing had been discontinued in August 1969, because of the appearance of tumors in the livers of rats. In October 1969, Squibb informed FDA that it was not considering followup. According to a letter of July 30, 1970, from the FDA Commissioner Edwards to Squibb, the question of followup had been raised by FDA with Squibb in a telephone conversation of December 9, 1969, with Dr. Lawrence Marks, a Squibb vice president. According to the letter, "he—Marks—stated that he would investigate and call back in a week. There was no reply."

Squibb continued to resist FDA's suggested followup procedures. As a result of Squibb's refusal, FDA medical officers recommended a full evaluation of Squibb's qualifications to be a sponsor of any investigational new drugs, because of its failure to fulfill its responsibility to patients placed in jeopardy.

After several FDA letters had gone unanswered, FDA officials visited the Squibb facility in New Brunswick, N.J., on June 26, 1972. As of November 17, 1972, the FDA still considered Squibb's followup on Cinanserin inadequate. It is noteworthy, however, that throughout this protracted and sometimes heated disagreement, FDA relied exclusively on persuasion in attempting to require a followup. In the absence of regulations requiring followup, FDA apparently felt itself powerless to act more vigorously. FDA could have at any point, however, required followup as a condition of IND approval or required followup by regulation. Thus, the agency's inability to require followup was a direct result of its own inaction.

Realizing that its lack of followup regulations was leaving patients unprotected and that drug companies would not voluntarily perform adequate followup, FDA contracted with the National Academy of Sciences for a study to be conducted by an NAS committee. The committee was formed in April 1972. Its chairman was Dr. Lawrence Marks, the Squibb vice president who had participated in the controversy over followup on Cinanserin.

As mentioned previously, after receiving no reply to a series of letters asking Squibb to undertake further followup, on June 26, 1972, FDA officials visited the Squibb plant in New Brunswick, N.J. According to a memorandum dated June 29, 1972, by an FDA inspector, Dr. Marks telephoned the inspector from Squibb headquarters in Princeton while the inspector was at the New Brunswick plant. According to the memorandum, Dr. Marks advised the inspector of his position as chairman of the NAS committee studying the very question of followup. The memorandum continuse:

> In view of this, Dr. Marks did not feel that as a representative of Squibb, he should commit the firm to a followup procedure until such a procedure is standard throughout the industry. He further supports this belief in that he feels that the FDA is not completely sure as to what followup should be made as evidenced by the fact that they set up the NAS Committee. Dr. Marks said that he had advised Dr. Marion Finkel (an FDA official) of his position several weeks ago and questioned the need for our assignment.

Dr. Marks confirmed to the subcommittee his conversation with Dr. Finkel and stated that he does not remember the conversation with the inspector. It was confirmed, however, by the two other FDA employees. At the time of the conversation, June 26, 1972, Dr. Marks was still Chairman of the NAS Committee. He subsequently resigned in August 1972, for reasons unrelated to the Cinanserin followup problem.

It was poor policy for FDA to tolerate a situation where the chairman of a committee established and financed by FDA for the purpose of recommending followup procedures is at the same time personally attempting, on behalf of his firm, to dissuade FDA from requiring followup examinations in a particular case. It is clear that responsible officials at the FDA were quite aware of Dr. Marks' dual role. . . .

Laetrile Controversy

Ban on laetrile continued. The importation and sale of laetrile, an alleged cure for cancer, would continue to be banned by the federal government, U.S. Food and Drug Administration chief Donald Kennedy said May 6, 1977. The controversial substance, also known as vitamin B-17 and the chemical amygdalin, occurred naturally in the pits of apricots and peaches, in bitter almonds and other plants. It was available in 26 countries and was currently being smuggled into the U.S. from Canada and Mexico. Amygdalin contained small amounts of the poison cyanide.

Promoters of laetrile use claimed that it could prevent and cure cancer. They contended that since there was no evidence of the chemical being harmful, the ban on it should be lifted. However, the FDA noted that laetrile was the most tested of all potential cancer cures and that five studies by the National Cancer Institute alone had indicated that it was therapeutically worthless. (According to the 1962 Kefauver-Harris amendments to the Food, Drug and Cosmetic Act of 1958, drug manufacturers were required to prove not only that a product was safe, but that it was also effective.) Some laetrile advocates maintained that it was a vitamin, not a drug, and should therefore be exempt from the legislation.

An FDA bulletin issued April 14 to physicians and other health professionals nationwide said supporters of laetrile use were "more vocal and better organized than in the past." The agency warned that early cancer patients who believed in laetrile's efficacy might be putting "their lives on the line" by failing to receive orthodox medical treatment.

Laetrile's background—It was in the days of Prohibition that a California doctor first used an apricot extract to improve the taste of moonshine whiskey. Later, the doctor experimented with the extract to treat tumors in animals. When the supposed anti-cancer agent did not prove effective, its use died out. But the San Francisco physician's son, Ernst Krebs Jr., isolated an alleged cancer-fighting substance from the apricot pit in 1949. He called the extract "laetrile." Since then laetrile has been a source of conflict in the field of medicine. Here is a chronology of the Laetrile controversy:

1920—The forerunner of laetrile was first used by Dr. Ernst T. Krebs Sr. in treatment of cancer.

1949—Dr. Krebs' son, biochemist Ernst T. Krebs Jr., isolated an extract from apricot pits and called it "laetrile."

1952—Biochemist Krebs claimed to have made laetrile safe for injection into humans.

1953—The California Medical Association's Cancer Commission investigated laetrile as a cancer treatment. The commission found it "completely ineffective" when used in large doses on cancer in laboratory animals.

Oct. 10, 1962—President John F. Kennedy signed into law the Drug Amendments of 1962. The law provided that the FDA has to certify new drugs to be effective as well as safe, thereby laying the legal basis for the ban on laetrile and other questionable cancer cures.

1962—Ernst T. Krebs Jr. and the John Beard Memorial Foundation pleaded guilty to violating the new drug provisions of Federal Food, Drug & Cosmetic act. Krebs was placed on probation provided he did not ship any new drugs interstate (specifically including laetrile) without an effective new drug application from the FWA.

1963—The California State Department of Public Health issued a regulation prohibiting the use of laetrile in the state.

March 1963—The FDA reported no evidence that laetrile is effective in cancer treatment.

May 15, 1965—The Canadian Medical Association Journal reported negative findings on laetrile in cancer treatment.

Aug. 2, 1965 Dr. Ernst T. Krebs Sr. agreed to a permanent court injunction against further distribution of laetrile.

Sept. 1965—Dr. Krebs pleaded guilty to criminal contempt of court for disobeying a restraining order prohibiting the shipment of laetrile.

Jan. 21, 1966—Dr. Krebs pleaded guilty to contempt of court for shipping Laetrile.

Feb. 3, 1966—Dr. Krebs was given a one-year suspended sentence by a U.S. District Court in California for failing to register as a producer of drugs.

April 20, 1970—FDA assigned an Investigative New Drug application number to the McNaughton Foundation on California for testing amygdalin-laetrile.

May 12, 1970—The application was terminated when the FDA found "serious preclinical and clinical deficiencies."

Sept. 1, 1971—FDA found "no acceptable evidence of therapeutic effect to justify clinical trials" of laetrile.

1976—Alaska became the first state to permit doctors to prescribe and administer laetrile. (Alaska law, however, prohibits the sale of the drug.)

Jan. 21, 1977—U.S. District Judge Gordon Thompson Jr. ruled in San Diego that terminally ill patients may import laetrile.

April 8, 1977—U.S. District Judge Luther Bohanon in Oklahoma City specified conditions under which patients may have access to laetrile.

Courts grant access to laetrile. Under a ruling by federal District Court Judge Luther Bohanon of Oklahoma City, some cancer patients had been importing laetrile from Mexico legally, it was reported April 17, 1977. Bohanon initially had ruled in favor of one cancer patient who sought the alleged cancer remedy. He later expanded the ruling to include about 20 other terminally ill persons.

Judge Bohanon April 8 issued a list of conditions under which patients could have access to laetrile, stressing that he had made no attempt to determine the drug's ability to fight cancer. Bohanon's order stipulated that laetrile be made available to terminal cancer patients who had sworn statements from a doctor on their condition. The physician's statement had to include "evidence of a rapidly progressive malignancy" and specify that recognized forms of cancer treatment would be administered in conjunction with laetrile.

Federal district court judges in New York and California also had ordered that terminally ill cancer patients be allowed to import laetrile. In San Diego, Calif., U.S. District Court Judge Gordon Thompson Jr. had said Jan. 21 that to deny a patient freedom of choice in the absence of a known remedy for his illness "would be grossly paternalistic of this court." Three doctors who had certified that no cure was available for the patient in question also had approved his use of laetrile.

FDA holds laetrile hearings—The Food and Drug Administration May 2 opened hearings on laetrile on behalf of a cancer patient seeking to obtain the substance. The hearings, in Kansas City, Mo. had been ordered by the 10th U.S. Circuit Court of Appeals in October 1976. The court had ruled in Denver that the FDA's laetrile records were "grossly inadequate."

The hearings were intended "to compile a record of the available evidence about the substance" rather than formulate a final policy on its use, according to Dr. John Jennings, associate FDA commissioner for medical affairs.

Supporters of laetrile use were represented by the Committee for Freedom of Choice in Cancer Therapy, whose spokesman called the hearings a "kangaroo court." An opponent of laetrile, Dr. Samuel C. Klagsbrun, a psychiatrist at St. Luke's Hospital in New York City, testified that the drug was a "hoax" and alluded to its use as "suicide."

States challenge FDA ban. The Indiana state legislature May 1, 1977 overrode a veto by Gov. Otis Bowen and made Indiana the first state to authorize the manufacture, sale and use of laetrile, which was banned from interstate commerce by the Food and Drug Administration. The bill, effective June 1, also legalized the use of the artificial sweetener saccharin.

The Florida state legislature approved a bill May 2 to allow doctors to administer laetrile when requested by a patient.

By June 23, with action by Louisiana, ten states had authorized the manufacture and sale of laetrile. Arizona, Nevada, Texas, Washington, Delaware and Oklahoma had taken such action by June 21.

At least one bill had been introduced in Congress to amend current federal law restricting the use of laetrile.

While the federal government and the scientific and medical communities contended that laetrile was worthless as an anticancer treatment, the National Cancer Institute (NCI) announced June 23 that it had agreed to conduct clinical tests of the substance on humans. The agency's acting director, Dr. Guy Newell, said that growing public interest and pressure had led the institute to reconsider its previous decision against human trials. The NCI assumed that definitive proof of the substance's ineffectiveness would discourage its use. Previous laetrile experiments had been conducted exclusively on animals.

The NCI also planned to assess claims that laetrile, which contained the poison cyanide, was harmless. A 10-month-old girl died June 11 at the Buffalo Children's Hospital of cyanide poisoning after accidentally swallowing an unknown number of laetrile pills her father was taking for cancer. The infant's death was believed to be the first linked to a laetrile overdose.

Sloan-Kettering finds laetrile useless—Researchers at Memorial Sloan-Kettering Cancer Center in New York City said at a press conference June 15 that laetrile did not possess preventative, tumor-regressing or curative anticancer powers. Their findings were based upon a four-year study of the chemical's effects upon cancerous tumors in animals. The scientists conceded that laetrile's alleged pain-relieving properties could not be evaluated by their study.

The Sloan-Kettering report stated that scientists had been unable to confirm experiments conducted by Dr. Kanematsu Sugiura in 1972–73 that had shown laetrile to be effective against lung cancer in mice. The authors of the report noted Sugiura's current contention that "laetrile is not a curative, but is a palliative agent."

Dr. Lewis Thomas, president of Sloan-Kettering, recommended human testing of laetrile and surveys of long-term laetrile users to determine if it had pain-killing, mood-altering or other effects on cancer patients.

AMA rejects laetrile proposal—A proposal by a special committee of the American Medical Association suggesting that laetrile be made available without a prescription was rejected June 21 by the AMA's policy-making body. The committee, which had not found any beneficial properties in laetrile, had recommended its over-the-counter sale in order to curtail the black market trade of the substance. It was estimated that laetrile smuggling had grown into a $20-million industry. Approximately 50,000 Americans were using laetrile as a cancer treatment.

Laetrile smugglers sentenced—Robert W. Bradford, 46, president of the Committee for Freedom of Choice in Cancer Therapy Inc., was fined $40,000 and put on three years' probation May 16 for smuggling laetrile into the U.S. from Mexico. Three co-defendants, Frank Salaman, Dr. John A. Richardson and Ralph S. Bowman, were also placed on probation and fined a total of $40,000.

All four defendants were sentenced by federal district court Judge William B. Enright in San Diego. Salaman, 52, was vice president of the Freedom of Choice committee, which claimed a membership of 35,000. Richardson, 54, was a physician whose medical license had been revoked in 1976 for treating cancer patients with laetrile, in violation of a 1969 California statute. Bowman, 52, was Richardson's business manager. Bradford and Richardson, like many of those in the laetrile movement, were members of the John Birch Society.

The convicted laetrile conspirators were the first of 19 defendants indicted on smuggling charges to stand trial. Andrew R. L. McNaughton, 60, a Canadian citizen living in Mexico, was described by investigators as the "kingpin" of the operation. McNaughton, who had been involved in several stock fraud cases in the U.S., admitted that his McNaughton Foundation in Tiajuana had once received $130,000 from Joseph Zicarelli, the alleged head of organized crime in Hudson County, N.J.

Action on DES

Drug linked to cancer in women. The Food & Drug Administration was accused Oct. 26, 1971 of sidestepping for four and a half months a decision on banning the use of synthetic estrogens by pregnant women.

A drug in the synthetic estrogen family—diethylstilbesterol (DES)—had been linked to several cases in which young women whose mothers had taken the drug during pregnancy had been afflicted with vaginal cancer.

According to an article in the Washington Post, the number of known cases tying vaginal cancer in young women to their mothers use of DES was 60.

The Post article said that the FDA was asked by the New York State Department of Health in June to "initiate immediate measures to ban the use of synthetic estrogens during pregnancy." The appeal was made after cancer researchers linked 13 cases of vaginal cancer to the drug. Dr. Hollis S. Ingraham, commissioner of health in New York, in a letter to the FDA commissioner, Dr. Charles Edwards, said his department had begun a program of "continuous surveillance and monitoring" to try to detect the disease as early as possible. Ingraham urged Edwards to initiate a similar program on a national basis.

The FDA replied Aug. 10 by asking for the records of five of the cases. At the same time, the FDA said it was "actively evaluating" eight other cases linking DES to vaginal cancer reported by physicians at the Massachusetts General Hospital in Boston.

Use in animals limited. The Agriculture Department Jan. 4, 1972 announced new regulations for the use of DES as a growth hormone in food animals.

Starting Jan. 8, no DES could be fed cattle or sheep within seven days of slaughter, compared with two days under the old rule, and animals brought to slaughter would now require certification of compliance. Large doses of DES had been found to induce cancer in test animals.

FDA curbs DES. The FDA Aug. 2, 1972 banned all further production of DES for use as a growth hormone in cattle feeds, but it allowed cattlemen to continue using DES in feeds until Jan. 1, 1973.

FDA Commissioner Charles C. Edwards said he acted under requirements of the 1968 Delaney amendment to the Food, Drug and Cosmetic Act, which banned all substances in foods that caused cancer in humans or animals, although, he said, "no human harm has been demonstrated in over 17 years of use."

The order permitted continued implanting of DES pellets in cattle and sheep. The pellets, which contained one-thirtieth the amount of DES in direct feed supplements, had not been known to leave detectible residues.

Secretary of Agriculture Earl L. Butz said Aug. 2 he regretted the FDA decision, which he said could add 3½¢ a pound to consumer beef prices.

A subcommittee of the Senate Health Committee approved an immediate ban on DES in feed and pellets Aug. 3. Edwards had opposed the bill in a July 21 hearing of the subcommittee. The FDA, he said, believed "piecemeal legislation directed at any given substance" was not "appropriate for making regulatory decisions that are to be based on scientific evidence," since "DES will not be the only substance to generate these kinds of issues."

Sen. Edward M. Kennedy (D, Mass), who chaired the hearing, noted that 21 countries, including Argentina and Australia, the leading beef producers, had banned DES.

Edwards had announced June 16 a formal proposal for a DES ban, in order to set in motion machinery for a public hearing, but at that time he repeated his belief that the hormone was "safe when used as directed." The FDA announcement noted that a ban would ultimately cost consumers $300 million–460 million in meat prices, because of increased feed requirements.

Such a ban was announced by the FDA April 23, 1973 (but federal courts later overturned the ban on the ground that hearings had not been offered to manufacturers as required by the law).

In a July 10 Washington Post interview, National Cancer Institute Director Frank J. Rauscher asked for a complete ban, saying "anything that increases the carcinogenic burden to man ought to be eliminated from the envirnoment if at all possible, and in this case it is possible."

Ban voided—The U.S. Court of Appeals ruled in Washington Jan. 24, 1974 that the FDA had acted illegally in banning DES in cattle feed. The court ruled that the drug could be marketed again until the FDA held the required hearings or the secretary of health, education and welfare concluded that "such marketing constitutes an imminent hazard to public health."

The court said the FDA had used "scare tactics" instead of sound regulatory procedures in banning the drug without hearings. Noting that "most drugs are unsafe in some degree," the court said that in light of the "acknowledged value" of DES in enhancing meat production, the FDA should consider the possibility of "meaningful restrictions" on the consumption of DES residues rather than an outright ban of the drug.

New study cuts DES cancer risk. Dr. Arthur L. Herbst, who in 1971 had been the first scientist to warn of the possible association between women who took DES during pregnancy and the incidence of cancer in their daughters years later, reported that the role of DES in the development of vaginal or cervical cancer was less than had been thought. He wrote in the May 1977 issue of the American Journal of Obstetrics and Gynecology that "this disease [cancer] is extremely rare among the DES-exposed group and, in fact, is more rare than had been assumed previously." The finding could affect the approximately 50 lawsuits seeking more than $3.5 billion in damages from present or former DES manufacturers, according to the Wall Street Journal May 3.

Herbst, currently chairman of the University of Chicago Medical School's department of obstetrics and gynecology, estimated that the odds of DES offspring developing vaginal or cervical cancer ranged from about one in 10,000 to about one in 1,000. The risk estimate varied so widely because scientists had no valid statistics on how many pregnant women had taken DES between 1947 and 1964, the period when it was prescribed to prevent miscarriages.

Following Herbst's initial report of the hormone-cancer link, the Food and Drug Administration (FDA) had banned the use of DES by pregnant women. Subsequent FDA efforts to ban DES from livestock feed, in which it was used as a fattening agent, failed. The drug continued to be available for treatment of prostate cancer, as an estrogen replacement in post-menopausal women and as a "morning after" contraceptive.

Women sue over DES experiment. Three women April 25, 1977 filed a $77 million class action lawsuit against the University of Chicago and Eli Lilly & Co. The plaintiffs charged that during pregnancy they and 1,078 other women had been given DES without their knowledge.

The women had been given the drug while receiving prenatal care at the school's Lying-In Hospital in Chicago in 1951 and 1952. The suit charged that none of the women had been advised that she was participating in a 20-month experiment to test the ability of DES to prevent miscarriages. In the experiment, an equal number of women had been given placebos.

The suit was filed in U.S. District Court in Chicago by attorneys for the Health Research Group, a unit of Ralph Nader's Public Citizen Inc. One of the three plaintiffs was Patsy Mink, a former Democratic congresswoman from Hawaii and currently an assistant secretary of state.

Ironically, the university had concluded as a result of its 1951–52 study that DES was ineffective in preventing miscarriages and discontinued hospital use of the drug.

The university April 26 said a National Institutes of Health-sponsored follow-up survey of 1,250 offspring of the DES mothers had found no evidence of vaginal or cervical cancer in their daughters nor any indication of genital deformity or sterility in their sons.

The university said it had begun contacting the women involved in the DES experiment in 1971 after the Food and Drug Administration banned its prescription for pregnant women.

Mink received a form letter of notification, dated Jan. 29, 1976, in Honolulu March 5, 1976. The letter urged her to have her daughter examined by a physician. It was later found that the 23-year-old woman was afflicted with adenosis, an often pre-cancerous condition also linked to DES offspring.

Lilly, the drug manufacturer, April 27 said its "only involvement" in the university study "was in furnishing the DES and placebos that were used."

Suit dismissed. Wayne County (Mich.) Circuit Court Judge Thomas Roumell May 16, 1977 rejected a $625 million damage suit filed by 144 women and 40 of their husbands. The suit charged that the women had contracted cancer because their mothers had taken DES during pregnancy.

Roumell dismissed the lawsuit because of each woman's inability to identify either a specific DES brand name or manufacturer responsible for her particular illness. The judge ruled in Detroit that the women could not jointly sue the 16 pharmaceutical firms named solely because they all had produced the carcinogenic hormone.

Since DES had not been patented by those who first had manufactured it, the product had been sold under its generic (chemical) name, not under brand names. As a result, lawyers for the women could not pin responsibility for a specific case of DES-related illness on a specific source of the drug. The lawsuit, filed in 1974, had contended that the drug manufacturers were jointly liable for any cancer or other medical problems the women had developed as a result of their mothers having taken DES.

Attorneys for the women had argued for industry-wide liability. They maintained that the drug firms had promoted and sold DES in a negligent manner, aware that it contained a cancer-causing agent called stilbene.

Michigan, with some 85,000 DES daughters, had been a test market for the drug, which had been prescribed to prevent miscarriages. All the female plaintiffs had undergone surgery for removal of cancerous or precancerous lesions.

Ban on Cyclamates & Saccharin

Cyclamates banned in all foods. The Food & Drug Administration Aug. 14, 1970 reinstated a total ban on the use of cyclamates, an artificial sweetener, in all foods, including those labeled "drugs" for diabetics or other persons needing to restrict intake of calories. The government had first banned cyclamates in October 1969, but had modified the order in February to exclude use of the sweetener as a drug.

The new order would make it illegal to sell any food, drug or soft drink containing cyclamates as of Sept. 1, 1970. The agency said its Medical Advisory Group on Cyclamates had "reviewed its recommendation" and decided on a total ban of the chemical "in the light of scientific evidence available to date."

The new evidence showed that much smaller amounts of cyclamates than previously tested produced cancer in rats. The agency said use of the chemical at a safe level would result in an "insignificant caloric reduction having no practical value for the obese or the diabetic patient."

Dr. Charles C. Edwards, FDA commissioner, had conceded in testimony before a House committee June 10 that cyclamates should have been withdrawn sooner.

(The Department of Health, Education and Welfare [HEW] had removed the artificial sweetener from the government list of substances recognized as safe in foods Oct. 18, 1969.)

Edwards told Rep. L. H. Fountain (D, N. C.), chairman of the House Committee on Government Operations, that "there is no question that it should have been done earlier," when asked about the government's ban. Edwards declined to say how much earlier.

Another health official who appeared before the committee, William W. Goodrich, assistant HEW general counsel, said that the government's action had not been taken sooner because of lack of agreement in the scientific study groups that advised the FDA about cyclamates.

Saccharin reported safe. A special study group of the National Academy of Sciences-Research Council reported to the FDA July 23, 1970 that the synthetic sweetener saccharin posed no known hazard to its users. The panel said its findings were made "on the basis of available information."

But the eight-man study group recommended further laboratory tests of the sweetener despite an "80-year history of saccharin use by man without evidence of adverse effects."

The panel's report was released by FDA Commissioner Charles Edwards. The FDA had requested the study in March 1969 after a University of Wisconsin researcher had reported that combinations of saccharin and cholesterol injected in the urinary bladders of mice caused cancers of that organ in some of the mice.

Saccharin curbed—The FDA Jan. 28, 1972 removed saccharin from its list of food additives "generally recognized as safe," after studies showed that mice fed large doses of the artificial sweetener developed bladder tumors.

Edwards said the action was taken to limit saccharine use to current levels while research continued. If the tumors were then found to be cancerous, and could be attributed to the saccharine, authorities would outlaw the product.

The Jan. 28 move would require food processors to list saccharine content on package labels. The FDA, following National Research Council advice, recommended a maximum adult daily use of one gram, the equivalent of seven 12-ounce bottles of diet beverage or 60 small tablets.

The FDA reported Jan. 9, 1975 that its study had been unable to determine whether saccharin caused cancer in test animals.

The FDA said that in the interim saccharin would continue to be marketed under current limitations.

FDA bans saccharin. The FDA March 9, 1977 issued a proposed ban on saccharin, the only artificial sweetener still available in the U.S. The agency based its decision in part on laboratory tests conducted by Canadian scientists that showed rats fed high dosages of the sweetener developed malignant bladder tumors.

Saccharin had been in use in the U.S. for about 80 years. Americans consumed about five million pounds of the substance each year, according to the government.

Saccharin was a staple of the diet-food industry, with low-calorie soft drinks accounting for three-quarters of the yearly consumption.

The FDA ban applied to all foods and beverages with saccharin additives. However, the agency indicated that existing inventories of saccharin products would not be recalled.

Action draws protests—The FDA ban on saccharin drew angry protests from consumers and representatives of the food industry March 9–10.

William P. Inman, a vice president of Sherwin-Williams Co. of Cleveland, the only U.S. manufacturer of saccharin, March 9 said his firm had not "seen anything that even [came] close to conclusively proving that saccharin [was] a health hazard." Inman's contention was supported the same day by a spokesman for Abbott Laboratories in Chicago, maker of a popular saccharin-based sweetener, Sucaryl. The spokesman said that "a number of other well-controlled studies" in addition to the Canadian experiments had "shown no harmful effects from saccharin used in equally high doses."

(The FDA, in announcing the ban, had admitted that a human would have to drink 800 12-ounce soft drinks sweetened with saccharin every day for a lifetime to match the doses given to the rats in the Canadian tests.)

Robert M. Kellen, president of the Atlanta-based Calorie Control Council March 9 criticized the FDA decision as "an example of colossal government overregulation in disregard of science and the needs and wants of consumers." Kellen charged that the results of the Canadian tests were inconclusive and that the risk to human health was minimal.

The executive vice president of Cumberland Packing Corp., maker of the nation's most widely used saccharin sweetener, Sweet 'n Low, March 9 called the ban "an outrageous and harmful action." Marvin Eisenstadt said the government, in effect, was telling diabetics they "can't taste anything sweet anymore."

Cumberland Packing March 10 announced plans to halt production for the immediate future and lay off 500 workers in New York City, 100 in Miami and 100 in Los Angeles. Sweet 'n Low was the company's sole product.

Both Coca-Cola Co. and PepsiCo Inc. March 10 said they probably would market diet soft drinks with sugar derivatives in the future. A PepsiCo spokesman said his company had a substitute product ready for production.

(It was reported March 10 that there were two artificial sweeteners awaiting federal approval. One was neohesperidine dihydrochalcone, a derivative of orange and grapefruit rinds. Discovered in 1967, it was 1,500 times sweeter than cane sugar and was reported to have demonstrated no ill effects on laboratory animals. The second product, Aspartame, had been approved by the FDA in 1974, but had not been marketed because discrepancies were discovered in the results of animal-feeding experiments. Aspartame currently was under re-review.)

A spokesman for the American Diabetes Association March 10 warned that the lack of sugar substitutes could have "very grave" effects for America's 10 million diabetics. Doctors considered diet control essential in the treatment of the disease. Most diabetics used an artificial sweetener as a substitute for natural sugar products.

Canada sets saccharin ban—The Canadian government March 9 announced that a broad ban on saccharin would take effect in that country June 1. As in the case of the U.S. action, the Canadian decision was based largely on the results of tests conducted by Canadian scientists that linked saccharin to cancer.

The Canadian ban would be more extensive than that of the U.S. The Ottawa government said saccharin would be forbidden in practically all its current applications. Beverages containing the substance would be outlawed after July 1. Drugs containing saccharin as a non medicinal ingredient would not be permitted after Dec. 31, 1978, with the exception of some "life-saving" drugs. Cosmetics, toothpaste and mouthwash containing saccharin would not be allowed after Dec. 31, 1979.

Canada planned to make saccharin available in pharmacies Sept. 1.

Trading reactions—Rumors of the impending U.S. and Canadian bans caused the common stocks of soft-drink manufacturers to drop sharply March 9. (The governments' announcements had been made after the close of trading in New York.) On the New York Stock Exchange composite tape, Coca-Cola Co. common stock fell $3 to $73 on a volume of 152,200 shares. PepsiCo Inc. common stock fell $2.62 to $68 on a volume of 50,600 shares.

FDA modifies saccharin ban. The FDA April 14, 1977 modified its proposed ban on saccharin to allow the artificial sweetener to remain on the market for limited use as a nonprescription drug. Under the new proposal, saccharin could be sold in tablet, powder or liquid form in pharmacies, food stores and restaurants, but its use still would be prohibited in commercially prepared foods and beverages. (Commercially prepared foods and beverages currently accounted for 90% of saccharin use.)

The new proposal would ban the use of saccharin in cosmetics likely to be ingested, such as lipstick, and in nonmedical additives used to make prescription drugs taste better. It also would allow the sweetener to be labeled as an over-the-counter drug. This would circumvent the legal ban on cancer-causing food additives—the so-called Delaney Clause of the 1958 Food, Drug and Cosmetic Act. The proposed drug classification would force manufacturers to show that saccharin was both safe and effective for the medical purpose for which it was intended, pursuant to the 1962 Harris-Kefauver amendments to the act.

Finally, the FDA proposal would require that packages containing saccharin be labeled: "Warning: saccharin causes bladder cancer in animals. Use of saccharin may increase your risk of cancer. For use as a non-caloric sweetener when sugar-restricted diets are medically indicated, as in patients with diabetes."

In the midst of a continuing furor over the proposed ban, FDA Commissioner Dr. Donald Kennedy defended the FDA action April 14, saying, "Our scientists now calculate that a moderate use of saccharin, the amount present in one large diet soft drink, if ingested daily over a lifetime by every American, might lead to 1,200 additional cases of bladder cancer per year."

OTA panel affirms cancer risk—A scientific panel named by the Office of Technology Assessment to review the saccharin controversy for Congress reported June 7 that the artificial sweetener was a weak carcinogen that should not be considered safe for human consumption. The group was unable to definitively measure saccharin's potential to cause cancer in humans but cited studies showing it had caused bladder cancer in rats.

Saccharin linked to human cancer. A new Canadian study reported June 17 directly linked the use of artificial sweeteners to bladder cancer in humans.

The as yet unpublished survey, conducted by the National Cancer Institute of Canada in conjunction with four Canadian universities, found that men who used saccharin or cyclamates had a 60% higher chance of developing bladder cancer thatn those who did not. The study showed no increased cancer risk among women who used artificial sweteners.

Previous concern about saccharin as a carcinogen had been based on evidence that it caused cancer in rats. The new study was the first to associate saccharin with human cancer. The survey, which involved 630 bladder cancer patients, also found that smoking was eight times more important as a determinant of bladder cancer than the use of non-nutritive artificial sweeteners.

FDA Commissioner Donald Kennedy said June 27 that the new study "raises serious questions about the wisdom of our present proposal," which would allow saccharin to remain on the market as a nonprescription drug. The recent findings raised doubts as to "whether saccharin should remain available for any purpose," Kennedy said.

Action on Amphetamines

FDA moves to curb 'pep pills.' The Food & Drug Administration Aug. 5, 1970 announced legal actions to sharply limit the use of amphetamines—drugs known as "pep pills." Food and Drug Commissioner Charles C. Edwards said the drug industry produced enormous amounts of the drug, which he said had only limited medical usefulness. He said the industry "has not faced its responsibilities with these drugs. . . . It is time for the manufacturers to accept the challenge of working closely with the FDA and the Department of Justice to stop unnecessary production of amphetamines."

The agency called for changes in amphetamine labeling to restrict claims of effectiveness and strengthen warnings of hazards. Labels could claim effectiveness for three medical uses: narcolepsy, an uncontrollable urge to sleep; hyperactivity in children with minor brain damage; and obesity, when short-term use of the drug would be allowed as an appetite suppressant in a weight reduction treatment based on restriction of calories.

The labeling changes would take effect 60 days after the guidelines were published in the Federal Register. The agency also ordered the drug industry to produce data within a year to validate claims made for amphetamine products. Although the FDA action would not limit a doctor's right to prescribe the drug, it would increase his exposure to malpractice suits if he deviated from the recommended uses.

The FDA estimated that drug companies manufactured 3.5 billion doses of amphetamines annually, with almost 40% sold illegally. In earlier testimony before a Congressional subcommittee, Dr. Sidney Cohen, a National Institute of Mental Health officer, cited three types of amphetamine abuse: occasional use by students, businessmen, truck drivers or athletes to stay awake or produce extra bursts of energy; daily use of large amounts of the drug to produce an emotional lift; and a comparatively new use by injection into a vein to produce an effect much like that of cocaine.

The FDA said the drug could induce "extreme fatigue and mental depression" after the initial effect wore off and continued use could produce "psychosis, often clinically indistiguishable from schizophrenia."

Thomas N. Rauch, president of Smith, Kline & French Laboratories, the leading manufacturer involved, said Aug. 5 that the company had been urging passage of more restrictive drug-abuse legislation. "As we have said before Congressional committees," Rauch added, "the company's amphetamine products are not supplying the illicit traffic."

Amphetamine cut set. John E. Ingersoll, director of the Justice Department's Bureau of Narcotics & Dangerous Drugs, signed an order Feb. 9, 1972 reducing the 1972 federal production quotas of amphetamine and methamphetamine by almost 82% of the 1971 total.

In December 1971, Justice Department officials had said that the proposed quotas would be near 60% of the estimated 1971 output, but recent developments had indicated that the final quota would be substantially lower.

Control of amphetamines and methamphetamines, two powerful types of stimulant drugs, was thought to be an important step towards reducing drug abuse by Americans. Improper use of the stimulants was considered to be a serious health hazard.

The order set production quotas at 1,564 kilograms of amphetamine, down 83% from the 9,356 kilograms produced in 1971 when there was no quota. The 1972 quota for methamphetamine was set at 969 kilograms, down 80% from the 4,926 kilograms produced in 1971.

Diet pills curbed. The Food & Drug Administration announced Dec. 14, 1972 that it would take a series of actions to restrict the use of amphetamine-related diet pills, because of their limited effectiveness and high risk.

Dr. Henry E. Simmons, director of FDA's Bureau of Medicine, told the Senate Monopoly Subcommittee that the agency would distribute the results of a recent test of the pills to 600,000 medical professionals, require manufacturers to stress the drug's limitations and hazards on labels, and might move to place most of the appetite-suppressants under the Controlled Substances Act, as had already been done with pure amphetamines.

Simmons reported that a study by an

advisory panel found that the drugs had an "extremely limited" effectiveness, and had caused side effects such as nervousness, insomnia and habituation in susceptible patients. He said, however, the agency would not ban the products, "because the treatment of obesity is particularly difficult," and "the physician should have the use of all adequately tested therapeutic aids."

Some 26 million prescriptions for weight-reducing drugs had been filled in 1971, earning drug companies about $65 million.

HEW asks amphetamine curb. The Department of Health, Education & Welfare (HEW) Jan. 18, 1973 recommended a series of restrictions on production of amphetamines that would reduce the low 1972 quota for the drug by at least a further 50%.

HEW asked the Bureau of Narcotics and Dangerous Drugs to bar all production of injectable amphetamines as unsafe, and of amphetamines combined with other drugs, used mostly as appetite suppressants.

HEW also recommended a 20% cutback in amphetamines to be taken by mouth. Taken together, the restrictions would reduce the year's quota by 50%–70% under the 1972 quota, which had itself been reduced by 80% from 1971 to combat a thriving black market in the stimulants.

Recall & quotas. The FDA and Bureau of Narcotics & Dangerous Drugs (BNDD) April 1, 1973 recalled all diet drugs containing amphetamines for the purpose of eliminating them from the market by June 30. The order applied to injectable amphetamines and all combination diet pills composed of amphetamines and other substances such as vitamins or tranquilizers.

In an attempt to further curb amphetamine abuse, the BNDD announced April 1 a 39% cut in the legitimate production quotas of amphetamines and methamphetamines. This cut from 1972 levels followed an 80% quota reduction from 1971. Since 1971, legitimate production quotas had been reduced from 9,356 to 992 kilograms for amphetamines and from 4,926 to 561 kilograms for methamphetamines.

The decision to recall the drugs was based on the FDA contention that injectable amphetamines had great potential for abuse and that combination pills did little to control against obesity. However, their use was still considered legitimate in treatment of a few rare diseases and some psychiatric and behavioral problems.

Diabetes Drugs Curbed

Doctors cautioned on tolbutamide. The American Medical Association (AMA), concurring with the Food and Drug Administration, warned physicians Oct. 23, 1970 to be cautious in prescribing a diabetes drug used by about 800,000 Americans. The drug, called tolbutamide, was taken orally in pill form. It was marketed by the Upjohn Co. under the trade name Orinase.

The AMA said its Council on Drugs had issued a statement to doctors in which it suggested that they try to control mild diabetes cases in adults by reliance on a regulated diet. If this was unsuccessful, the statement said, the council recommended diet and insulin injections. The AMA's statement said that "the consideration of treatment with oral hypoglycemic agents should be secondary to the use of insulin."

The AMA's action represented an evaluation of an 8½ year study conducted at 12 hospitals by the University Group Diabetes Program. In the study, more than 800 adult patients with mild cases of diabetes were treated with various combinations of insulin, tolbutamide and a strict diet. One conclusion made by the study group was that the combination of diet and tolbutamide was no more effective in prolonging a patient's life than control of the diet alone. The FDA had endorsed the report early in 1970.

Diabetes drugs curbed. The FDA announced in a letter to doctors (reported May 26, 1972) that it had approved new labeling for all oral diabetes drugs warning against "apparent increased cardiovascular hazard," and recommending use only when the condition could not be controlled by diet and weight reduction or by insulin injections.

The ruling was the result of a 1961–1970 study by the National Institute of Arthritis and Metabolic Diseases of 823 diabetes patients, which found that those using oral drugs had a cardiovascular death rate 2½ times greater than those using diet or insulin alone. Furthermore, after two or three years of use the oral drugs tended to lose their effectiveness in reducing blood sugar.

About 1.5 million U.S. patients used the oral drugs daily, under the trade names Orinase, Tolinase, Diabinese, Dymelor, Meltrol-50 and DBI.

Second oral diabetes drug linked to heart deaths. The second major type of oral drug used to fight diabetes was found to have been linked to excessive deaths from heart diseases (reported Feb. 27, 1975). The report was part of a study of oral diabetic drugs by the University Group Diabetes Program (UGDP), which evaluated 1200 diabetic patients over 8½ years. The latest report focused on the drug phenformin, showing a death rate from heart attacks that was three times greater than for those patients treated with insulin (a hormone) alone. It also linked the drug with high blood pressure and rapid heart rate. An earlier UGDP study recommended the banning of tolbutamide and later extended the recommendation to most oral drugs after finding dangers of heart disease.

The UGDP studies cast serious doubt on the use of oral drugs for lowering blood sugar in diabetics. Aside from the dangerous side effects, it was found that a change of diet or the use of diet and insulin, appeared more efficacious than the oral drugs alonc in prolonging the lives of diabetics whose troubles began when they were adults. This was backed up in the report on phenformin. The 1970 study had lead to a warning to physicians by the FDA against prescribing such drugs. Nevertheless the drugs were reported still being prescribed to about 1.5 million Americans by physicians who contested the findings.

A study by a special panel of the internationally prestigious Biometrics Society, reported Jan. 28, confirmed the validity of the 1970 UGDP study. The group declared, in the American Medical Association (AMA) journal, that in light of the findings it was "the responsibility of the proponents of oral agents to conduct scientifically adequate studies to justify the continued use of such agents." The FDA was reported Feb. 1 considering new labeling that would sharply cut back the approved uses for the pills.

Tolbutamide was being sold under the trade name Orinase, phenformin as DBI and Meltrol. Other drugs in question included tolazamide (trade name Tolinase) and acetohexamide, (trade name Dymelor). Chlorpropamide, sold as Diabinese, was not part of the UGDP study but had been linked to the others by the FDA and was included in its letters of warning on oral diabetes drugs sent to physicians in 1972.

Phenaformin sale banned. Secretary of Health, Education & Welfare Joseph A. Califano Jr. July 25, 1977 ordered phenformin, a prescription drug used by some 385,000 diabetics, off the market. Califano called the drug an "imminent hazard to public health." In withdrawing phenformin, Califano invoked for the first time in the department's history an emergency provision of the Food, Drug and Cosmetic Act that allowed him to summarily halt the sale of a drug, bypassing hearings or appeals on the matter.

Phenformin, marketed by Ciba-Geigy Corp. as DBI and DBI-TD and by USV Pharmaceutical Corp. (a subsidiary of Revlon Inc.) as Meltrol, had been prescribed since 1959 to lower blood-sugar levels in adults suffering from so-called onset diabetes.

Califano acted on the basis of overwhelming evidence that phenformin was a prime cause of lactic acidosis, a metabolic disorder in which lactic acid accumulated in the blood in abnormal amounts. The condition was fatal in half of the 245 cases reported to the Food and

Drug Administration. In October 1976, when the FDA knew of 190 phenformin-related cases of lactic acidosis, a special advisory panel had unanimously recommended removal of the drug from the market.

Califano's action came ten weeks after the Health Research Group, an affiliate of Ralph Nader's Public Citizen Inc., petitioned for a phenformin ban, claiming the drug killed more people than it saved. (Only the HEW secretary had the authority to issue the imminent-hazard order; all other drug regulatory actions were handled by the FDA.)

In a 66-page statement, Califano noted that the death rate among phenformin users was "far higher than has been regarded as acceptable for any other drug approved for use in the U.S. for a broad patient population." The marketing ban provided a 90-day phaseout period that would permit physicians to transfer their diabetic patients to other available medications, such as insulin.

Salk drug licensing criticized. Licensing procedures for a new diabetes drug developed by the Salk Institute came under Justice Department criticism.

According to a report appearing in the Wall Street Journal March 19, 1975, report in the Wall Street Journal, Salk had proposed to grant patent licenses for the drug, somatostatin, to four companies for clinical testing necessary before the drug could be approved for sale by the Food and Drug Administration. Additional licenses would not be granted for three years to provide incentive for investing in the testing procedures, according to the institute. But the Justice Department contended that the three-year head start would discourage other companies from buying the patent rights.

Tests reportedly had shown that human diabetics given somatostatin, together with insulin, had lowered blood sugar far below that achieved with insulin alone. The medication, a brain hormone, was said to work by inhibiting the release of glucagon, another natural hormone thought to be responsible for maintaining high levels of sugar in the blood of diabetics.

Warning on pills proposed. The Food & Drug Administration July 7, 1975 published a proposal to require a label for widely-used diabetes pills—oral hypoglycemic drugs—warning that the drugs "may be associated with increased cardiovascular mortality as compared to treatment with diet alone or diet plus insulin." The drugs were used by 1½ million adult diabetics, it was estimated, for a $100 million market value. A warning label for oral diabetes drugs had been approved by the FDA in 1972 but had been blocked by litigation. A hearing on the new labeling was scheduled for public comment.

The proposal was based on a controversial study completed in 1971 that concluded that patients who used the pills had a death rate from heart disease twice as high as that of comparable patients using diet or diet plus insulin. The warning label would report the study and state that "despite controversy regarding the interpretation of these results, the findings . . . provide adequate basis for this warning."

The proposed label also would recommend to doctors that the drugs be used only for patients who cannot be treated effectively with diet or diet and insulin. Doctors also were to be told on the label that "patients should be informed of the advantage and potential risks of the [oral antidiabetic] drug and alternative modes of treatment and should participate in the decision to use the drug."

The controversy over the study involved technique—whether the individuals were properly selected and assigned to treatment groups—and applicability—whether the fixed dosage administered accurately reflected that of actual practice, where the dosage varied according to patient need.

AMA aide's letter minimized danger—The New York Times reported July 8 that Dr. James H. Sammons, executive vice president of the American Medical Association, had permitted Upjohn, the largest manufacturer of the controversial drug, to use a letter he wrote in their sales talks for the drug. The letter had been sent to local AMA officials about the Feb.

10 issue of the AMA's own magazine, The Journal of the American Medical Association, and its article and an editorial raising questions about the drugs. The letter minimized the questions and said "diabetic patients should not be influenced by press reports, and should continue on whatever diabetic management program their own physician had prescribed."

Other FDA Actions & Powers

FDA acts vs. antibiotics. FDA Commissioner Charles C. Edwards announced June 24, 1970 that his agency had completed legal actions needed in order to remove from the market 48 combination antibiotic drugs that were ruled ineffective more than a year earlier. The action—affecting all fixed combinations of penicillin and various sulfa drugs and penicillin with streptomycin—was in line with previous steps the agency had taken against combination drugs, following results of a study conducted by the National Academy of Sciences-National Research Council.

(In a ruling reported July 25, the FDA said that after July 31, it would no longer certify Signemycin—an antibiotic combination manufactured by Pfizer Co.—as safe and effective. The agency said the company had failed to produce studies supporting use of the drug, which had been prescribed for severe, acute infections.)

According to an Aug. 24 report, the FDA ordered 13 nasal sprays and drops removed from the market within 30 days. Commissioner Edwards said there was no reason to believe that the preparations—combination products mostly sold by prescriptions—could produce the results claimed. He said the preparations included antibiotics combined with steroids, vaso-constrictors, decongestants and antihistamines. The order applied to products of the Upjohn Co., Kalamazoo, Mich.; Merck & Co., West Point, Pa.; Smith, Kline & French Laboratories, Philadelphia; Warner-Lambert Pharmaceutical Co., Morris Plains, N.J.; and Lemon Pharmacal Co., Sellersville, Pa.

FDA approves L-dopa use. The Food and Drug Administration June 4, 1970 cautiously authorized the marketing of L-dopa as a prescription drug for treating persons afflicted with Parkinson's disease. The FDA approved L-dopa, clinically known as levo-dihydroxyphlenlalanine, in an unusually short time as a result of heavy public pressure.

In announcing approval of the drug, FDA Commissioner Dr. Charles C. Edwards stressed that L-dopa was to be used with caution because it was known to have dangerous side effects. He said that the FDA, for the first time, was requiring the two companies that would market the drug to continue their studies of patients who use it.

Edwards said that L-dopa "shows promise of being one of the major drug discoveries of recent years" despite its dangers. He added that "possibly as many as a million Americans" suffered from Parkinson's disease.

The commissioner said that the compound would be reviewed yearly by the FDA.

Uncertified drugs barred. The FDA told two drug companies Feb. 1, 1971 to stop selling a pair of medicines that had been marketed in violation of a law governing "new" drugs. At issue was a law that no drug legally classified as "new" could be sold without FDA approval of a new-drug application.

The two companies—Smith Kline & French Laboratories, maker of a non prescription decongestant and painkiller called Ornex, and Ayerst Laboratories, producer of a glaucoma treatment called Epitrate—had claimed their products were legally "old drugs" whose active ingredients had been medically accepted for years. The FDA acted on the basis of a letter Jan. 28 from Rep. L.H. Fountain (D, N.C.), who complained that the agency had taken no action although he had brought the matter to its attention two months before.

(The FDA also told Cord Laboratories and Linden Laboratories to recall their versions of chlorpromazine, a tranquilizer, because the products lacked approved new-drug applications.)

In another case involving the "new drug" provisions of the federal Food, Drug and Cosmetic Act, the Justice Department announced Jan. 19 that Dow Corning Corp. (Midland, Mich.) had entered pleas of nolo contendere in a 1967 indictment charging violations involving a silicone fluid, best known for its use to augment women's figures. The government charged that the drug was shipped illegally and misbranded for its use as an injection into human beings. In not contesting the charges, the company and officials indicted were liable to a maximum fine of $1,000 on each of two counts, or imprisonment for a year, or both.

Combination drug rules. The FDA proposed new regulations Feb. 1, 1971 to ensure the safety and effectiveness of fixed combination drugs, those containing two or more active ingredients in a fixed dosage form.

The FDA standards would require that each active ingredient in a combination drug contribute to the medicine's effectiveness. The agency statement said the action would insure that combination drugs were used only when the product offered advantages over any one or more of its ingredients taken separately. FDA Commissioner Dr. Charles C. Edwards said the agency recognized that some combinations had a legitimate role in medical treatment.

The agency announcement said, "The new policy affects up to 40% of the most widely sold prescription drugs and most [about 50%, an FDA officer said later] over-the-counter drugs—those sold without prescription."

FDA scientific work criticized. An advisory panel criticized the FDA May 27, 1971 for "poorly managed laboratories" and other inadequacies in the agency's scientific effort. The panel of five professors from leading medical schools, in a report based on a one-year survey requested by FDA Commissioner Dr. Charles C. Edwards, said, however, that the agency "does an extraordinary job in many ways" to protect the public, given budget and manpower limitations.

The report said some of the agency's laboratories were excellent, but it said facilities in Chicago and Philadelphia were antiquated, crowded and unsafe and labs in Denver were only barely adequate. The panel said, "one can also find laboratories so poorly managed that scientists seem to be unable to describe their work coherently or to produce interpretable data books containing their findings." The commission also complained of lack of sound data, "a curious aura of secrecy" and an "unhurried atmosphere."

The panel said the responsibilities of FDA laboratories "are literally overwhelming" and that the agency had "limited resources." Edwards, in a news conference announcing the report, said much had been done to implement many of the panel's 50 recommendations but that the FDA's $85 million budget would have to be dramatically increased to allow complete reform.

Specifically, the panel urged "overall surveillance at the source" of food and drug products to insure quality and safety. The report said the panel members were "dismayed to learn" that the FDA had no continuously up-to-date data on the identity and amount manufactured of all drugs on the U.S. market. The report pointed to one area of "possible danger to the public" in the wide use of antibiotics in livestock and poultry feed despite "the fact that the public health significance of drug residues in meat and poultry is not well understood."

The panel asked that sound science be the basis of the agency's decisions rather than "economic or political factors."

Adverse-findings rule. The FDA announced June 7, 1971 that prescription-drug labels and advertisements would have to include adverse findings on their effectiveness by the National Academy of Sciences-National Research Council. The ruling took effect in October. It applied only to prescription drugs, usually advertised only in medical journals.

Cold remedies questioned. The FDA July 7, 1972 published a three-year-old report of the Science-National Research

Council (NAS-NRC) that found most claims on cold remedy labels to be unsubstantiated.

Twenty-seven representative cold remedies were reviewed in the study. Of 45 claims, the NAS-NRC said manufacturers had provided substantial evidence for only four, while 14 were found "probably effective," five "effective, but," when some doubts were expressed, 14 "possibly effective" and eight "ineffective as a fixed combination," in which cases the combination of singly effective ingredients was considered unsafe or unnecessary for must users.

The remedies included pills, capsules, inhalers, jellies and nose drops, all marketed before 1963. After that date new non-prescription drugs could not be sold without proof of efficacy. In 1970, $580 million was spent by consumers on nonprescription cold remedies.

The study was part of a long-term program to regulate the safety, effectiveness and labeling of nonprescription drugs.

Smith, Kline and French, manufacturer of Contac, which the study found only possibly effective for two of three claims, replied in a July 7 statement that the NAS-NRC had based its study on data submitted prior to September 1966. Since then, the company claimed, it had submitted further, more conclusive verification for the efficacy of Contac.

Hexachlorophene curbed. The FDA Sept. 22, 1972 ordered curbs on the use of the germicide hexachlorophene.

The FDA, which had originally proposed curbs on the product in January, issued the considerably more stringent rules after 39 babies died in France in August after being treated with talcum powder containing an accidentally high 6% level of hexachlorophene.

The new order would ban all production or shipment of 400 categories of over-the-counter products containing less than .75% of the chemical, a dose widely considered ineffective as a germicide. The ban would not apply to products already on retail shelves, or those containing minute amounts of hexachlorophene as a preservative.

The January proposal would have permitted the sale, with a cautionary label, of these over-the-counter products, which included deodorants, soaps, shampoos, toothpastes, cosmetics and cleansers with annual sales of about $200 million.

Medical products containing over .75% hexachlorophene, used mostly to treat skin outbreaks and dandruff, would continue to be sold, but only by prescription. But all baby powders containing the chemical were recalled, "because they are not rinsed off, are applied repeatedly and are covered by diapers."

The FDA said the action was taken because "under certain circumstances and at higher concentrations hexachlorophene is a very, very potent neurotoxin," although there was no evidence that products containing limited amounts of the chemical were health hazards. The order would serve to ban unnecessary exposure "to assure continued safe use of this effective germ fighter" in special cases.

Vertigo drug recalled. The FDA withdrew marketing approval in December 1972 for a controversial drug against vertigo, Serc, after hearing evidence that the drug increased episodes of the ailment.

Drugstore stocks of Serc would be recalled, although drug bureau director Dr. Henry E. Simmons said the drug was safe.

FDA defends tough rules. Commissioner of the Food and Drug Administration (FDA) Dr. Charles C. Edwards, and FDA drug bureau director Dr. Henry E. Simmons told the Senate Monopoly Subcommittee Feb. 5, 1973 that their cautious policy on licensing new drugs had probably prevented thousands of deaths and deformities among Americans. They cited some 25 harmful drugs that had been marketed abroad but never reached the U.S. public because of the policy.

The agency was responding to criticism that amendments to the Pure Food and Drug Act in 1962 had decreased the number of beneficial new drugs appearing on the market. Subcommittee Chairman

Sen. Gaylord Nelson (D, Wis.) cited a Jan. 8 Newsweek magazine column by economist Milton Friedman charging that the amendments "condemn innocent people to death." Nelson expressed his "dismay" at attacks on the FDA by "certain elements of the medical profession."

Simmons cited the well-known case of thalidomide, in which over 10,000 babies were born deformed in European countries to mothers who had used the drug during pregnancy in the early 1960s.

"Of even more concern," he said, was a report that an aerosol spray for bronchial asthma had probably led to the death of 3,500 children in England and Wales alone in the mid 1960s. The drug, Simmons claimed, could not have been licensed in the U.S. without extensive animal and human testing. In another case, an appetite suppressant called aminorex, which the FDA had barred from further human tests in 1968 because of safety problems, might have caused an "epidemic" of a type of fatal high blood pressure of the lungs among German, Austrian and Swiss citizens in the late 1960s.

The amendments required evidence of effectiveness before a drug could be marketed, informed consent from participants in new drug tests and generally stronger safety measures.

FDA power upheld. In a series of rulings, the Supreme Court June 18, 1973 unanimously upheld the FDA's power to remove ineffective drugs from the market.

The court upheld 1962 Congressional legislation authorizing the FDA to require prescription drug manufacturers to prove their products' effectiveness as well as their safety. The decision was also extended to uphold a part of the 1962 law that gave the FDA power to regulate drugs that previously had been cleared for safety but not for effectiveness.

Reversing an appellate court ruling, the Supreme Court said the FDA could, without going to court, remove "me too" drugs from the market. "Me too" drugs were never approved by the FDA on the grounds they contained the same ingredients as other prescription preparations already being marketed.

The FDA was also held to have the jurisdiction to decide administratively, subject to judicial review, whether a product had to be cleared as a "new drug" before marketing.

The court ruled the FDA could deny a hearing to a drug manufacturer when it failed to provide evidence its product met requirements.

Justice Douglas wrote: "If the FDA were required automatically to hold a hearing for each product whose efficacy was questioned . . . even though many hearings would be an exercise in futility, we have no doubt that it could not fulfill its statutory mandate to remove from the market all those drugs which do not meet effectiveness requirements."

Non-prescription drugs sold over the counter were not affected by the rulings.

FDA to control medical devices. Congress May 13, 1976 voted to expand the FDA's regulatory powers over medical devices of almost all varieties. Both houses approved the bill by voice votes, and the President signed it May 28. The new legislation would allow the FDA to promulgate certain controls applicable to all devices and to require pre-market testing for certain classes of devices.

Pre-market testing for safety and effectiveness would in general be required for life-support devices and for those implanted in the body. Devices in those categories which had been on the market before the legislation was cleared would have to be approved before they could continue to be sold.

Without the powers contained in the new legislation, the FDA had to wait until a device had been marketed, then seek a court order against it. The agency's statutory authority was restricted to seeing that devices were neither adulterated nor incorrectly labeled.

The legislation required that medical devices be classified into one of three categories, subject to different degrees of FDA oversight. Devices in the first category would be subject only to general controls, allowing the government to set manufacturing and distribution standards and to order manufacturers to repair, replace, or give refunds for items that were risky because of faulty manufacturing.

Devices in the second category would be subject to construction, testing and performance standards and would also come under the first category's general controls.

The third category would be for those devices that required premarket approval. Manufacturers would have to file test reports and other information with the FDA, and generally would have to provide sample devices. The devices also would be subject to the general controls of the first category.

Devices subject only to general controls would essentially be those which, by virtue of their simplicity and long-standing record of safe use, were not considered to pose hazards to health (e.g., tongue depressers, thermometers). The category of devices subject to performance standards as well as to general controls was described as a 'gray' area; it comprised devices that were more vital to a person's health, and less time-tested, than the devices subject only to general controls, but still not so critical to health as those requiring pre-market testing. Prosthetic limbs could fall into the category of devices required to meet performance standards.

Other Developments

Antibiotic misuse charged. Dr. Henry E. Simmons, director of the FDA's Bureau of Medicine, told the Senate Monopoly Subcommittee that antibiotic misuse caused tens of thousands of deaths in the U.S. each year (reported Dec. 8, 1972).

Simmons said the drugs were properly used only to treat serious illnesses like typhoid and meningitis, but had been used for such routine discomforts as the common cold. The overuse of antibiotics, Simmons said, had led to development of immune strains of bacteria, and had caused a major wave of hospital blood poisoning from superinfections, which occurred when the antibiotic "kills off one set of microorganisms, thereby allowing another group to flourish."

Witnesses testifying before the subcommittee said at least 60% of antibiotic patients in hospitals could do without the drugs, and that U.S. antibiotic production had more than tripled in 10 years, reaching an annual average of 50 doses for every person in the country.

AMA drug policy criticized. Three former top advisers to the American Medical Association (AMA) accused the organization of being "a captive of and beholden to the pharmaceutical industry." The charge was made Feb. 6, 1973 in testimony they gave before the Senate Monopoly Subcommittee of the Small Business Committee. The advisers were the last two chairmen and a former vice chairman of the AMA's Council on Drugs, an independent group of scientists and doctors established by the AMA in 1905 to advise the medical profession on drugs. The council was abolished October 1972 in what the AMA called an economy move.

Dr. John Adriani, council chairman from 1968 to 1970, and Dr. Harry C. Shirkey, Adrian's successor, both of Tulane University, and former vice chairman Dr. Daniel L. Azarnoff, of the University of Kansas testified before the subcommittee. The following summary of their combined testimony was reported by the Feb. 7 Washington Post and New York Times:

> The AMA had committed itself to publish a complete, unbiased guide to prescription drugs. Drawing on over 300 experts, the Council on Drugs completed the report in 1971 at a cost of over $3 million and readied the report for distribution to members. In January 1971, Max H. Parrott, chairman of the board of directors of the AMA, told the council that publication of the study would have to be delayed for a few months so the book could be reviewed by people he called "our friends,"—the Pharmaceutical Manufacturers Association (PMA). Actually the PMA had already been given draft copies. Although the council initially demurred, it later accepted. Soon after, the PMA submitted "three or four crates" of proposed revisions, which the council dealt with by making about 35 token revisions in areas such as dosage sizes and revised formulations. The council stood fast against any substantive revisions, especially against condemnations of heavily advertised drug combinations.
>
> When the book appeared, Dr. Parrott attempted to tone down the report by adding a cover letter that said that some of the condemned combination drugs "may be justifiable."
>
> A second clash came in September 1972, when the AMA board was given an advance look at the second edition of "AMA Drug Evaluations." Many medicines had been evaluated as "not recommended," a

rating that board representative Dr. Richard Palmer asked be deleted. The council instead proposed that an explanation accompany each appearance of "not recommended," a compromise that was unacceptable to the board.

One month later the council was abolished and the task of completing the second drug manual was turned over to paid employes of the AMA.

Dr. Adriani testified that the "not recommended" designation left the AMA board with "no choice but to appease the pharmaceutical industry." The alternative he said, was to sacrifice ad revenues in the AMA Journal of Medicine.

Prescription drug panel—The PMA and Sen. Edward M. Kennedy (D, Mass.) Nov. 30, 1976 announced the establishment of the Joint Commission on Prescription Drug Use, which would devise a system of monitoring the safety and effectiveness of drugs after they had been marketed. The independent panel would report on adverse drug reactions and analyze the drug-prescribing habits of American physicians.

The 18-member commission, established on a three-year trial basis, would be largely financed by the pharmaceutical association, which had expressed concern about the abuse and misuse of medicinal drugs. The annual budget of $250,000 would be provided through a trust designed to protect the commission's autonomy.

Krebiozen ban upheld. The Supreme Court Oct. 15, 1973 let stand a ruling that the drug Krebiozen was not recognized as a safe and effective cure for cancer and therefore could be banned from the market.

Needless X-ray use charged. Dr. Karl Z. Morgan, professor of health physics at the Georgia Institute of Technology in Atlanta, told the American Cancer Society's seminar for science writers in St. Augustine, Fla. March 27, 1974 that Americans received harmful overdoses of radiation from diagnostic X-rays. Asserting that most U.S. doctors and dentists "didn't have the remotest concept of the risks associated with exposure to diagnostic X-rays," Morgan charged that 3,000 Americans died each year from cancer resulting from unnecessary exposure to diagnostic X-rays.

Morgan, director of health physics at the Atomic Energy Commission's Oak Ridge (Tenn.) National Laboratory 1943–72, urged that outmoded, high-dose X-ray equipment be replaced with new low-dose apparatus; that radiation technologists be appropriately educated, trained and certified; and that dentists reserve use of X-rays for special needs only.

Stricter rules issued—The FDA July 29, 1974 published a new set of standards designed to reduce public exposure to unnecessary radiation. Under the new rules, which were effective for medical and dental diagnostic equipment manufactured after July 31, X-ray beams were limited to the smallest size necessary to produce an acceptable picture. The rules also contained provisions to minimize film retakes by requiring improvement in equipment reliability.

Curb on breast X-rays—The National Cancer Institute Aug. 23, 1976 issued new guidelines on the use of X-ray techniques, known as mammography, to detect breast cancer. NCI recommended that routine mammography be discontinued for women aged 35–50 unless they showed specific symptoms of breast cancer or otherwise were classified as "high risk."

The guidelines, which would have no regulatory force, were distributed to the 27 detection centers participating in a nationwide screening project, which was jointly sponsored by NCI and the American Cancer Society. NCI acted after recent studies indicated that the risk from irradiation during mammography might outweigh the benefits of the procedure for women under 50. Doctors estimated that an average woman had a 7% chance of developing breast cancer and that each mammogram increased that chance by 1% for women aged 35–50.

Dr. John Bailar 3rd, editor of the Journal of the National Cancer Institute, concluded in a paper published in January that "the routine use of mammography" in screening symptomless women could "eventually take almost as many lives as it saves."

Defending the X-ray screening, NCI

Director Dr. Frank J. Rauscher Jr. said Aug. 22 that one-third of all breast cancers were detected in the 35–50 age group. Of these, he said, one-third could not have been detected without the use of mammography. The figures were based on 259,000 women screened for breast cancer at the 27 detection centers.

The NCI May 10, 1977 announced more stringent guidelines on the use of mammograms in its nationwide breast-cancer detection project. The institute restricted mammograms for women under 50 to those with a history of breast cancer or with such a history in the immediate family.

A cancer institute panel May 3 cited figures showing that despite recommendations to discontinue the procedure, issued in August 1976, 75% of the women in the detection project between ages 35 and 49 were still undergoing mammographies. The new guidelines were endorsed by the American Cancer Society, which jointly sponsored the country's 27 breast cancer screening centers.

Breast cancer surgery debate. Breast cancer surgery on Betty Ford, wife of President Ford, and on Margaretta Rockefeller, wife of Vice President-designate Nelson A. Rockefeller, resulted in widespread public discussion of the disease, which afflicted 90,000 U.S. women and resulted in the deaths of 30,000 others in 1973.

Mrs. Rockefeller, 48, underwent surgery for the removal of her left breast, 32 adjacent lymph nodes and part of the underlying chest muscle Oct. 17, 1974 after doctors at a New York City hospital had confirmed that one large and two small nodules in her breast were malignant.

In announcing the surgery on his wife, Rockefeller said she had been prompted to examine herself for possible malignant lumps because of the heightened "consciousness" that followed Mrs. Ford's operation.

Despite the high incidence of occurrence of breast cancer, its treatment remained in dispute. A study released by the National Cancer Institute Sept. 29 found that a radical mastectomy, the operation performed on Mrs. Ford, was unnecessary in many cases. The study also found that chemical therapy could "drastically" reduce the incidence of recurrence of breast cancer.

The institute was reporting the results of studies involving 1,700 women at 37 U.S. hospitals since 1971. The report showed that radical mastectomies, which produced life-long pain, weakness and periodic swelling of the arm, were not required for patients whose lymph nodes were cancer-free. By changing normal procedures, surgeons could order immediate laboratory tests on the lymph nodes, the report said. If the tests failed to show malignancy in the nodes, the surgeons could limit treatment to the less disfiguring, less traumatic simple mastectomy—amputation of the breast only. (Normal procedure was to remove the lymph nodes and conduct tests afterward.) "I would estimate that well over half of those [undergoing breast cancer surgery] would be candidates for the less radical procedure," Dr. Frank J. Rauscher, director of the institute, said. Currently, 95% of all women undergoing breast cancer surgery received radical mastectomies.

(The almost universal use of the radical mastectomy had been criticized by some women's rights groups, who suggested that surgeons, most of whom were men, would be less likely to perform such a radical procedure to treat a comparable male affliction.)

The American Cancer Society Oct. 17 took a cautious view of the institute study, pointing out that it had three more years to run before anything definitive could be said about the relative effectiveness of the simple mastectomy. The society said it would continue to recommend radical mastectomy for most cases of breast cancer.

Another study, reported in the Oct. 14 issue of Time magazine, indicated that chemotherapy had been found effective in controlling and preventing cancerous tumors in the lymph nodes. Among 67 premenopausal women who had undergone surgery for breast cancer, only one of 30 given the oral drug L-phenylalanine mustard (L-PAM) had recurrence of cancer, while 11 of 37 women receiving no drug treatment had recurrences.

2 tranquilizers put under control. The Drug Enforcement Administration and the Health, Education and Welfare Department announced June 1, 1975 that Valium and Librium, widely used tranquilizers, would be under federal control, effective July 2. The action was taken to prevent abuse of the drugs, which had retail sales in 1974 of $670 million (Valium $550 million, almost three billion tablets; Librium $120 million, more than one billion capsules).

The agencies cited evidence the drugs had a potential for abuse and could produce physical and psychological dependence.

The federal control was extended also to some less well-known drugs: Dalmane, a sedative; Tranxene and Serax, both tranquilizers; and Clonopin, an anticonvulsant, which was not on the market as yet.

All these products, placed under the 1970 Controlled Substances Act, would be limited to five prescription refills within a six-month period with a new prescription needed after that. Records on production and distribution and a tightened security against theft also were required.

Polio-vaccine warning. The live-virus, oral polio vaccine was responsible for more than half the cases of the disease in the U.S. between 1973–75, the government's Center for Disease Control (CDC) reported Sept. 23, 1976. Dr. Jonas Salk, discoverer of the killed-virus, injected vaccine, told a Senate hearing Sept. 23 that the live-virus vaccine, discovered by Dr. Albert Sabin, was "the principal if not the sole cause" of the 140 polio cases reported in the U.S. since 1961.

"At present," Salk told the Labor and Public Welfare Committee's subcommittee on health, "the risk of acquiring polio from the live-virus vaccine is greater than from the naturally occurring viruses."

Salk and other scientists who testified at the hearing criticized the "informed consent statement" used by parents to permit the immunization of their children with the live-virus vaccine. The form acknowledged neither its risk nor the existence of the alternative vaccine that used killed viruses, they said.

The CDC had said Sept. 21 that a nationwide shortage of live-virus vaccine had developed at a time when the drug was in demand for public-health programs to immunize school-age children.

CDC officials blamed the shortage on the insistence of one supplier, Lederle Laboratories, a division of American Cyanamid Co., that all persons receiving the vaccine through public-health facilities sign an informed consent statement warning of the vaccine's possible risks. Lederle had stopped distributing the drug in June because of the contractual dispute.

The concern over who accepted responsibility for adverse reactions to vaccine administration stemmed from a 1974 court ruling upheld by the Supreme Court that a drug manufacturer was liable when an infant contracted polio after being given the vaccine.

The contractual dispute was resolved Sept. 21. The agreement stated that the CDC would take "all appropriate steps" to provide patients or their parents or guardians with "meaningful warnings" about the vaccine's use.

Prescription drug deaths reported. Approximately 10,000 U.S. hospital patients who were not chronically ill died from adverse drug reactions each year, according to data reported in the Feb. 28, 1977 Journal of the American Medical Association. The Boston University Medical Center's latest survey was based on the monitoring of 26,462 patients admitted to 21 acute-disease hospitals between 1971–76. Ten of the hospitals were in the U.S. and the other 11 were in Canada, Scotland, West Germany, Italy, Israel and New Zealand.

The study found that 24 of the observed patients (0.9 per 1,000), had died from a drug reaction and concluded that one-fourth of the deaths could have been prevented by better administration of the drug. Internationally, the rate of deaths varied from a low of zero in Israel and Italy to a high of 1.4 per 1,000 in New Zealand.

Previous figures compiled in 1971 by the same researchers—Jane Porter and Dr. Hershel Jick—had indicated that 29,000 hospitalized Americans died annually from drugs. However, that study had included a disproportionately large number of chronically ill patients who were particularly susceptible to the toxic drugs they often had to receive. The newly figured percentage of deaths did not reflect any chronically ill patients.

In a telephone interview reported in The New York Times Feb. 28, Dr. Jick said the most reasonable approximation of the total number of drug-related deaths in U.S. hospitals was 18,000 a year, based upon the combined findings of the earlier and later reports. Jicks headed the 10-year-old Boston Collaborative Drug Surveillance Program, a federally funded project to measure drug-induced injury.

Nevada legalizes acupuncture. A bill setting up a system for state licensing of practitioners of the ancient Chinese medical art of acupuncture was signed by Nevada Gov. Mike O'Callaghan (D) April 20, 1973.

In related news developments, the Internal Revenue Service ruled that acupuncture was a deductible medical expense for income tax purposes, it was reported Jan. 18.

Doctors at the Washington (D.C.) Hospital Center reported April 22 that they had used acupuncture as anesthesia in four abortion cases. Its use was expected to be confined to cases in which patients had adverse reactions to conventional anesthetics, they said.

Nevada authorizes Gerovital. The Nevada legislature May 20, 1977 authorized the manufacture of the controversial drug Gerovital (GH3). Gerovital was hailed by its proponents as a powerful antidepressant and rejuvenator. The measure was passed as part of the bill legalizing the manufacture and sale of the purported anticancer drug laetrile. The chemical Gerovital, discovered and popularized in Europe, had never been licensed by the U.S. Food and Drug Administration.

The so-called "fountain of youth" drug consisted mainly of procaine hydrochloride, which was used by dentists as a local anesthetic under the trade name Novocain. It allegedly relieved depression, tension and reversed physical degeneration. Its developer, Dr. Ana Aslan, director of the Institute of Geriatrics in Bucharest, Rumania, claimed it could extend the human life span.

American researchers who had tested Gerovital's efficacy had found it to be an effective antidepressant with fewer side effects than expected from drugs currently available. Marvin Kratter, 61, controlling stockholder of Rom-Amer Pharmaceuticals Ltd., which had the U.S. rights to market Gerovital, had withdrawn the company's application for FDA approval, the Wall Street Journal reported June. 2

AMA eases peer review opposition. Delegates to the American Medical Association's (AMA) semiannual convention in Chicago, voted to cooperate with the federal government in establishment of Professional Standards Review Organizations (PSRO) to monitor the quality of care under the Medicaid and Medicare programs. By 185–57 vote June 26, 1974, delegates agreed to not to wage, as some had demanded, a campaign of outright opposition to PSROs, but to work for the programs' success while seeking to amend portions of the law creating the organizations.

The AMA board of trustees and its Council on Medical Services had spent much of the meeting warning the delegates that fighting PSROs would be futile. A continuance of efforts to seek repeal of the PSRO law could seriously weaken AMA impact on pending health legislation and destroy its public credibility, they said. One trustee said, "I believe the federal government, which purchases care for 38% of our population, is entitled to assurances that that care is efficient, effective and economical."

Utah PSRO begins operation—The peer review system became operative June 18 with the signing of a $951,000 contract by the Utah PSRO. In existence for two years, the Utah organization had served as a model for peer review legislation.

Doctors had warned that the PSRO would be costly to administer, would add hours of paperwork to a doctor's day, allow the federal government to interfere in medicine and lead to "cookbook medicine" by discouraging innovative practices. But the Utah doctors involved in the pilot project asserted that none of these fears was valid.

Only 5.5% of all cases required additional review by the PSRO, and in only 24 of 20,000 cases was payment denied. Dr. Alan R. Nelson, chairman of the Utah PSRO, said there was "zero paperwork" and most physicians in Utah had agreed to participate in the program. The cost of review, Nelson said, was about $2 a year for each Medicare and Medicaid patient.

Sex-change funds denied. The New York state Court of Appeals April 6, 1976 upheld, 4–3, the Department of Social Services's refusal to pay for a Brooklyn man's sex-change operation. The man, identified as Denise R., was said to have been living as a female for 18 years. In 1972 he had applied to a New York City agency asking it for funds for the operation under the state law which allowed anyone to apply for funds to "correct or cure" a condition that interfered with a person's "normal activity."

The city and then the state had refused to pay for the operation. It was estimated that the operation would cost between $2,000 and $15,000.

Unnecessary Surgery

Congressional Report

In 1975 the Oversight & Investigations Subcommittee of the House Interstate & Foreign Commerce Committee conducted an investigation that, Subcommittee Chairman John E. Moss reported, focused "upon an in-depth examination of unnecessary surgery, particularly to the extent to which the Medicare and Medicaid Programs contribute to overutilization and support unnecessary surgical procedures." The report, as issued under the date of Jan. 19, 1976, is reproduced on the following pages. Portions of Rep. Moss' letter of transmittal follow on this page:

The report concludes that second consultations before surgery can cut down on unnecessary surgical procedures. This report reommends that the Department of Health, Education, and Welfare (HEW) should promptly institute a program of independent second professional opinions to confirm the need for elective surgery underwritten by Medicare and Medicaid. The Subcommittee found that surgical payments by the fee-for-service mechanism encourages surgery in questionable situations. It recommends that a comprehensive study be undertaken to examine this situation in depth. The report determines that HEW has a totally inadequate data and information system and recommends that HEW remedy this situation promptly.

The report spells out concern that Professional Standards Review Organizations (PSRO's) are being developed too slowly and do not encourage a review of the entire gamut of health care. It recommends that this situation be corrected.

The report finds that the Secretary of HEW is not fulfilling his obligations under the mandatory provisions of the Social Security Act that call for establishing appropriate utilization control standards to protect consumers of health care. The report recommends that this situation be corrected forthwith.

Finally, the report indicates that unnecessary surgery has deleterious effects upon the American public. It estimates there were approximately 2.4 million unnecessary surgeries performed in 1974 at a cost to the American public of almost $4 billion, and it further estimates that these unnecessary surgeries led to 11,900 deaths last year.

UNNECESSARY SURGERY

I. Introduction

Public and private expenditures for health care are projected to reach $118.5 billion for 1975 as opposed to expenditures of $69.2 billion in 1970 and $42.1 billion in fiscal year 1966.

This explosive rise in medical care costs significantly impacts upon the Federal budget, since the Federal Government is the nation's largest purchaser of personal health services. Medicaid and Medicare—the two major programs underwritten by the Federal Government—are administered by the Department of Health, Education, and Welfare (HEW). HEW now estimates that expenditures for these two programs will climb from $25 billion in fiscal year 1976 to $30.4 billion in fiscal year 1977—a 20 percent increase. Since these programs have existed for over a decade without any significant review and since the costs of these programs far exceed original estimates, the Subcommittee on Oversight and Investigations has undertaken an in-depth study of the cost and quality aspects of these programs.

The Subcommittee has underway a major study to determine the gaps, loopholes, and inequities in the current health care delivery system and to examine in detail the cost and quality issues of health care in this country.

One area identified for in-depth examination is unnecessary surgery. The Subcommittee is trying to determine the volume and nature of unnecessary surgery within the health care delivery system and to what extent Medicare and Medicaid programs encourage over-utilization and unnecessary surgical procedures.

In 1972, Congress passed legislation (Pub. L. No. 92–603 § 207, 237, 86 Stat. 1379, 1415) calling for quality of care review for the health care rendered under Federal programs. These quality review programs are to set standards for treatment and utilization control to prevent unnecessary procedures.

Focusing specifically on Medicaid expenditures, the Subcommittee undertook to evaluate the role that HEW plays in implementation of the quality control programs required under the Social Security Act. The Subcommittee's hearings on unnecessary surgery were part of a broader study that will provide information on health insurance legislation.

These hearings marked the first time since the Committee on Interstate and Foreign Commerce acquired jurisdiction over portions of the Social Security Act that oversight hearings have been planned covering the health care delivery system. It is the intent of the Subcommittee, through hearings and staff investigations, to gather information that will assist the full Committee on Interstate and

Foreign Commerce, and the Subcommittee on Health and the Environment as they begin to consider national health insurance legislation.

II. Methodology

Information received from a variety of sources spurred the Subcommittee to investigate unnecessary surgery. First, a number of articles appeared in technical journals in the last few years indicating that many surgical operations performed in the United States need not have been performed.[1-7]

Second, the General Accounting Office (GAO) examined utilization review systems for all services provided by Medicaid. GAO concluded in a report published April 1975 that certain states had systems that were ineffective[8] and that the Social and Rehabilitation Service (SRS), the HEW arm which administers Medicaid,[9] was not vigorously enforcing the utilization review provisions of the Social Security Act.

A third impetus was the surgical community itself which had just completed its three-year "Study on Surgical Services for the United States" (SOSSUS) under the auspices of the American College of Surgeons and the American Surgical Association.[10] SOSSUS concluded that there were significant regional differences in the amount of surgery performed in the United States and identified six categories of surgical abuse.

A fourth source of information was the material gathered by Congressional committees with jurisdiction over health care programs, particularly reports by the House and Senate Appropriations Committees.[11] [12]

Finally, inquiries were made of HEW for additional information concerning surgical utilization. Requests for information and data were made to the Federal Medicaid officials, state Medicaid officials,

---

[1] J. P. Bunker, "Surgical Manpower, A Comparison of Operations and Surgeons in the United States, England, and Wales," *New England Journal of Medicine*, 285 : No. 3 (January 1970), 135–44.

[2] E. Vayda and G. D. Anderson, "Comparison of Provincial Surgical Rates in 1968," *The Canadian Journal of Surgery*, 18 (January 1975), 18–26.

[3] J. E. Wennberg and A. Gittleson, "Small Area Variations in Health Care Delivery. A Population-based Health Information System Can Guide Planning and Regulatory Decision-making," *Science*, 182 (1973), 1102–08.

[4] J. E. Wennberg and A. Gittleson, "Health Care Delivery in Maine, I: Patterns of Use of Common Surgical Procedures," *Journal of Maine Medical Association*, 66 (May 1975), 123–49.

[5] E. G. McCarthy and G. W. Widmer, "Effects of Screening by Consultants on Recommended Effective Surgical Procedures," *New England Journal of Medicine* (December 1974), 291–25, 1331–35.

[6] E. F. X. Hughes, E. M. Lewit, and E. H. Rand, "Operative Work Loads in One Hospital's General Surgical Residency Program," *New England Journal of Medicine*, 289 (September 18, 1973), 660–66.

[7] E. F. X. Hughes, E. M. Lewis, R. N. Watkins, and R. Handschin, "Utilization of Surgical Manpower in a Prepared Group Practice," *Surgery*, 77 (March 1975), 371–83.

[8] Report to the Subcommittee on Health, Committee on Finance, United States Senate, No. MWD–75–74, *Improvements Needed in Medicaid Program Management Including Investigations of Suspected Fraud and Abuse, Social and Rehabilitation Service, Department of Health, Education, and Welfare*, by the Comptroller General of the United States, at 44 (Apr. 14, 1975).

[9] The Medicaid program, authorized by Title XIX of the Social Security Act, as amended (42 U.S.C. § 1396 et seq.), is a grant-in-aid program under which the Federal Government pays part of the costs incurred by states in providing medical services to persons who are unable to pay for such care. The Federal Government pays from 50 to 81 percent (depending on the per capita income in the state) of the costs incurred by states in providing medical services under the Medicaid program.

[10] *Study of Surgical Services for the United States* (*SOSSUS*) (Draft mimeographed, publication forthcoming). Baltimore, Md. (July 1975).

[11] H.R. Rep. 93–1140, 93d Cong., 2d sess. (1974).

[12] S. Rep. No. 92–1230, 92d Cong., 2d sess., 217 (1972).

Federal regional HEW personnel, and Medicaid providers. There were also site visits and telephonic interviews.

Specific information regarding the number and types of surgical procedures performed in each state was requested from HEW. When the Department replied that the information was not available, the Subcommittee undertook its own survey. Fifty-three commissioners of state Medicaid programs were asked to furnish information for 1974 on the numbers of surgical procedures and the populations at risk for (1) all surgical procedures, (2) tonsillectomies, (3) hysterectomies, and (4) cholecystectomies.[13] Thirty states were able to furnish the data requested in a useable form....

Hearings were then held by the Subcommittee to supplement the information it had obtained. The hearings were designed to determine the magnitude of unnecessary surgery, the extent to which Government funding and regulations contribute to the volumes of unnecessary surgery performed, current efforts at quality control by HEW, and implications for a comprehensive national health insurance program. These hearings were held by the Subcommittee on July 15, 17, and 18, and September 3, 1975.

The Subcommittee sought information on the following issues, among others:

The effect that second consultations or pre-surgical screening programs can have in reducing the frequency of certain operations.

The correlation that exists between fee-for-service/individual practice/pre-paid group practice and surgical procedures.

Variability in performance of surgery by specific procedure nationally, regionally, and intrastate.

Whether surgeons are underemployed and whether there may be too many surgeons.

The need for surgical standards including possible certification, recertification, and restriction of hospital privileges or Government reimbursement to individuals who are board-certified.

The need to collect data on surgical procedures in order to obtain regional profiles, hospital profiles, and individual practitioner profiles for comparative purposes.

The extent to which the Department of Health, Education, and Welfare is implementing the quality control provisions of the Social Security Act.

III. Summary of Findings

A. SECOND CONSULTATIONS

Testimony by experts studying elective surgery indicates that second consultations can lower surgical abuse as well as concomitant costs. This applies to both voluntary and mandatory consultative programs.

B. SURGICAL PAYMENTS BY FEE-FOR-SERVICE VERSUS SALARIED ARRANGEMENTS

The fee-for-service payment mechanism absent adequate professional controls may encourage and provide financial incentives for

[13] Letter to the Commissioner of the Medicaid Program—Each State, from Honorable John E. Moss, Chairman, Oversight and Investigations Subcommittee, June 22, 1975.

surgeons to perform surgery in equivocal situations and may encourage the performance of more extensive procedures in questionable situations.

C. DATA NEEDS AND INFORMATION SYSTEMS

The Medical Services Administration (MSA) of HEW has failed to collect the most rudimentary information necessary to monitor significant portions of the Medicaid program and still does not require the states to furnish data on the volume or type of surgery performed.

D. SURGERY ON AN OUTPATIENT BASIS

The evidence suggests that up to one-fourth of surgical procedures now performed in hospitals might be performed without hospitalization. If up to 25 percent of surgical procedures can be performed with equal safety on an ambulatory basis, this would mean substantial savings for both consumers and taxpayers.

At least three factors contributing to this excess hospitalization include—

(1) Consumers receive little, if any, insurance reimbursement if the surgery is not done on an inpatient basis,

(2) Hospitals receive no compensation for unfilled beds and unused operating rooms, and

(3) Physician fee-for-service reimbursement discourages use of the ambulatory mode for minor surgical procedures.

E. SURGICAL MANPOWER

There appears to be a correlation between the volume of unnecessary surgery performed and the number of physicians performing surgery. In some geographic areas, the number of surgeons is excessive.

Many of the surgical procedures are being performed by non-certified specialists who have failed the certification examination and by general practitioners.

F. PROFESSIONAL STANDARDS REVIEW ORGANIZATIONS

Professional Standards Review Organizations (PSRO's) should be considered as an adjunct to but not as a replacement for second consultations before elective surgery. The PSRO machinery as currently constituted will not (1) routinely provide consumers with protection against unnecessary surgery, (2) encourage procedures to be done on an ambulatory basis, or (3) be established at a rapid enough pace to insure high-quality care to consumers in the near future.

G. MANDATORY NATURE OF THE LAW

Section 1903(g) of the Social Security Act requires the Secretary of Health, Education, and Welfare to monitor state methods and procedures to review utilization of care and services under Medicaid. It is unambiguous, mandatory, and self-executing, and the Secretary of HEW is legally bound to implement that section of the law. Proper implementation would save millions of taxpayer dollars through curtailment of unnecessary procedures.

H. HEW POLICY OF SLIPPAGE AND DELAYS

HEW has been obligated since September 30, 1973 to undertake validation surveys in order to establish that cost controls and quality procedures for Medicaid are in effect. The Secretary has been obligated since that time to make findings in order for states to receive incentive payments. The Secretary has failed to comply with these obligations.

I. MALADMINISTRATION

HEW, since July 1, 1973—

(1) designed and undertook a sample validation survey, commencing October 1973, which the Department later claimed to be invalid;

(2) undertook a second validation survey in the same fiscal year (commencing June 1974), although the HEW General Counsel claimed this was unnecessary;

(3) asked for a "plan of correction" from states but has not indicated the purpose of this "plan," nor has HEW undertaken adequate followup of the "plan" implementation; and

(4) has not yet undertaken fiscal year 1975 or 1976 validation surveys which are required to be conducted by HEW for states to receive full Medicaid funding.

J. METHODOLOGY

The methodology employed by HEW for the validation survey was developed without appropriate coordination between the Medicaid officers and the HEW General Counsel, a fact which has led to delays of two years and doubt about the validity of the surveys. The surveys emphasized patient records and gave inadequate attention to other aspects of the utilization control review that are required for compliance, such as single-state agency requirements and committee utilization review activities.

HEW procedures on reducing state payments unless quality provisions are met require clearance by the Office of the General Counsel. The workload in that office leads to inordinate delays in mandated requirements.

K. EXAMINATION OF REDUCTION PROVISIONS

A review of penalties, sanctions, and incentives by HEW, such as that announced in September 1975 by Secretary Mathews, is appropriate and important. However, failure to carry out the law during this period of review cannot be excused or justified.

L. COST ISSUES

There are significant costs associated with unnecessary surgery. The Subcommittee estimates that 2.38 million surgical procedures were unnecessarily performed in 1974 at a cost to the American public of $3.92 billion. . . .

Medicare support of unnecessary procedures is estimated to be $816 million, while Medicaid support is estimated to be $272 million. Medicaid also spent approximately $150 million for hospital procedures that could have been performed on an out-patient basis....

M. QUALITY ISSUES

It is estimated that unnecessary surgeries led to 11,900 deaths last year. Medicaid support was involved in an estimated 1700 deaths....

There were striking variations in surgical length of stay by region and wide variations in the rates of surgical removal by organs within small geographic areas studied.

At this time, PSRO's are not a viable substitute for mandated utilization review programs. The effect the present functioning PSRO's have had upon unnecessary surgery needs to be examined fully before they are accepted as a substitute for the mandatory requirements under utilization control.

Specific deficiencies in public accountability are widespread within HEW and include—

(1) a complete lack of information on the incidence, prevalence, and costs of surgery financed under Medicaid;

(2) a lack of coordination in the information requested of the states on financial and statistical matters; and

(3) a lack of timely requirements for state reporting. For example, at the beginning of fiscal year 1976, the most recent statistical report available by HEW was for fiscal year 1972.

Public accountability must be improved by HEW to avoid squandering taxpayer dollars.

IV. RECOMMENDATIONS

On the basis of the above findings, the Subcommittee makes the following recommendations:

A. With respect to second consultations—

(1) The Subcommittee recommends that HEW promptly mandate second professional opinions to confirm the need for elective or non-emergency surgery under Medicare and Medicaid.

(2) The Subcommittee recommends that such a program be carefully evaluated to determine the (a) impact upon quality of care, (b) containment of health care costs, (c) percentage of surgical procedures deemed to be unnecessary, and (d) cost of administering such a program compared with the cost of paying for unnecessary procedures.

B. With respect to salaried arrangements—

(1) The Subcommittee is impressed with the evidence presented that pre-payment plans for consumers and salaried surgeons help reduce surgery in equivocal situations. More evidence is needed, however, to determine the extent to which this result can be achieved nationally. The Subcommittee is also interested in determining what factors other than the payment and salary mechanisms help account for the differences in surgery in different areas,

e.g., scarcity of beds, population mix of the pre-paid plans, ratio of surgeons to population, etc.

The Subcommittee, therefore, recommends that HEW immediately undertake a comprehensive study to determine the differences in health indices, costs and the surgical procedure rates between salaried surgeons and fee-for-service surgeons.

(2) Further, the Subcommittee recommends that HEW utilize Section 402 (a) of the Social Security Amendments of 1967 to provide for demonstration projects concerning innovative arrangements for reimbursement to providers utilizing experimental arrangements to provide surgical services in a more cost-effective manner. These arrangements should be monitored carefully for cost containment and quality control.

(3) An annual report should be required of HEW concerning the comprehensive study cited above and the demonstration projects under Section 402 (a) to the following congressional committees:

Senate: Labor and Public Welfare, Finance, Government Operations, Appropriations, and Budget.

House of Representatives: Interstate and Foreign Commerce, Ways and Means, Government Operations, Appropriations, and Budget.

C. With respect to outpatient surgery—

The Subcommittee is impressed with evidence presented that up to 20 or 25 percent of surgical procedures can be performed without the need for hospitalization. More evidence is needed to determine what factors—such as types of surgical procedures or reimbursement mechanisms—retard outpatient surgery.

The Subcommittee will request that the Office of Technology Assessment (OTA) undertake a study projecting the available data on outpatient surgery to the population as a whole, project the savings, and evaluate the impact this increase in outpatient surgery would have on quality of care.

D. With respect to data and information needs—

The Subcommittee is convinced that the Medical Services Administration (MSA) needs to improve its data collection systems immediately. At a minimum, major topical categories, such as the extent of surgery and dollars spent for surgery, must be enumerated.

The Subcommittee recommends and will request promptly from the Secretary of HEW a suggested protocol for data collection that will include the above-listed items.

E. With respect to Surgical Manpower—

The Subcommittee recommends that Congress consider legislation that will require states to adopt uniform minimum standards, to be prescribed by HEW, for certification and recertification for physicians performing surgery.

F. With respect to Professional Standards Review Organizations—

(1) The Subcommittee believes that PSRO's have been implemented by HEW at a pace far slower than Congress intended. The Subcommittee recommends that HEW submit a revised timetable providing for implementation of PSRO's not later than

January 1, 1977 to the Congressional committees listed in paragraph B. (3) above.

(2) The Subcommittee recommends that the lack of emphasis by HEW in requiring PSRO's to develop quality control programs for non-hospital care be corrected immediately. HEW should require all designated PSRO's to submit a plan indicating their procedures for determining that care be provided in the most cost-effective manner—especially in cases when hospitalization is unnecessary.

G. With respect to administrative and legal issues—

(1) The Subcommittee recommends that the Secretary of HEW implement the utilization control requirements under Section 1903 of the Social Security Act *immediately*. Further delay shall be considered by the Subcommittee as an intentional failure to carry out the law by the Secretary.

(2) The Secretary of HEW has failed to make compliance findings under Section 1903(g) of the Social Security Act on a quarterly basis as required by law.

If this willful inaction of the Secretary continues uncorrected, the Subcommittee recommends that Congress review its own powers of enforcement to compel compliance with its statutory mandates and request that the GAO invoke sanctions available against the Department of Health, Education, and Welfare and the appropriate HEW officers under the Budget and Accounting Act of 1921 and the Accounting and Auditing Act of 1950.

(3) The Subcommittee recommends that Congress consider legislation that will provide effective remedies to prevent departmental and agency heads from acting in contravention of specific statutory provisions.

(4) The Subcommittee notes the lack of coordination among health services within HEW. It considers the current system of separate statistical units, different standards, multiple inspections, and overlapping auditing procedures an unnecessary, bureaucratic burden upon providers and a substantial waste of taxpayer dollars.

The Subcommittee, therefore, recommends the need for new legislation to coordinate the health service programs now scattered under the control of the Assistant Secretary for Health, the Administrator of the Social and Rehabilitation Service, and the Commissioner of the Social Security Administration.

(5) The Subcommittee recommends that HEW, wherever possible, take steps promptly to streamline portions of the overlapping bureaucratic process that can be remedied administratively.

(6) The Subcommittee further recommends the need for new legislation that will coordinate the Public Health Service (PHS), Medicaid, and Medicare health service programs under a new administrative framework.

H. With respect to cost and quality issues—

(1) The Subcommittee recommends that HEW take immediate steps to rectify the appalling lack of information on the incidence, prevalence, per capita utilization, resource supply rates, and costs

of surgery financed under Medicaid. It further recommends that the lack of coordination in information-gathering be rectified and that data collection be accelerated.

(2) The Subcommittee recommends that the excessively burdensome procedures for states be streamlined and made more relevant to program planning and operative needs. The Subcommittee recommends that new procedures be implemented by June 30, 1976 and that a draft of the new procedures be submitted to those Congressional committees cited in paragraph B(3) above.

V. The Current Situation

There has been a general lack of public discussion about "unnecessary surgery." However, there is clearly a growing professional and societal concern regarding the proper utilization of surgical services. Clear-cut and widely accepted standards distinguishing "necessary" from "unnecessary" surgery are not yet formulated. In this report, the Subcommittee will utilize the six categories of unnecessary surgery developed by Dr. George Zuidema and presented in testimony before the Subcommittee:

Category I. Completely discretionary operations for asymptomatic non-pathologic, non-threatening disorders;

Category II. Operations where no pathologic tissue is removed;

Category III. Operations where indications are a matter of difference in judgment and opinion among experts;

Category IV. Operations to alleviate endurable or tolerable symptoms;

Category V. Operations formerly performed in large numbers, now considered outdated, obsolete, or discredited;

Category VI. Operations done primarily for the personal gain of the surgeon, wherein the weight of informed opinion would deny any indication to the present.[14]

Most of the studies published to date focus upon utilization and length of stay differences. Such studies provide information on the volume and nature of surgery among different segments of the population.

Bunker and Wennberg summarize this situation well—

> The quality of surgical care remains unmeasured. We are not yet even certain how to define the quality of care, let alone how to measure it. But we do know that there are large quantitative differences in the surgical care received by different populations, and it is reasonable to assume, a priori, that there are also differences in quality.[15]

Statistical variation studies have the obvious disadvantage that individual cases cannot be studied in detail. However, more recent studies, such as those done by McCarthy and Widmer, begin to compile data that will allow for individual case studies.[16]

During the hearings, the Subcommittee heard first-hand accounts of consumer experiences with elective surgery.

---

[14] Statement of George D. Zuidema, M.D., Chief, Department of Surgery, Johns Hopkins University School of Medicine, *Hearings on Getting Ready for National Health Insurance: Unnecessary Surgery* before the Subcommittee on Interstate and Foreign Commerce, U.S. House of Representatives, 94th Congress, 1st session, at 33–4 (1975).

[15] J. P. Bunker and J. E. Wennberg, "Operations Rates, Mortality Statistics and the Quality of Life," *New England Journal of Medicine,* 289 (1973), 1249.

[16] Note 5 supra at 1331–35.

A. CONSUMER CASE STUDIES

Witnesses focused attention upon two elective procedures—hysterectomy and tonsillectomy.

In January of 1963, Mrs. Dorothy O'Grady of Lauderhill, Florida entered a Florida hospital for treatment of chronic backaches. At the hospital, her general practitioner performed a series of tests and called in a gynecologist as a consultant. At no time did Mrs. O'Grady have X-rays taken of her back, which was the site of her pain. The gynecologist recommended that Mrs. O'Grady undergo an operation that would put her presumably "misplaced" uterus back in the correct position and thereby relieve her back pain. After the operation, Mrs. O'Grady discovered that what had been planned as a simple corrective procedure ended with the removal of her uterus and one ovary.

Subsequently, Mrs. O'Grady suffered severe discomfort, complications, and added health expenses. At a malpractice trial, the court determined that the gynecologist had inadvertently injured her bladder during the operation. The bladder injury led to obstruction of her urinary tract, kidney infections, and the need for surgical repair of her bladder.

This iatrogenic bladder injury also led to financial difficulties. The insurance carrier for Mrs. O'Grady would not pay for any of the subsequent care, refusing payment on grounds that the health problem was a pre-existing condition.[17]

Subsequent to the hysterectomy, but during the period of medical complications, Mrs. O'Grady's backache persisted. Her lawyer recommended that she see an orthopedic specialist. This resulted in a diagnosis of a structural back deformity which causes her left leg to be approximately a quarter of an inch shorter than the right leg. Insertion of a heel lift in her left shoe alleviated her backache.

Another personal case study was presented by Mrs. Marie Valenzuela from Woodland, California, accompanied by her daughter, Linda. In the winter of 1969, Mrs. Valenzuela brought her youngest child, who had been running a high temperature, to a physician who informed her that the child would need a tonsillectomy.

On a return visit, following treatment of the daughter with penicillin, Mrs. Valenzuela brought her other three children, at the doctor's request, so that he could examine their previously healthy throats. The physician determined that all the children needed their tonsils removed. Mrs. Valenzuela had brought along a young niece who had been experiencing nosebleeds on occasion. After a brief examination, the physician indicated that this child would need her tonsils removed as well.

The surgeries began, and one of Mrs. Valenzuela's children experienced brief respiratory difficulty but had no serious complications. Linda Valenzuela did not fare as well. Six days after being discharged from the hospital, she began bleeding profusely from the neck and required three different surgical procedures. The operations left Linda with half the normal cerebral blood circulation. She was very near death from the bleeding, developed pneumonia, required a tracheot-

---

[17] Statement of Dorothy O'Grady, Lauderhill, Fla., *Hearings on Getting Ready for National Health Insurance: Unnecessary Surgery* before the Subcommittee on Oversight and Investigations of the Committee on Interstate and Foreign Commerce, U.S. House of Representatives, 94th Congress, 1st session, at 2 (1975).

omy, and subsequently became anemic and contracted hepatitis.[18] The loss of carotid circulation on one side increases the likelihood that sometime in the future Linda might experience brain damage.[19] Laboratory tests determined that the operating physician had removed healthy tissue from each of the five children.[20]

B. HYSTERECTOMIES AND TONSILLECTOMIES

The Subcommittee heard testimony from experts and examined various studies in an attempt to determine the extent to which these case studies are illustrative of the experience of the general population undergoing elective surgery. Testimony was presented concerning a study of employees of the American Federation of States County Municipal Employees (AFSCME) Health Security Plan of District Council 37 (New York City). This plan allows for second consultations before elective surgery.

Mrs. Mary Barber, a member of the New York City plan, described her experiences under the plan. Mrs. Barber had been told by a physician that she needed a hysterectomy because of profuse bleeding and occasional pain during menses. Mrs. Barber took advantage of the Health Security Plan's consultation services, saw a second physician, and was offered alternatives to a hysterectomy. As a result, Mrs. Barber did not have the surgery[21] and became one of 594 cases where hospitalization was prevented.[22]

Statistics were presented by Dr. Eugene McCarthy, Professor of Public Health, Cornell Univerity Medical College, New York City, that he had developed from case histories of union employees in New York who had received an original opinion to operate and a second opinion arranged through the plan. The voluntary program permitted a consumer to request a second consultation. The mandatory program requires a second opinion prior to hospital admission for elective surgery.[23]

Forty-six percent of the recommendations for hysterectomies were not confirmed under the voluntary program; 26 percent were not confirmed under the mandatory program.[24]

Tonsillectomies as a routine surgical procedure have become highly questionable. Dr. Zuidema testified that tonsillectomies should be included in the category of "operations where indications are a matter of difference in judgment and opinion amongst experts." [25]

[18] Statement of Marie Valenzuela, Woodland, Calif., *Hearings on Getting Ready for National Health Insurance: Unnecessary Surgery* before the Subcommittee on Oversight and Investigations of the Committee on Interstate and Foreign Commerce, U.S. House of Representatives, 94th Congress, 1st session, at 12 (1975).

[19] *Id.* at 13.

[20] *Id.*

[21] Testimony of Mary Barber, Manhattan, N.Y., *Hearings on Getting Ready for National Health Insurance: Unnecessary Surgery* before the Subcommittee on Oversight and Investigations of the Committee on Interstate and Foreign Commerce, U.S. House of Representatives, 94th Congress, 1st Session, at 12 (1975).

[22] Statement of Eugene G. McCarthy, M.D., M.P.H., Professor of Public Health, Cornell University Medical College, New York City, *Hearings on Getting Ready for National Health Insurance: Unnecessary Surgery* before the Subcommittee on Oversight and Investigations of the Committee on Interstate and Foreign Commerce, U.S. House of Representatives, 94th Congress, 1st session, "Table 1.—Participation in Elective Presurgical Screening Program, February 1972 through December 1974," at 110 (1975).

[23] *Id.* at 108–109.

[24] Id., "Table 3.—Percent Not Confirmed for Elective Surgery According to Most Frequently Screened Procedures," at 110.

[25] Note 14 *supra* at 33.

Dr. Zuidema further testified that—

> . . . Some segments of informed otolaryngological opinion would hold that a number of tonsillectomies could be avoided with little hazard to the child or the young adult, many of which are performed by non-certified Otolaryngologists.[26]

National data substantiates a major shift in the rates of tonsillectomies. In 1965, the rate per 100,000 population was 635.9 in the United States.[27] In 1973, the rate per 100,000 population was 400.9, a drop of 23 out of every 100 people.[28] The data also point out wide variations. John E. Wennberg, Physician, Waterbury Center, Vermont, documented in his Vermont study that "for the tonsil, the probability of removal by age 26 ranges from 8 percent to 62 percent across 13 Vermont areas." [29]

George S. Perrott reported in 1966 that data for 1961–62 showed a tonsillectomy rate for the Government-wide Blue Shield plan over 2.5 times that of the group practice plans.[30]

The Federal Employees Health Benefit Program Utilization Study, published in January 1975, included tonsillectomy data for 1970. It found that the probability of tonsillectomy varied from 41.3 percent for Blue Cross subscribers to 10.5 percent for prepaid group subscribers.[31]

These case studies and variations in elective surgery raised questions about the broader health issues.

VI. Specific Health Issues

The Subcommittee feels, as a result of its investigation, that health issues need to be examined in detail. These are (A) second consultations, (B) surgical payment mechanisms, (C) data needs and information systems, (D) outpatient surgery, (E) surgical manpower, and (F) Professional Standards Review Organizations.

A. Second Consultations

The concept of providing a second consultation to a consumer before elective surgery was discussed by a number of witnesses. Dr. George Zuidema, Chief, Department of Surgery, Johns Hopkins School of Medicine, served as a coordinator of the Study on Surgical Services for the United States (SOSSUS), undertaken by the American College of Surgeons and the American Surgical Association.[32] Dr. Zuidema stated before the Subcommittee that a program of presurgical screening has as its objective the curtailing of diagnostic and unnecessary admissions.[33] Dr. Zuidema testified that this program in the State of Maryland provided evidence that the frequency of certain operations could be markedly reduced.[34] Zuidema stated that—

---

[26] *Id.*

[27] Hospital Discharge Survey Data, National Center for Health Statistics, Public Health Service, HEW, Washington, D.C. (1973 data) (May 1975).

[28] *Id.*

[29] J. E. Wennberg, M.D., Waterbury Center, Vt., *Hearings on Getting Ready for National Health Insurance: Unnecessary Surgery* before the Subcommittee on Oversight and Investigations of the Committee on Interstate and Foreign Commerce, U.S. House of Representatives, 94th Congress, 1st sess. at 76 (1975).

[30] G. S. Perrott, "Utilization of Hospital Services," *American Journal of Public Health*, 56 (1966), 62.

[31] Federal Employees Health Benefit Program Utilization Study, Public Health Service, HEW, Washington, D.C. (January 1975).

[32] Note 10 *supra.*

[33] Note 14, *supra* at 32.

[34] *Id.* at 34.

> . . . MARP [Maryland Admission Review Program] has resulted in a saving of 2.5 to 3.0 million dollars and it is estimated that this is a saving of 1 to 2% in actual dollars, over and above the cost of the Program's administration, for the 1974/75 year.[35]

Dr. Zuidema testified that the SOSSUS study, as previously mentioned, identified six categories of unnecessary surgery.[36] He tied the relationship of unnecessary surgery to second consultations by concluding, "In all of the . . . six categories any tendency to surgical abuse is reduced by frequent consultation." [37]

Dr. Sidney Wolfe, Director of the Public Citizens Health Research Group, strongly urged inclusion of second consultations as a nationally-accepted requirement. He recommended that a program of second consultations be handled by independent practitioners and be mandatory for Medicare and Medicaid.[38]

Dr. Eugene McCarthy presented data from union programs in New York City which called for second consultations and in which all surgical consultants were board-certified specialists. He said he would "strongly endorse the idea that second opinion programs be a part of Medicare and Medicaid." [39] Dr. McCarthy added that when he queried the American College of Surgeons concerning consultations, a poll of their members indicated that approximately 75 percent of the board-certified surgeons endorsed second opinions.[40]

On December 3, 1975, Blue Cross and Blue Shield of Greater New York instituted a program of second professional opinions to confirm the need for non-emergency surgery.[41] In announcing this program, the plan declared—

> . . . Studies have indicated that when an independent second professional opinion was obtained regarding elective surgery, a significant proportion of proposed surgical procedures were considered to be unnecessary.[42]

B. SURGICAL PAYMENT MECHANISMS

Several expert witnesses at the hearings stated that the reimbursement method for surgeons was an important factor in unnecessary surgery.

Dr. William M. Stahl, Professor of Surgery at New York University School of Medicine, who has worked as a solo fee-for-service surgeon, as a member of a group practice on a fee-for-service basis, and as a member of a group practice on a prepaid patient basis, provided insight into the psychological differences between these type of practice:

> My own experience in the solo fee-for-service practice is that there is this pressure on the solo fee-for-service surgeon. The practice in a group lessens the

[35] Letter from George D. Zuidema, M.D., to Elliot Segal, Special Assistant, Subcommittee on Oversight and Investigations of the Committee on Interstate and Foreign Commerce, U.S. House of Representatives, July 21, 1975, received for the hearing record, at 55.

[36] Note 14 *supra*.

[37] *Id.* at 34.

[38] Statement of Sidney Wolfe, M.D., Director, Public Citizens Health Research Group, Washington, D.C., *Hearings on Getting Ready for National Health Insurance: Unnecessary Surgery* before the Subcommittee on Oversight and Investigations of the Committee on Interstate and Foreign Commerce, U.S. House of Representatives, 94th Congress, 1st sess. at 60 (1975).

[39] Note 22, *supra* at 113.

[40] *Id.* at 114.

[41] News Release, Blue Cross and Blue Shield of Greater New York, N.Y. (Dec. 3. 1975).

[42] *Id.*

pressure somewhat but the only way that you can practice without the economic pressure is in a prepaid group practice system.

* * * * * * *

. . . there are many instances where the question of proper treatment is not absolutely clear cut. . . . It is a condition like hernia, varicose veins, small fibroid, many of these back problems, pain, where the patient could be treated medically or could be treated surgically and there is very little hard evidence to indicate that he is better off significantly one way or the other.

I think that under fee-for-service . . . there isn't any question in my mind but there is an intense pressure to choose the surgical method rather than the nonsurgical method . . .[43]

Dr. Stahl indicated that in a prepaid salary system, he felt much freer to look at the question objectively: " . . . there are many . . . patients on whom I did not operate that I am sure I would have operated on in previous years under the other system."[44]

Another surgeon who testified on this subject was Dr. Edward F. X. Hughes, an Assistant Professor at Mt. Sinai School of Medicine and Research Associate at the National Bureau of Economic Research in New York City. He has published studies comparing practices in a prepaid setting and the workloads of a population of 19 general surgeons in suburban practices in the New York metropolitan area.[45–49] Dr. Hughes testified, ". . . insofar as a surgeon derives his income from performing surgery, . . . the pressure is on him in an equivocal situation to maintain his income by operating on patients."[50]

Dr. George Crile, Jr., Emeritus Consultant in General Surgery at the Cleveland Clinic, also described the issues relating to fee for service:

I think in surgery we have a prime example of conflict of interest in that if a patient comes to you with a symptom or sign of some disease and it can be treated surgically or it could be treated not surgically, and the surgeon benefits by the fee, $200, $500, whatever it may be, if he decides for that, and he gets only a consultation fee, $20 perhaps, if he decides against it so immediately a conflict of interest comes up.[51]

As the remedy, Dr. Crile proposed hospital-based surgery:

If the surgeons were employed by the hospitals, you immediately have your hospital acting as a group, you have a surgical group there and they would not tolerate one of their group, which they are responsible for, performing a type of surgery which they did not approve of.

* * * * * * *

---

[43] Statement of William M. Stahl, M.D., Professor of Surgery at New York University School of Medicine, *Hearings on Getting Ready for National Health Insurance: Unnecessary Surgery* before the Subcommittee on Oversight and Investigations of the Committee on Interstate and Foreign Commerce, U.S. House of Representatives, 94th Congress, 1st session, at 91, 100–01 (1975).

[44] *Id.* at 101.

[45] E. F. X. Hughes, V. R. Fuchs, J. E. Jacoby, and E. M. Lewit, "Surgical Work Loads in a Community Practice," *Surgery,* 71 (March 1972), 315–327.

[46] Note 6 *supra.*

[47] Note 7 *supra.*

[48] E. F. X. Hughes, E. M. Lewit, and F. V. Lorenzo, "Time Utilization of a Population of General Surgeons in Community Practice," *Surgery,* 77 (March 1975), 371–83.

[49] Statement of Edward F. X. Hughes, M.D., M.P.H., Assistant Professor, Department of Community Medicine, Mount Sinai School of Medicine, and Research Associate, National Bureau of Economic Research, New York City, *Hearings on Getting Ready for National Health Insurance: Unnecessary Surgery* before the Subcommittee on Oversight and Investigations of the Committee on Interstate and Foreign Commerce, U.S. House of Representatives, 94th Congress, 1st session, at 184 (1975).

[50] *Id.* at 188.

[51] Testimony of Dr. George Crile, Jr., M.D., Emeritus Consultant, Department of General Surgery, Cleveland Clinic, Cleveland, Ohio, *Hearings on Getting Ready for National Health Insurance: Unnecessary Surgery* before the Subcommittee on Oversight and Investigations of the Committee on Interstate and Foreign Commerce, U.S. House of Representatives, 94th Congress, 1st session, at 191 (1975).

. . . I think the time has come in our country where surgery should be hospital based. It has to be hospital based. You can't operate except in a hospital, so why shouldn't they be salaried from the hospital? [52]

In describing prepaid plans, Dr. Zuidema added a cautionary note. He observed that some operations that should be carried out are occasionally omitted for economic reasons. This might be called, he said, the "converse of 'unnecessary operations' and might be called the 'unjustified withholding of surgical care'." [53]

An HEW study by Gaus, Cooper, and Hirschman studied Health Maintenance Organizations (HMO's and fee-for-service performance.[54] It found that "hospital use in group practice plans was significantly lower, 2½ times, than in the fee-for-service system." [55] This research data was collected during fiscal 1975 on over 8,000 Medicaid families.

Surgical rates revealed similar patterns. There were half as many surgeries performed for group practice plans, where surgeons are salaried, than for those control groups where surgeons were remunerated on a fee-for-service basis. The HMO group practices had 12 admissions per 1,000 persons for surgery, while the corresponding control groups where surgeons were on a fee-for-service basis had 25 admissions per 1,000.[56] This evidence suggests that salary arrangements for surgeons are important in controlling surgical procedures.

C. DATA NEEDS AND INFORMATION SYSTEMS

Dr. Wennberg recommended development of data-gathering systems in order to inform surgeons about the differences in rate of specific procedures among defined populations.[57] For example, in the State of Vermont, there was a range of probability of removal of tonsils by age 26 from 8 percent to 62 percent, depending on what part of the state one lived in.[58]

Dr. Wennberg testified that here should be thorough exploration of the possible uses of small-area data, particularly as an instrument of feedback to the professionals:

. . . In cases where variations cannot be attributed reasonably to differences in access or illness of the population, they should be interpreted as an indicator of the range of differences in professional opinion about using specific technologies.[59]

Regional differences in length of stay for Medicare patients were not just confined to surgery but appeared for all diagnoses.[60] HEW presentation of Medicare data indicated that there were often 50 percent more length-of-stay days in the Northeastern portion of the country as in the West. For example, the mean length of stay for patients supported by Medicare is 15.0 days in the Northeast and 10.0 days in the West.[61]

---

[52] *Id.* at 192, 193.
[53] Note 14 *supra* at 34.
[54] C. R. Gaus, B. S. Cooper, G. C. Hirschman, *Contrasts in HMO and Fee-for-Service Performance,* Office of Research and Statistics, SSA, HEW, Washington, D.C. (mimeographed Dec. 30, 1975).
[55] *Id.* at 11.
[56] *Id.*, Table 4.
[57] Note 29 *supra* at 77.
[58] *Id.* at 83.
[59] *Id.* at 77.
[60] Marian Gornick, "Medicare Patients: Regional Differences in Length of Hospital Stays, 1969–71," *Social Security Bulletin* (July 1975), at 16, 26.
[61] *Id.* at 17.

The Medicare program collects data that can help describe the dimensions of a service such as surgery. HEW's Office of Research and Statistics (ORS), within the Social Security Administration, revealed that $4.7 billion was spent in 1974 by Medicare for surgical cases.[62] An HEW study done by Marian Gornick presented information that regions vary considerably in surgical rates. Surgical procedures accounted for 34–36 percent of discharges in the Northeast and 25–27 percent in the South.[63]

While the HEW Medicare administrators were able to supply the Subcommittee with relevant data, the Medicaid administrators were not. Neither the Medical Services Administration (MSA) nor the National Center for Social Statistics (NCSS) gathered or compiled sufficient data to allow for comparisons or analysis of utilization of surgical procedures paid for by the Medicaid program.

To obtain the information necessary to do such an analysis, the Subcommittee queried the 53 individual state Medicaid program administrators on the numbers of surgical procedures and the population at risk (see Appendix A). The data indicated that the Medicaid rate of surgical procedures was more than two times the rate for the rest of the population. The higher proportion of surgery among the Medicaid population than the population as a whole strongly suggests that there is also a significantly higher rate of unnecessary surgery among the Medicaid population (see Appendix A). It should be noted that there was unevenness in the States' responses. The determination by some states of eligible population at risk seems to be at variance with other data collected by HEW. While this determination of eligibles by some states casts doubts about the validity of their population base, it underscores the need for better recordkeeping.

D. OUTPATIENT SURGERY

Testimony was presented that a significant number of surgical procedures could be done on an outpatient basis. This could lead to substantial cost savings to the Government.

In comparing a prepaid salaried situation and general-practice fee-for-service surgeons, Dr. Hughes found that—

> Perhaps the most substantial economy in the utilization of surgical resources in the prepaid group practice was the fact that almost one in every four general surgical operations was performed on an ambulatory basis.[64]

The ambulatory modality was used much less frequently for surgery in the fee-for-service community.[65]

Dr. Hughes concluded, "The prepaid reimbursement mechanism would seem to foster ambulatory surgery as it results in cost savings to the prepaid plan and to the consumer."[66] A systematic problem exists, he said:

> . . . In fee-for-service settings . . . hospitals can receive no compensation for unfilled beds and unused operating rooms, and patients may receive little, if any,

[62] Insert 1, Estimated Medicare Benefit Expenditures for Surgery-related Services, Calendar Year 1974," Office of Research and Statistics, Social Security Administration, July 14, 1975, prsented at *Hearings on Getting Ready for National Health Insurance: Unnecessary Surgery* before the Subcommittee on Oversight and Investigations of the Committee on Interstate and Foreign Commerce, U.S. House of Representatives, 94th Congress, 1st session, at 203 (1975).

[63] Note 57 *supra* at 19.

[64] Note 49 *supra* at 185.

[65] *Id.*

[66] *Id.* at 185–6.

insurance reimbursement for elective surgical work performed in a doctor's office. The pressures from both directions may work toward the hospitalization of patients for minor surgical problems.[67]

Hughes testified that—

> The amount of money a surgeon gains from ambulatory care in his office is far less than that gained from operative fees. The pressure is thus terrific on surgeons with low operative workloads. The fee-for-service system contributes to this pressure.[68]

Based on this complexity, Dr. Hughes concludes that 20 to 24 percent of the surgical procedures now being done in hospitals could be done on an out-patient basis and that major cost savings could be realized if such incentives could be broadly developed.[69]

One ambulatory surgical program that incorporates incentives is the Surgicenter in Phoenix, Arizona, described by Dr. Hughes as a "path-breaking development in the delivery of American medical care."[70] A recent article describes the Center as follows:

> When Surgicenter opened in 1970, charging an average of $70 for an operation ($120 average now), four hospitals in the Phoenix area lowered out-patient surgery fees 30 to 50 percent. The center then charged $95 for a D and C (with an additional $10 charge made by the pathologist for laboratory fees). The usual charge for the same operation, with a two-day stay in a Phoenix hospital, was about $300 at that time. (Surgicenter has recently raised its fees, and a D and C now costs $121.)
>
> The center has had an impact not only on the cost of ambulatory surgical care in Phoenix but also on the way such care is delivered. It is forcing hospital administrators to take a closer look at the high cost of their inpatient ambulatory surgery. If it is assumed that at least 75 percent of Surgicenter's patients would have been hospitalized for two days if the facility had not been available, then it follows that Surgicenter allowed Phoenix to use 34,500 fewer hospital days, from February, 1970, to September, 1974.[71]

E. SURGICAL MANPOWER

Several experts raised the issue of surgical manpower as an important component of unnecessary surgery.

Dr. Zuidema indicated that the SOSSUS area studies included research into who was performing surgery and the professional credentials of operating surgeons. Tonsillectomies were performed in most instances by non-certified surgeons or non-surgical specialists, the study concluded.[72]

Dr. Zuidema testified that 40 percent of operations performed in this country were performed by non-certified individuals who come from two groups—

(1) non-certified specialists (two thirds of whom have taken their certification examinations and failed them); and

(2) general practitioners.

When Zuidema was asked about limiting reimbursements only to certified surgeons, he expressed the opinion that this would be ill-advised at this time. Instead, he suggested establishing hospital accrediting standards regulating residency numbers and limiting surgery to current, competent surgeons and those surgeons who pass an educa-

---

[67] *Id.* at 186.
[68] *Id.* at 188.
[69] *Id.* at 189.
[70] *Id.*
[71] Felicia A. Holton, "What Future Now for Surgical Centers," *Prism* (March 1975), 52.
[72] Note 14 *supra* at 35.

tional and certification process over the next five to seven years.[73] Congressman Andrew Maguire (D–N.J.) suggested certification and recertification every five or ten years.[74] The issue, he said, was one of competence and judgment, and the certification process may well be the tool necessary to protect the public.

Some surgeons may be underworked, according to Dr. Hughes. His published studies measuring surgical workloads of surgeons in the Greater New York area indicated that the average workload of these surgeons was approximately 43 percent of the postulated full workload and the median was approximately one-third of the postulated workload.[75] These findings, he said, suggest inefficient use of surgical skills in this community, leading to pressure to increase workloads by operating in equivocal situations. Again, the result is higher-than-necessary costs for health care borne by consumers and the Government.[76]

Currently, 22 percent of all residency physician slots in this country are for surgical specialties when well organized health care systems indicate that only 10 percent of the trainees should be in these specialties, said Dr. Stahl. He concluded that we are training twice as many surgeons as we need.[77]

One of the causes of variations of surgical procedures in his area study was the supply of physicians in that area, Dr. Wennberg found. He said that this factor appeared—

> more important than consumer behavior in determining the relative rates of use of medical care among neighboring geographic areas. Studies in Kansas, Vermont, and across Canadian Provinces show that overall supply of surgeons and hospital beds strongly affect the incidence rates of surgery. In Vermont we see that areas with more surgeons have greater rates of surgery . . .[78]

F. PROFESSIONAL STANDARDS REVIEW ORGANIZATIONS

HEW testified that Professional Standards Review Organizations (PSRO's) are the vehicles which can and will affect the utilization of health services such as surgery in this country.[79]

Robert Van Hoek, M.D., Acting Administrator, Health Services Administration, HEW, said that a PSRO program sets "criteria" for surgical procedures.[80]

In a letter to seven Subcommittee Congressmen, Dr. Theodore Cooper, Assistant Secretary for Health, HEW, presented HEW's current position that PSRO's can take the place of a second consultation program. Nevertheless, Cooper acknowledged that—

> unnecessary procedures, including elective surgical procedures, is detrimental to the provision of high quality care, and promotes the inefficient utilization of health care facilities and resources.[81] . . .

---

[73] *Id.* at 59.
[74] Question by Honorable Andrew Maguire (D., N.J.) *Hearings on Getting Ready for National Health Insurance: Unnecessary Surgery* before the Subcommittee on Oversight and Investigations of the Committee on Interstate and Foreign Commerce, U.S. House of Representatives, 94th Congress, 1st session, at 58 (1975).
[75] Note 49 *supra* at 184.
[76] *Id.*
[77] Note 43 *supra* at 91–2.
[78] Note 29 *supra* at 76.
[79] Statement of Robert Van Hoek, M.D., Acting Administrator Health Services Administration, Department of Health Education, and Welfare, et al., *Hearings on Getting Ready for National Health Insurance: Unnecessary Surgery* before the Subcommittee on Oversight and Investigations of the Committee on Interstate and Foreign Commerce, U.S. House of Representatives, 94th Congress, 1st session, at 259 (1975).
[80] *Id.* [81] *Id.* at 196.

Dr. Van Hoek testified—

> The purpose of the PSRO program is to assure that there is full and adequate review by physicians of the performance of their peers. This performance is measured prospectively as well as retrospectively by the use of professionally established criteria and standards of medical practice. As part of implementation of the program, we have supported the development of area-wide criteria and standards, based upon accepted practice patterns, and these criteria and standards are in the process of being disseminated to the professional organizations, to hospitals, to PSRO's and to our committees in order that they may carry out their responsibilities.
>
> . . . the hospital review system includes three integrated components: Concurrent review, medical care evaluation, and profile anaysis. Hospitals and long-term care facilities are required to use criteria standards that review the appropriateness of all admissions under the medicare, medicaid, maternal and child health and crippled children's programs. If there is a decision [that] the admission was not appropriate, there will be no reimbursement for that care. This includes admissions for postsurgical procedures either on an emergency or elective basis.[82]

HEW's position on unnecessary surgery appears to concentrate upon the hospital review system and raises three significant issues. These relate to (1) public protection, (2) ambulatory reviews, and (3) time slippage.

(1) Public protection

PSRO's are designated to review for payment purposes the medical necessity, appropriateness, and quality of institutional care. HEW has chosen to focus on hospital reviews. This would lead a hospital utilization review committee to focus on the care and services provided to the patient while in the hospital—an emphasis which does little to protect the consumer-patient. There is little solace after undergoing an unnecessary surgery to learn that reimbursement for that procedure was denied to the physician, especially if that physician turns around and bills the patient. This situation is probably exacerbated because HEW has indicated that "medical care evaluations are short-term *retrospective* studies . . . [Emphasis added.][83] This leads to unnecessary procedures being discovered after the fact and does not protect the consumer before the unnecessary procedure takes place.

(2) Ambulatory reviews

Dr. Van Hoek testified that—"The legislation authorized but did not require the review of ambulatory care by PSROs . . .",[84] but Section 1155(a)(1)(C) of the Social Security Act, in describing duties and functions of PSRO's, states—

> In case such services and items are proposed to be provided in a hospital or other health care facility on an inpatient basis, such services, and items could, consistent with the provision of appropriate medical care, be effectively provided on an outpatient basis or more economically in an inpatient health care facility of a different type.[85]

Moreover, Section 1155(a)(2) states—

> Each professional standards review organization shall have the authority to determine, in advance, in the case of—
>
> (A) any elective admission to a hospital or other health care facility, or
>
> (B) any other health care service which will consist of extended or costly courses of treatment,

[82] *Id.* at 196, 197.
[83] *Id.* at 200.
[84] *Id.* at 199.
[85] 42 U.S.C. § 1320c-4(a)(1)(C).

whether such service, if provided, or if provided by a particular health care practitioner or by a particular hospital or other health care facility, organization, or agency, would meet the criteria specified in clauses (A) and (C) of paragraph (1).[86]

Several experts could be done on an ambulatory basis with significant cost savings. Hughes, for example, said—

> . . . I think there are incentives in prepaid group practice plans for a surgeon to utilize the ambulatory modality for surgical care. Major cost savings could be realized if such incentives could be broadly developed within the American health system. This would especially appear to be true in view of the large number of operations less complex than an inguinal herniorrhaphy we found being performed on an inpatient basis in our community study.[87]

Hughes testified that the complexity of elective surgical procedures would allow for 20 to 24 percent of these procedures to be done on an ambulatory basis without detriment to the patient and with increased savings to consumers.[88]

Since PSRO's are focusing upon inpatient admissions, there is little evidence to suggest that PSRO reviews will provide the incentives needed to perform surgery on an ambulatory basis.

(3) Time slippage

Congress intended the Medicaid utilization control program to be operative on July 1, 1973. Regarding Section 207 of the Social Security Amendments of 1972, the report of the Committee on Finance declared—

> The Committee is concerned over the fact that there exists in many areas of the country a substantial degree of unnecessary and avoidable utilization of costly institutional care under Medicaid, accompanied by insufficient usage of less costly alternative out-of-institution health care. This has been repeatedly demonstrated by investigations of the General Accounting Office, in HEW audit agency reports, and in other testimony.[89]

The report further states that while Federal dollars should be used to match state Medicaid dollars for the coverage of necessary institutional services under Title XIX, those Federal dollars should not be used to pay for unnecessary or inappropriate institutional services.[90]

In explaining Section 249F. of the Social Security Amendments of 1972 that established professional standards review, the Committee on Finance report declared—

> Witnesses testified that a significant proportion of the health services provided under Medicare and Medicaid are probably not medically necessary. In view of the per diem costs of hospital and nursing facility care and costs of medical and surgical procedures, the economic impact of this overutilization becomes extremely significant. Aside from the economic impact, the Committee is most concerned about the effect of overutilization on the health of the aged and the poor. Unnecessary hospitalization and *unnecessary surgery* are not consistent with proper health care. [Emphasis added] [91]

Congress intended the Medicaid utilization control program to be operative on July 1, 1973.[92] HEW was required to tentatively designate PSRO areas (but not the functional agencies) throughout the country by January 1, 1974.[93] Since it would not be possible for

---

[86] 42 U.S.C. § 1320c–4(a)(2).
[87] Note 49 *supra* at 189.
[88] *Id.*
[89] S. Rep. No. 92–1230, 92d Cong., 2d sess., 217 (1972).
[90] *Id.*
[91] *Id.* at 254.
[92] *Id.* at 219.
[93] *Id.* at 258.

PSRO's to be in place before the implementation of the Medicaid utilization control program, it is obvious that Congress intended functional utilization control programs to be operating under Medicaid, beginning July 1, 1973, and that these programs would subsequently be transferred to PSRO's when such entities became operative.

These time delays by HEW were a major subject of House Report 93–1140, issued June 24, 1974, by Chairman Daniel Flood (D-Pa.) of the Subcommittee on Labor, Health, Education, and Welfare of the House Committee on Appropriations. That committee report declared—

> The committee received information as late as May 28 to the effect that none of the 1974 funds available for PSRO contracts had been obligated as of that date. It appears to the committee that there is considerable slippage in the program and thus the 1975 budget request for PSRO programs was reduced by $7,000,000 from the requested level of $57,900,000.[94]

In view of the long delay in developing PSRO's the rapid implementation of faithful execution of utilization control under the Medicaid program becomes even more important.

VII. Administrative and Legal Issues

Utilization control is the system used to determine the appropriateness of medical care provided and to prevent excessive use of medical services, including surgery. Utilization control has two basic purposes: (1) to insure that consumers receive high-quality medical care, and (2) to control program costs by preventing unnecessary use. These two programmatic issues will be dealt with in greater detail in Section VIII.

Section 1902 (a) (30) of the Social Security Act requires states to have methods and procedures to review the utilization of care and services provided under the state Medicaid plan.[95] The regulations require state-wide surveillance and utilization control systems to safeguard against unnecessary or inappropriate utilization of the care and services provided. The regulations also require that there be a basis for assessing the quality of these services.

The Social Security Amendments of 1972 were passed by Congress on October 30, 1972. Among these amendments was Section 207 which calls for the provision of "Incentives for States to Establish Effective Utilization Review Procedures Under Medicaid.[96] This section stipulates that as of July 1, 1975, states must have institutional utilization review systems which provide that—

> (1) the physician certify at the time of admission that the patient requires inpatient, institutional services;
>
> (2) the physician recertify every sixty days that the patient continues to require inpatient, institutional services;
>
> (3) medical and professional personnel not directly responsible for the care of the patient and not employed by or financially interested in any similar institution conduct authorization review of the necessity for admission and the continued stay of each patient;

---

[94] H.R. Rep. No. 93–1140, 93rd Cong., 2d sess. (1974).
[95] 42 U.S.C. § 1392(a)(30).
[96] Public Law 92–603, § 207, 86 Stat. 1379.

(4) the medical review of the care of patients in mental hospitals, skilled nursing homes, and intermediate care facilities is reviewed and evaluated at least annually by independent, professional review teams; and

(5) a utilization review in hospitals and skilled nursing homes meet the requirements of the Medicare system unless the Secretary of HEW waives this requirement because the state has a utilization review system better than Medicare's system.[97]

The law further provides that if these requirements are not met, HEW is to reduce Federal payments to states by one-third for the cost of institutional care provided to individuals for more than 60 days during a fiscal year (90 days in a mental hospital). This reduction must be made unless the state makes a satisfactory showing to the Secretary of HEW that the state has, in fact, an effective system in operation (see Section 207 at Appendix C).

A. CONGRESSIONAL INTENT

The need for this law and the purpose for its enactment is contained in the report by the Senate Committee on Finance in considering H.R. 1 (Senate Report 92–1230). It states:

> . . . Both the General Accounting Office and the HEW audit agency have found substantial unnecessary and overutilization of costly institutional care under medicaid accompanied by insufficient usage of less costly alternative out-of-institution health care. There is no provision in present law which places affirmative responsibility upon states to assure proper patient placement.[98]

The purpose of this law is unambiguous—to prevent unnecessary institutional stays and services and to provide quality medical care under Medicaid. A second purpose is to control program costs by preventing unnecessary use.

However, implementation of this law by HEW has been inconsistent with purposes of the law. The extent of this maladministration became clear during the hearings and may be summarized as follows:

(1) Mandatory nature of law

One legal issue raised was the mandatory nature of Section 1903 (g) of the Social Security Act. The self-executing nature of the section was verified by Deputy Comptroller General R. F. Keller in a letter to Chairman Moss on July 3, 1975. He said:

> . . . Since the substantive portions of the statutorily enumerated criteria which help make up the satisfactory showing of an effective utilization control are clear and do not require implementing regulations to be effective, those States which wish to take advantage of maximum Federal assistance must have started making such a showing effective July 1, 1973. In our view, in the absence of such a showing by a State, the Secretary of HEW has no choice but to decrease the Federal medical assistance percentage by 33⅓ per centum [see Appendix D].

In a Subcommittee hearing on July 17, 1975, Director of Manpower and Welfare Division of the General Accounting Office, Gregory J. Ahart, reiterated GAO's position. Ahart testified that—

> . . . if the Secretary determines that the State has not made a satisfactory showing of an effective system in operation, it is mandatory on the Secretary

---

[97] *Id.*

[98] Note 88 *supra* at 44.

to decrease the Federal percentage for the excess services beyond the 60- or 90-day limits.[99]

Representatives of HEW testified before the Subcommittee on July 18, 1975 and again on September 3, 1975. On July 18, Dr. Robert Van Hoek, Acting Administrator, Health Services Administration, HEW, was asked whether the Secretary of HEW acknowledged that Section 1903 (g) of the Social Security Act is not discretionary. Dr. Van Hoek replied,

> It is my understanding that that provision is not discretionary, that it is a requirement that, if institutions are found not to be in compliance, a fiscal penalty[99a] is to be imposed.[100]

The same position was reiterated by HEW General Counsel John B. Rhinelander during the September 3 hearing before the Subcommittee. Rhinelander testified—

> . . . I advised the Secretary that the reduction procedure in 1903 (g) is mandatory. I also advised him that I think it would be wise that it be done in a way which is legally supportable if and when we are challenged in the courts after taking a reduction, but Secretary Mathews fully understands that the present statute has a mandatory provision with respect to reduction.[101]

(2) Clearly determined policy of slippage and delays

The legislative purpose of the statute as well as its mandatory character are not questioned by HEW officials. Why then has HEW failed to impose the reductions called for under Section 1903 (g)? A chronology of the actions taken by HEW pursuant to the statute provides some insight.

On June 8, 1973, the Department's Social and Rehabilitation Service (SRS), which has been delegated authority by the Secretary of HEW to administer the Medicaid program, issued an Information Memorandum to state agencies administering approved medical assistance programs.[102] The stated purpose of the memorandum was—

> . . . to advise State Medicaid agencies concerning their utilization review responsibilities until such time as Sections 207 and 237 [of Public Law 92–603] are fully implemented by new or revised regulations.[103]

The memorandum also specifically provides that the State agencies should send copies of the memorandum to each provider of institutional services since they may be affected by the provisions of Section 207 and 237.

---

[99] Testimony of Gregory J. Ahart, Director, Manpower and Welfare Division, General Accounting Office, et al., *Hearings on Getting Ready for National Health Insurance: Unnecessary Surgery* before the Subcommittee on Oversight and Investigations of the Committee on Interstate and Foreign Commerce, U.S. House of Representatives, 94th Congress, 1st session, at 121 (1975).

[99a] NOTE: HEW officials continue to apply the misnomer "penalty" to this program. Section 1903 (g) is in reality an "incentives" program and is so labeled in Section 207 of Public Law 92–603.

[100] Note 78 *supra* at 224.

[101] Statement of John B. Rhinelander, General Counsel, Department of Health, Education, and Welfare, et al., *Hearings on Getting Ready for National Health Insurance: Unnecessary Surgery* before the Subcommittee on Oversight and Investigations of the Committee on Interstate and Foreign Commerce, U.S. House of Representatives, 94th Congress, 1st session, at 284 (1975).

[102] Memorandum, dated June 8, 1973, from Commissioner of Medical Services Administration, HEW, to State agencies administering approved medical assistance programs, re utilization review requirements under section 207 and 237 of Public Law 92–603, included in *Hearings on Getting Ready for National Health Insurance: Unnecessary Surgery* before the Subcommittee on Oversight and Investigations of the Committee on Interstate and Foreign Commerce, U.S. House of Representatives, 94th Congress, 1st Session, at 227–31 (1975).

[103] *Id.* at 227.

The June 8 memorandum put the states on notice regarding the new statute and explained its application. HEW fully envisioned that decreases would be made as the memorandum declares:

. . . The reduction in FFP will apply to expenditures for all days beyond the 60th in each fiscal year for each patient in an SNF and hospitals (including TB), and for all days beyond the 90th in each fiscal year for each patient in a mental hospital. For the former the reduction can be effective as early as August 30, 1973; for the latter, September 29, 1973.[104]

The states were thus adequately informed of the requirements the statute dictates as well as the mandate of HEW to make Federal fund reductions for noncompliance with those requirements.

GAO officials agree with the advice given in the June 8 Information Memorandum, as testimony before the Subcommittee indicates.[105] Between October and December 1973, the SRA (HEW) conducted its first validation survey, as provided in Section 1903 (g) (2) of the Social Security Act. That survey judged State compliance in the five areas enumerated in the statute. The 1973 evaluations determined that nine states did not meet the requirement of physician certification at the time of admission.[106] Thirty-two states failed to require the recertification by a physician at least every 60 days.[107] The statute also requires that services be furnished under a plan established and periodically reviewed and evaluated by a physician. The SRS validation survey detected fifteen states in which the plans of care were not in place.[108]

The survey found that 26 states did not have—

. . . in effect a continuous program of review of utilization . . . whereby the necessity for admission and the continued stay of each patient in such institution is periodically reviewed and evaluated . . . by medical and other professional personnel who are not themselves directly responsible for the care of the patient and who are not employed by or financially interested in any such institution . . . (42 U.S.C. 1396b(g)(1)(B)).[109]

Each state must likewise have an effective program of medical review of the care of patients in mental hospitals, skilled nursing facilities, and intermediate care facilities, in order that the professional management of each case be reviewed and evaluated at least annually by independent professional review teams. SRS found that such a program of medical review did not exists in 11 states, based on the 1973 survey.[110] However, no reductions of Federal funds were made by HEW based on the 1973 evaluations.

A report by the Comptroller General of the United States issued April 14, 1975 on "Improvements Needed in Medicaid Program Management Including Investigations of Suspected Fraud and Abuse," discussed HEW's actions in implementing Section 1903 (g) and the fact that no reductions have been made pursuant to it.[111] The report states—

---

104 *Id.* at 230–1.
105 Note 99 *supra* at 119.
106 *Report to the Subcommittee on Health of the Committee on Finance,* U.S. Senate, "Improvements Needed in Medicaid Program Management including Investigations of Suspected Fraud and Abuse, Social and Rehabilitation Service, Department of HEW," by the Comptroller General of the United States, MWD–75–74, Apr. 14, 1975, at 43.
107 *Id.*
108 *Id.*
109 *Id.*
110 *Id.*
111 *Id.* at 122–76.

> The Administrator, SRS, informed us that SRS had limited capability with respect to validating the effectiveness of State institutional utilization review systems in 1973. He stated that the 1973 evaluation was a preliminary sample of States' systems to allow SRS to refine its techniques for evaluating State compliance. According to the Administrator, SRS did not penalize any State as a result of this sample because SRS criteria for compliance were not specific. However, SRS obtained commitments from States to improve their systems when evaluations disclosed problems.[112]

At that time, GAO recommended SRS ". . . assess penalties on States that fail to comply with utilization review requirements."[113]

(3) HEW maladministration

In hearings before the Subcommittee, held June 18, 1975, Dr. Keith Weikel, Commissioner of Medical Services Administration (MSA), HEW, testified as to why HEW did not reduce Federal funds based on the 1973 surveys:

> The first survey *did not utilize a statistically valid sample.* They looked at every State's utilization review or control system. They looked at, however, a much smaller number of facilities and patient records. I believe 13,000 patient records during the 1973 survey. They indeed did find a number of States that were not in compliance, just based on the limited sample.
>
> The States were then asked to develop a plan of correction to come into compliance with that regulation. [Emphasis added][114]

The legal status of "plans of correction" required by HEW of the States is not clear to this Subcommittee. Were these plans of correction to be considered by HEW as an acknowledgement by the Senate that they did not make a satisfactory showing under Section 1903 (g)? Did HEW wish to waive the mandatory nature of the noncompliance reduction? Did HEW wish to ask Congress for a change in statute? HEW has not provided evidence that demonstrates any follow-through to the plans of correction.

SRS undertook a second set of validation surveys from June to December 1974. As with the 1973 surveys, this survey likewise discovered several states who were not in compliance with the statutory requirements. These states' survey results were compiled on the basis of the five criteria enumerated in the statute. Five states were not in compliance with the physician certification requirement, and seven states were not in compliance with the physician recertification requirement.[115] Six states did not have adequate plans of care as required, and 23 states did not meet the required facility utilization review.[116] For the requirement of medical review by the state, five states were not in compliance based on the 1974 surveys.[117]

HEW failed to act upon the results of the 1974 evaluation. An HEW memorandum, dated April 3, 1975, from Galen Powers, Assistant General Counsel, to Dr. Keith Weikel, stated that in his

[112] *Id.* at 174.
[113] *Id.* at 175.
[114] Testimony of M. Keith Weikel, Ph. D., Commissioner, Health Services Administration, Department of Health, Education, and Welfare, *Hearings on Getting Ready for National Health Insurance: Unnecessary Surgery* before the Subcommittee on Oversight and Investigations of the Committee on Interstate and Foreign Commerce, U.S. House of Representatives, 94th Congress, 1st Session, at 232 (1975).
[115] Note 106 *supra* at 174.
[116] *Id.*
[117] *Id.*

opinions, SRS did not supply sufficient legal backing for the recommendations.[118]

SRS had recommended that reductions, for approximately $47 million, be applied to 10 states based upon the surveys of single-state agencies and patients' medical records. This reduction was for one quarter in fiscal year 1974. The Powers memorandum fails to point out that General Counsel Rhinelander, in testimony before the Subcommittee on September 3, 1975, stated that reductions for states out of compliance must be for the entire year. Rhinelander stated, ". . . the fiscal reduction provided for in section 1903(g) applies for the entire fiscal year and not for just the quarter in which the state has failed to make a satisfactory showing.[119]

(4) Methodology criticism

In the April 3, 1975 memorandum Mr. Powers states—

> . . . It is our judgment that the penalties proposed to be taken for nonadherence to the medical records criteria are legally indefensible. The penalties based upon failure to meet single state agency requirements, while not legally indefensible, present serious problems.[120]

The basis of that contention is due primarily to the methodology employed in the examination of the patients' medical records. SRS previously determined that 75 percent of the patients' medical records must fully meet the requirements of certification, recertification, and plan of care. This 75 percent figure was to be based upon a review of medical records for a period of one month. In some cases, the records were reviewed for a longer period of time, thus, increasing the possibility that the records would be found to be in non-adherence.

The memorandum also questioned the uniformity of the survey based on the particular findings. The Powers memorandum states—

> It is disturbing to note that the ten states now being recommended for penalties come from only three regions—two in Region I, five in Region V, and three in Region VIII. Thus, in three regions with a total of eighteen jurisdictions, ten states are being penalized, while in stark contrast, in seven regions with a total of thirty-eight jurisdictions, no states are being penalized.[121]

The Powers memorandum raises serious questions concerning the methodology employed by HEW. It points out the lack of uniformity among the regions, wide-ranging regional discrepancies, and standardization problems for examining patient records. The SRS should have assumed legal enforcement was going to be necessary and cleared the methodology beforehand through the Office of the General Counsel.

The compliance check by HEW relied upon the use of patient records almost exclusively. This raises very serious questions about the judgment used by SRS. It appears from the results of some states that a very detailed examination of medical records need not have been done at all. There were states that did not present an effective utilization control program to HEW as is required. On December 18, 1975, the Subcommittee learned that some states did not even file the

---

[118] Memorandum, dated Apr. 3, 1975, from Galen D. Powers, Assistant General Counsel, HEW, to M. Keith Weikel, Ph. D., Commissioner of Medical Services Administration, re Medicaid-utilization control penalty (Section 1903 (g)), included in *Hearings on Getting Ready for National Health Insurance: Unnecessary Surgery* before the Subcommittee on Oversight and Investigations of the Committee on Interstate and Foreign Commerce, U.S. House of Representatives, 94th Congress, 1st sess., at 245–54 (1975).

[119] Note 101 *supra* at 276.

[120] Note 118 *supra* at 245.

[121] Id. (footnote 9) at 253.

required utilization control certification. Evidence of this was gathered by GAO, and this information was brought to the attention of HEW in a letter from Chairman Moss (see appendix E).

There were several important measures that could have been utilized in lieu of the very time-consuming and expensive methodology employed by SRS—examining patient records. For example, checking the organization of utilization review committees and their minutes, as well as tissue committee activities, could provde a much less expensive and more detailed review of utilization activities with better results than the long, drawn-out check of patient records. The utilization committee review and tissue committee review could have eliminated, in some cases, the need for the validation surveys to require a patient check altogether.

(5) *General Counsel as policymaker*

The Powers memorandum causes significant impact on the actions of HEW with regard to the mandatory reductions required by Section 1903 (g) In particular, the memorandum raised questions concerning the role of the Office of General Counsel within HEW. In testimony before the Subcommittee on July 18, 1975, it was asserted that once the recommendations were made by the General Counsel, the entire matter remained dormant until the recomputations were initiated. It appeared to Chairman Moss that the General Counsel was determining policy, since lengthy delays in the General Counsel's Office caused the program to come to a complete standstill.[122] The Commissioner of MSA recommended on March 27, 1975,[123] and the Administrator of SRS recommended on August 26, 1975,[124] that the reductions be made based upon the second 1974 survey, but delay in the General Counsel's office has kept the Secretary from making his findings.

Given the leading role the General Counsel was playing in policy formulation, he was called to testify before the Subcommittee. That hearing was held on September 3, 1975. General Counsel John Rhinelander prepared a statement originally scheduled for presentation on July 30, 1975. Disparities between that statement and his September 3rd testimony can only be explained by the fact that the new Secretary of HEW, Dr. F. David Mathews, was sworn into office in the interim and that Secretary Mathews chose to further delay implementation of the law. In the July 30 statement, Mr. Rhinelander stated—

> The delays that the Department has experienced in implementing section 1903 (g) are indeed regrettable, but I want to emphasize that no legal rights have been lost to the Government. The provision will be applied with full force for the entire period since it became effective. The SRS survey for the last quarter of fiscal year 1974 is currently being recomputed. When that is done—and I understand that it will be done soon—the reductions will be made for the entire fiscal year 1974, the first year for which the reduction provision became effective.[125]

---

[122] Question by Chairman John E. Moss (D-Calif.) *Hearings on Getting Ready for National Health Insurance: Unnecessary Surgery* before the Subcommittee on Oversight and Investigations of the Committee on Interstate and Foreign Commerce, U.S. House of Representatives, 94th Congress, 1st session, at 288–89 (1975).

[123] Information Memorandum, dated Mar. 27, 1975, Department of HEW, Social and Rehabilitation Service.

[124] Information Memorandum, dated Aug. 26, 1975, Department of HEW, Social and Rehabilitation Service.

[125] Note 101 *supra* at 275.

On September 3, Mr. Rhinelander testified—

Since Dr. Weikel's previous testimony, the new Secretary of Health, Education, and Welfare, Dr. Mathews, has taken office and has decided to suspend the imposition of the utilization control reductions of matching funds pending a review of all reductions or penalties under the Social Security Act.[126]

Mr. Rhinelander also acknowledged the Department's understanding as to the mandatory nature of the statute:

Indeed, we believe that the Department is legally obligated to take the one-third decrease provided for in section 1903 (g) if a state has failed to make a showing satisfactory to the Secretary that it has in operation an effective utilization control program with respect to each calendar quarter.[127]

(6) *Examination of reduction provisions*

The August 29, 1975 letter from Secretary Mathews to Chairman Moss reflects a new attitude by HEW toward Section 1903 (g) and other sections which involve reductions in Federal monies to the states.[128] In that letter, Secretary Mathews informed the Chairman that he was instructing his staff to make an in-depth review of the penalty provision to see if more appropriate incentives could be designed that would result in the improvement of state utilization control programs. Secretary Mathews further stated, "I am not planning to impose the 1903 (g) sanctions until this review is completed.[129]

This new approach by HEW was reenforced by the General Counsel in his testimony before the Subcommittee on September 3, 1975. During those hearings, Mr. Rhinelander stated:

While Dr. Mathews clearly recognizes that the statute requires imposition of the reductions when a satisfactory showing of an effective utilization control program is not made, he is also aware that the statute mandates no date certain when the reductions must actually be imposed. Accordingly, he has directed that an intensive study be made of the problems in this area and of possible alternatives which would better effectuate the purposes of the various reduction or penalty provisions.[130]

Mr. Rhinelander indicated that he thought the study of sanctions "would be completed *before* the end of the year." [131] [Emphasis supplied] Furthermore, Mr. Rhinelander stated that the review of the data—known within HEW as "recomputations"—was separate and distinct from the study of 1903 (g). Thus, this review should not be considered as an alternative or in lieu of faithfully executing Section 1903 (g).

B. SUMMARY

Section 1903 (g) of the Social Security Act is unambiguous, mandatory, and self-executing, and the Secretary of HEW must implement that section of the law as of July 1, 1973. Proper implementation of the section would save millions of taxpayer dollars.

---

[126] *Id.* at 272.
[127] *Id.* at 275.
[128] Letter, dated Aug. 29, 1975, from David Mathews, Secretary, HEW, to Chairman John E. Moss re Additional views of HEW re Implementation of the utilization control program mandated by Congress in 1972, included in *Hearings on Getting Read for National Health Insurance: Unnecessary Surgery* before the Subcommittee on Oversight and Investigations of the Committee on Interstate and Foreign Commerce, U.S. House of Representatives, 94th Congress, 1st session, at 269–70 (1975).
[129] *Id.* at 270.
[130] Note 101 *supra* at 272.
[131] *Id.* at 286.

HEW has been obligated since September 30, 1973 to undertake validation surveys and make findings of compliance based upon those surveys. The Secretary has failed to comply with these obligations.

Review of penalties, sanctions, and incentives by HEW is appropriate and important. However, all reasonable time for HEW to comply with the mandatory provisions has been exhausted, and failure to carry out the law during this period of review cannot be excused or justified.

VIII. Policy Issues

The Subcommittee investigation and hearings on unnecessary surgery point out three problem areas that require specific focus—cost, quality, and public accountability. In each of these areas, there were major deficiencies requiring better execution of existing laws and, possibly, remedial legislation.

A. COST ISSUES

The Subcommittee investigation turned up convincing evidence that unnecessary surgery wastes lives and dollars.[132] Data presented during the hearings indicate that the benefit cost ratio may be as favorable as six or eight dollars saved for every dollar spent in second consultation programs to reduce unnecessary surgery such as those undertaken by New York unions.[133]

The financial cost of unnecessary surgeries is clearly immense. This cost is borne in large measure by consumers and by payors such as Government through Medicare and Medicaid vendor payments. The cost is also borne by private insurance carriers and by Blue Cross and Blue Shield and is ultimately passed on to consumers through increased premiums.

(1) Number of surgical procedures

Dr. Wolfe, in hearing testimony, and the Health Resources Administration (HRA), HEW, used 18.4 millon procedures as their base number of surgical procedures.[134] This figure was derived from the number of procedures performed on inpatients discharged from non-Federal general and special short-stay hospitals during 1973.[135] The estimates are also based on data collected by the Hospital Discharge Survey (HDS). This study of short-stay hospital utilization in the United States was done by the National Center for Health Statistics (NCHS), a unit of the HEW's Public Health Service. The latter estimate includes all listed surgical operations for inpatients discharged from short-stay hospitals, by surgery class and selected operations, sex, and age in the United States for 1973.[136]

The American Hospital Association developed a "Hospital Indicators Panel Survey" which compiled utilization data in community hospitals. This summary indicates that for 1973 there were 15.96 million surgical operations in community hospitals.[137]

---

[132] Note 22 *supra* at 113; Note 38 *supra* at 67.

[133] Note 38 supra at 68.

[134] *Id.* at 65.

[135] U.S. Department of Health, Education, and Welfare Monthly Vital Statistics Report: Hospital Discharge Survey Data, from the National Center for Health Statistics (May 30, 1975). Supp. Vol. 23 (No. 3).

[136] *Id.*, "Table 4."

[137] Hospital Indicators Panel Survey, American Hospital Association, Selective Utilization Data and Percentage Charge Community Hospitals, 1972–75.

The Subcommittee will use a lower estimate, namely 14 million procedures, for two reasons. First, neither the 18.4 million procedures identified by the HEW estimate nor the 16 million procedures classified by the American Hospital Association can all be classified as elective. Secondly, the 18.4 surgical operations were for 13.5 million patients, indicating the average number of operations and procedures per patient with surgery was 1.4 operations. Certain procedures such as biopsies are included within the surgical operations listed and serve to increase the overall total.

If there were 13.3 million patients undergoing surgery in 1973, then 14 million patients appears to be a reasonable estimate for 1974. This estimate is reenforced by the Commission on Professional and Hospital Activities (CPHA) which found that 7.6 million patients were operated upon during the first six months of 1975—an annualized estimate of 15.2 million. The Subcommittee believes that to use 14 million surgical procedures insures that the projected cost estimates will be conservative.

The Subcommittee chooses to use 17 percent as the rate of unnecessary surgical procedures. The primary source for this estimate is the HEW-funded study conducted by Dr. McCarthy. He found that 24 percent of all procedures recommended were not confirmed. The proportion not confirmed in each surgical specialty, in descending order of frequency utilization, were— [138]

	Percent
General surgery	16.4
Gynecology	16.4
Orthopedic	40.3
Ear, nose, and throat	16.3
Opthalmology	28.2
Urology	35.8

Seventeen percent represents the percent of surgical procedures not confirmed for those participating in the elective presurgical screening program (February 1972 through December 1974) undertaken by the Storeworkers Union Welfare Fund. In this program, 81 percent of the union members had received a second opinion prior to admission for in-hospital elective surgery.

Asked whether 17 percent was considered a representative figure, Dr. McCarthy testified—

> I think it is an approach to that figure [17 percent] because I think we are talking here about a substantial number of cases. As I said, we saw approximately 80 to 85 percent of the cases involved.[139]

Utilizing 17 percent of the procedures as unnecessary and 14 million as the total number of elective surgeries, the Subcommittee concludes that approximately *2,380,000 surgeries were unnecessarily performed last year.*

One of the major unanswered questions at this point is how many of the patients, whose operations were not confirmed later, had or will need to have an operation for the condition screened and how many required continuing medical treatment. In order to receive more definitive information about unnecessary surgery, we need to know what proportion of the 17 percent nonconfirmed cases will never require

---

[138] Note 22 *supra* at 133.
[139] *Id.* at 111.

surgery, what proportion will have the surgery at a later date, and what are the consequences of that postponement. In addition, a cost analysis needs to be performed comparing the costs of operating a typical pre-surgical screening program to the substantial costs of unnecessary surgery.

(2) Costs of unnecessary surgery

The Subcommittee attempted to ascertain the costs of a typical surgical procedure In that regard, Dr. McCarthy commented:

> . . . Obviously we focused on hospital, anesthesia fee and surgery fees. Keep in mind when someone does not have surgery, he can be working, there is no disability payment which in total dollars would be more significant.
>
> In terms of direct savings . . . surgery, anesthesia, hospitals, we project now $2500. That is how we came up with the figure this morning of roughly over a billion dollars savings. You must add to that the disability funding . . .[140]

This estimate may be understated because in some cases the consumer has to pay a physicians' fee which is not included within the hospital surgical and anesthesia fees.

The McCarthy study published December 19, 1974, in the *New England Journal of Medicine*, contained more detailed estimates of the average payment per hospital. It stated:

> If the average payment per hospital day by Blue Cross to hospitals in the lower 17 counties of New York State to date in 1974, $141, is multiplied by a weighted average of a length of stay for the nine most frequently unconfirmed diagnoses, 7.3 days, an average cost per stay of $1,029 is obtained. To this must be added the surgeons fee and estimated average of $500 per procedure and an estimated average anesthesiologist fee, $125.[141]

This results in total cost of hospital stay at $1,654, Using the estimate of $1,650 per procedure and the Subcommittee estimate of 2.38 million unnecessary surgeries, the Subcommittee determined that *the American public spent $3.92 billion* in 1974 on unnecessary surgery. This represents about twice the amount of dollars spent by this country for all of its health research funded through the National Institutes of Health (NIH). Moreover, it represents approximately 16 per cent of the amount of dollars that the Federal Government spent for Medicare and Medicaid for fiscal year 1975.

(3) Cost to Medicare

Medicare underwritten surgical procedures were supported by $4.66 billion Federal Government dollars.[142] Making the same assumptions as above—namely that 17 percent of the procedures were unnecessary—$816 million of Federal money was spent on unnecessary surgery last year under Medicare by the Federal Government. This does *not* include out-of-pocket expenditures by senior citizens to meet the coinsurance and deductibles not covered by the Medicare program.

(4) cost to medicaid

Medicaid cost estimates for surgery in 1974 was $1.6 billion dollars according to staff projections. HEW was asked but indicated it could

---

[140] *Id.* at 112.

[141] Note 5 *supra* at 1334.

[142] "Estimated Medicare Benefit Expenditures for Surgery-related Services Calendar Year 1974," Office of Research and Statistics, Social Security Administration, July 14, 1975, included in *Hearings on Getting Ready for National Health Insurance: Unnecessary Surgery* before the Subcommittee on Oversight and Investigations of the Committee on Interstate and Foreign Commerce, U.S. House of Representatives, 94th Congress, 1st session, at 203 (1975).

not supply an estimate of total dollars spent on surgery. The staff estimate was built upon two HEW estimates—namely, that $3.5 billion was spent on hospital costs and $1.3 billion was spent on physician costs under the Medicaid program in 1974.[143] It is estimated that one-third of the hospital and physician costs are related to surgery. This amounts to $1.17 billion for hospital costs and 0.43 billion for physician costs. Cumulatively, therefore, $1.6 billion is considered the surgical expenditure estimate for Medicaid.[144]

Using 17 percent as the percent of unnecessary procedures and $1.6 billion as the Medicaid surgical cost, the unnecessary cost to the Medicaid program would be $272 million.

Combined, the cost of unnecessary surgery for Medicare ($816 million) and Medicaid ($272 million) is, therefore, estimated to be $1.088 million or almost $1.1 billion. To the extent that HEW has failed to implement cost control procedures mandated by Congress, it can be said that HEW is responsible for *waste* of more than $1 billion.

(5) Cost savings through changes in location for surgical procedures

Hughes presented a detailed study showing that 24 perecnt of surgical procedures done in conjunction with a pre-paid program were done without inpatient hospitalization.[145] Hughes testified that 20 to 24 percent of procedures currently performed on in-patients were simple enough to be completed on an out-patient basis.[146]

Testimony presented by Crile and Stahl, two prominent surgeons, indicated that the fee-for-service system compared to a salaried arrangement led to surgeons undertaking of more complicated procedures in equivocal situations. With fee-for-service arrangements, there is no financial incentive to prevent individuals from being hospitalized for simple procedures.[147] Crile suggested that surgeons be required to be salaried in order to hold hospital-surgical privileges.[148] His contention is that this procedural change will remove the financial incentive to do the more expensive operation and will remove the financial incentive to do the procedure when indications are marginal.

There appears to be enormous potential for cost savings in non hospitalized surgery. For example, there were at least 2.4 million surgical procedures financed by Medicaid last year and if approximately 500,000 (20 percent) of the procedures could have been performed on an outpatient basis, the savings would have been substantial. If as little as $300 could have been saved per procedure, the overall savings in this area alone would approximate $150 million.

(6) Cost-benefit opportunities

There was a broad consensus among the expert witnesses that second consultations before elective surgery would improve quality and cut down unnecessary procedures.[149] The cost savings of second consulta-

[143] Understanding Medicaid: An Introduction to the Medical Services Administration (MSA), HEW, May 1975, p. IV. 2.

[144] Statement of John A. Svahn, Acting Administrator, Social and Rehabilitation Service, Department of Health, Education, and Welfare, *Hearings on Getting Ready for National Health Insurance: Unnecessary Surgery* before the Subcommittee on Oversight and Investigations of the Committee on Interstate and Foreign Commerce, U.S. House of Representatives, 94th Congress, 1st session, at 281 (1975).

[145] Note 49 *supra* at 188–89.

[146] *Id.* at 189.

[147] Note 43 *supra* at 92–3; Note 50 *supra* at 193–194.

[148] Note 51 *supra* at 195.

[149] Notes 1 through 7 *supra*.

tions, although substantial as demonstrated in the New York union studies, must be balanced off against the cost of administrative mechanisms devised for implementation.[150] The McCarthy study concluded:

> The expense of operating the presurgical programs and providing the consultations during the study period includes the cost per consultation and the average ancillary service charges, totaling $28 per patient (this figure has risen to $33 since the reporting period), and the direct administrative office costs for both programs of approximately $37,300. Thus, the overall operating costs of the programs, $75,268, compared to the total savings, $581,873, represents a return of almost *eight dollars for every dollar spent.*[151]

B. QUALITY ISSUES

(1) Mortality due to unnecessary surgery

On July 15, 1975, Dr. Wolfe testified:

> Bunker has estimated that the mortality rate for elective surgery is 0.5 percent (it is higher for emergency surgery). If this rate is applied to unnecessary operations, the U.S. mortality due to unnecessary surgery may be 16,000 deaths per year.[152]

This estimate of 16,000 deaths was based upon the 3.2 million surgical procedures deemed to be unnecessary by Dr. Wolfe.[153]

The Bunker estimate was contained in a study published in the *New England Journal of Medicine*, December 6, 1973. Bunker and Wennberg stated:

> Discretionary operations all carry a discrete and measurable risk of death. The operative and postoperative mortality for all operations in the United States is approximately 1.4 percent (National Center for Health Statistics, unpublished data). For discretionary operations one might conservatively assume a mortality of 0.5 percent.[154]

HEW's Office of Research and Statistics published in 1975 an extensive study of Medicare recipients demonstrating a much higher mortality rate. This study, using 1967 data on hospital discharges, found that of 1,609,539 discharges *with surgery*, 85,222 patients were discharged dead representing a mortality rate of 5.2 percent.[155]

The study one in 1967 utilized an elderly population, a mixture of discretionary and non-discretionary procedures, including procedures that were necessary as well as unnecessary. All these factors tend to make the 5.2 percent figure an underestimate of the total population. The fact that 85,000 patients died out of 1.6 million procedures performed makes it probable that at least 100,000 patients were discharged dead as a result of the 12,000,000 surgical procedures performed in 1967—a mortality rate exceeding 0.8 percent.

The Commission on Professional and Hospital Activities (CPHA) of Ann Arbor, Michigan gathers data jointly with IMS, America, Ltd., on hospital stays. Dr. Virgil Slee, President of CPHA, estimated that of the 7,600,000 patients operated upon during the first six months of 1975, 105,000 patients were discharged dead. That estimate represents a mortality rate for all surgery of 1.4 percent.

---

[150] Note 5 *supra* at 1334.
[151] *Id.*
[152] Note 38 *supra* at 67.
[153] *Id.*
[154] Note 1 *supra*.

[155] U.S. Social Security Administration, Office of Research and Statistics, *Medicare: Health Insurance for the Aged, 1967, Section 4.1: Short-Stay Hospital Utilization,* Washington, D.C. (1975), at 4.1–9.

Three operations: hysterectomy, tonsilectomy, and cholecystectomy were examined for the relationship between unnecessary procedures and mortality rates. Dr. Slee provided the following estimates:

1ST 6 MONTHS (1975)

	Operations	Discharged dead	Mortality rate (percent)
Hysterectomy, abdominal	276,000	[1] 500	[1] 0.2
Tonsilectomy:			
(a) Tonsilectomies	115,000	(2)	
(b) Tonsilectomies and adenoidectomy	257,000	(2)	
Cholecystectomy	226,000	2,000	1.0

[1] Approximately.
[2] Virtually none.

These date serve to confirm the reasonableness of the Bunker mortality rate estimate of 0.5 percent, the estimate used by the Subcommittee.

CPHA and IMS, America, Ltd., collect data for 30 percent of all hospitals in the United States. They obtained their estimates of mortality rates by projecting data from their 30 percent sample to the population as a whole.

The Subcommittee used a conservative estimate for the volume of unnecessary surgical procedures—2.38 million. Utilizing this figure and the estimated surgical mortality rate developed by Bunker and Wennberg, 0.5 percent, *the number of deaths from unnecessary surgeries approximates 11,900 for* last year.[156]

(*1*) *Medicaid mortality*

The Subcommittee staff undertook to determine the extent of surgical procedures underwritten by Medicaid. It found that 26 states paid for 1.9 million surgical procedures last year (see Appendix A). Utilizing the 17 percent unnecessary surgery rate and the surgical mortality rate estimated by Bunker, this would mean that in those 26 states, 240,000 unnecessary procedures resulted in *1,700 unnecessary deaths to Medicaid recipients.*

(*2*) *Utilization differences*

Evidence was presented during the hearings using an epidemiological approach to estimate the extent of unnecessary surgery. Wennberg reported wide variations in use of health care among neighboring communities of Vermont.[157]

The Gittleson technique, using a "probability of organ removal by a given age" was examined. This showed that the probability of tonsils removal ranged from 8 to 62 percent across 13 Vermont areas.[158] By age 75, the probability of uterus loss ranges were from 24 to 52 percent.[159]

Wennberg observed that in those areas of Vermont with more surgeons, there were higher rates of surgery.[160] He testified:

That physician characteristics help determine variations in aggregate use of medical care is not surprising. The market for health care is characterized by

[156] Note 1 *supra.*
[157] Note 29 *supra.*
[158] Note 3 *supra.*
[159] Note 29 *supra.*
[160] *Id.* at 76.

uncertainty. In seeking care, patients are uncertain about what they should purchase and depend in large part on the recommendation of the physician they contact. Physicians chose treatments from alternatives whose end results are incompletely evaluated. It is easy to believe that the intrinsic uncertainties concerning effectiveness lead an individual specialist to recommend one type of therapy more often than would a physician of another specialty.

What I believe more surprising is the range in differences of opinion about using specific types of procedures. Although the overall rate of surgery may be identical between neighboring areas, the rates of specific procedures vary markedly. Patterns of variation observed in a recently completed study in Maine illustrate this point.[161]

In the HEW study by Gornick study patterns of surgery among Medicare patients similarly striking regional differences were found for even broader geographic areas.[162] The Gornick study concluded that consistent regional differences were found in hospital stay that "are not explained by variations in the patient characteristic examined."[163] Specifically, this HEW study found thta regions of the country varied considerably in their surgery rates. In the Northeast, a surgical procedure was recorded for 34 to 36 percent of all discharges. In the South the proportion of all discharges with surgery was 25 to 27 percent.

The Gornick study also showed large variations in the mean length of patient stays in hospitals. For appendectomies, for example, the mean length of stay in the Northeast section of the country was 16.1 days; in the West the mean length of stay was 11.2 days—a difference of 44 percent.[164] Such variability raises significant questions about the quality of care differences between these two regions.

HEW's analysis concludes that consistent regional differences "suggest that factors other than the medical ones for which the patient was hospitalized affect the duration of stay."[165]

The Gornick study concludes that there is a need for extensive investigation of the regional variations used in managing medical problems of the elderly under Medicare.[166]

(3) Professional standards review organizations

Professional Standards Review Organizations (PSRO's) have been established to help assure that medical care delivered to Medicare and Medicaid beneficiaries is of high quality and is provided in a manner which reflects the most appropriate and efficient utilization of our nation's health care institutions.[167] The Subcommittee is hopeful that the PSRO program may eventually be able to assist in that goal. To date, however, the PSRO program has been hobbled by the lack of appropriate ambulatory reviews, lack of appropriate prospective reviews, and inordinate time delays.

Dr. Van Hoek testified that it is through quality assurance review systems that we can ultimately affect the costs of medical care:

It is the intent of both the PSRO program and utilization review to establish effective peer review systems in hospitals and long-term care facilities to assure that Federal and State expenditures for Medicare and Medicaid services are spent on medically necessary, high-quality medical care. While these programs have frequently been characterized as cost-containment measures, I should like

---

[161] *Id.*
[162] Note 60 *supra* at 16.
[163] *Id.*
[164] *Id.* at 22.
[165] *Id.* at 26.
[166] *Id.* at 31.
[167] Note 79 *supra* at 198.

to emphasize that they are primarily mechanisms to assure the appropriateness and quality of medical care. It is through quality assurance review systems that we can ultimately affect the costs of medical care. These are the systems that assess and reduce such factors as unnecessary surgery and medically unnecessary admissions. PSROs will use explicit, areawide medical care criteria in their review systems. These criteria will include, for example, indications for surgery, and it is through the use of such written criteria that the system may affect the amount and quality of care delivered. By reducing the volume of unnecessary services, we thereby reduce the expenditures for medical care and provide higher quality care.[168]

HEW has indicated that it considers the implementation PSRO's as an alternative to establishment of required second consulations under utilization review.

While both PSRO and utilization review have the same intent, and they share many common characteristics in the conduct of peer review, they differ significantly in their approach and organizational arrangements for carrying out such review. PSRO introduces new approaches to the concept of utilization review which should significantly improve the quality and effectiveness of such review for the Medicare, Medicaid, and Maternal and Child Health programs. In particular PSROs carry out review as voluntary community or area-wide physician organizations, whereas utilization review is carried out under the auspices of an individual hospital or nursing home.

As physician organizations, PSROs are given authority by legislation to make decisions for the Medicare and Medicaid programs on issues of medical necessity and the appropriateness of care which are binding for payment purposes. Under the U. R. system, such final decision-making authority is vested with the Medicare intermediaries and Medicaid fiscal agents. Giving physicians the *responsibility* as well as the authority to review care in an organized fashion should significantly improve the quality of care and efficiency with which health services are delivered.[169]

The Subcommittee does not feel that PSRO's are a total substitute, for two reasons:

(a) *Timing*—It is clear that Congress fully intended utilization control programs for Medicaid to be in place on July 1, 1973. Section 1903 (g) provides for this in unambiguous language.[170] The Comptroller General has held that the section is mandatory and self-executing.[171] It is clear that Congress intended this program to provide quality controls to Medicaid recipients as of that date, and that the subsequent implementation of PSRO's would suplement these cost and quality controls.

Premature transfer of utilization controls to PSRO's before they become functional will leave cost and quality controls by the Government in a state of limbo. The fact that PSRO implementation has been very slow only increases the need for effective utilization control in place now. As early as June 24, 1974, the House Labor—Health, Education and Welfare Appropriations Subcommittee stated in its report that there is "considerable slippage in the PSRO program." [172]

There were 203 PSRO areas designated in late 1974. Dr. Theodore Cooper, Assistant Secretary for Health, HEW, testified before the Labor-HEW Appropriations Subcommittee on April 8, 1975 on the implementation of PSRO's:

We have 91 in planning now. We have 13 conditional and 13 support centers. Maybe Mr. Weinman can comment on the projections for the following years and when we will reach 203.

---

[168] *Id.* at 198.

[169] *Id.*

[170] 42 U.S.C. § 1396b(g).

[171] Note 99 *supra* at 121.

[172] Note 94 *supra* at 52.

Mr. WEINMAN. I would guess it would probably be calendar year 1977 or 1978 based on the present financing and the speed of implementation.

I think we are making good progress. In June we will convert somewhere between 35 and 40 of the present plans which will give us a total of about 55 conditional professional standards review organizations. We also hope to let another 20 planning contracts in order to keep the momentum. It is very clear, based on our present available resources and what we estimate the cost of the program to be, that we will not be able to implement the 203 PSRO's as hoped, certainly not as soon as January 1976. I think it will go to 1977 or 1978 based on present projections and the present administration request.[173]

(2) *Functions.*—The establishment of PSRO's does not mean that Government responsibility for cost and quality controls from Medicare and Medicaid are automatically transferred to these agencies. The Senate Committee on Finance report describes this relationship:

. . . The Government has a responsibility to establish mechanisms capable of asuring effective utilization review. Its responsibility to millions of persons dependent upon medicare and medicaid, to the taxpayers who bear the burden of billions of dollars in annual program costs, and to the health care system.[174]

The Senate Finance Committee report declares in unequivocal terms that PSRO's must demonstrate they can improve upon existing utilization programs before such efforts are terminated.

In a number of areas of the country, carriers and intermediaries—even though their activity is limited to retrospective review—are doing a reasonably effective job of controlling unnecessary utilization of health care services. Such efforts should not be terminated in any area until such time as a PSRO has satisfactorily demonstrated the willingness, operational capacity, and performance to effectively supplant and improve upon existing review work. Even where the PSRO becomes the paramount review organization, the existing review, if it is efficient and effective, should not be dismantled, if the PSRO can benefit by utilizing its experience and services.[175]

The Senate Finance Committee report is most emphatic in declaring

. . . *The Committee does not intend any abdication of public responsibility or accountability* in recommending the professional standards review organizations approach [Emphasis supplied] [176]

HEW has not been able to provide evidence that PSRO's have demstrated they have the operational capacity to reduce unnecessary surgical procedures. In fact, HEW has acknowledged that it does not have such evidence.

During House Appropriations hearings, HEW presented information that the Colorado admissions program, a PSRO program, found the number of admissions per 1,000 eligibles dropped by 10 percent in 1974. HEW says, however, that the drop in unwarranted admissions primarily represented short-stays for diagnostic tests.[177]

C. PUBLIC ACCOUNTABILITY: INADEQUATE INFORMATION COLLECTION BY HEW

Despite the size and importance of the program, HEW administers Medicaid with very serious gaps in information. These gaps extend to operations of program management and planning for future

[173] Statement of Dr. Theodore Cooper, Acting Assistant Secretary for Health, and Mr. David Weinman, *Hearings on Departments of Labor and Health, Education and Welfare Appropriations for 1976* before the Subcommittee on the Department of Labor and Health, Education and Welfare of the House Committee on Appropriations, 94th Congress, 2d session, pt. 2, at 459 (1975).
[174] Note 89 *supra* at 256.
[175] *Id.* at 258.
[176] Id.
[177] Note 94 *supra* at 52.

changes. These informational gaps make it difficult to evaluate the Medicare and Medicaid programs in relation to proposals for national health insurance.

One major deficiency is that HEW does not know how many persons are eligible for Medicaid. Equally striking is the fact that at the beginning of Fiscal Year 1976, i.e., July 1, 1975, it was not known by HEW how many persons received a particular type of service, e.g. hospital surgery, paid for by Medicaid during any year later than fiscal year 1972.[178]

HEW's inability to account for the dollars expended under these programs is truly shocking when one considers that the Medicaid program in fiscal year 1972 paid out $4.6 billion, and in 1976 will pay out an estimated $7.8 billion. These are Federal dollars and do not include the state and local shares.

Federal responsibility for collecting data on Medicaid lies with the National Center for Social Statistics (NCSS).[179] Information on the Medicaid program comes primarily from two sources—(1) the grant award procedures, and (2) statistical reporting by the states.

Under the grant award procedures, an award is made quarterly to states to meet the Federal share of state program requirements for the upcoming quarter. HEW regional offices recommend the grant award for each state. However, these quarterly reports do not include even rudimentary breakouts of the expenditures by type of service, nor any kind of data on the recipients of these services.[180]

States are required to file the statistical reports on Medicaid to NCSS on a monthly and yearly basis. The current reporting system required by NCSS presents major problems. The lack of coordination among the reporting elements of SRS frequently results in data which is often meaningless and not comparable. For example, family planning is not included as a type of service. Also, basic information on intermediate care facilities (ICF's) is required to be reported under cash assistance programs, while expenditures for ICF's are included under "other care."

Current Medicaid reporting does not collect vital and necessary information from the states. Such information is needed at the Federal level in order to help determine program policies and insure better public accountability. Needed, and not yet available, is information by diagnosis as well as data concerning the number of surgical procedures underwritten by Medicaid.

In testimony before the Subcommittee, John A. Svahn, HEW's Acting Administrator of the Social and Rehabilitation Service (SRS), indicated that NCSS collects reports from the states on a "periodic basis or on an as-needed basis." [181] Mr. Svahn testified that he did not have information concerning the number of dollars spent on surgical costs last year. He stated that his agency does not collect information indicating how many surgical procedures were paid for under Medicaid and said he is not aware that such information is collected at all.[182]

[178] Note 143 *supra* at 278.
[179] *Id.*
[180] *Id.*
[181] Note 144 *supra.*
[182] *Id.*

"In terms of knowing how much surgery is done, I am not sure that just knowing how many operations were conducted would give us any information in terms of how much of it was unnecessary," Svahn testified.[183] The Subcommittee finds that position of HEW totally unacceptable. The Subcommittee feels that knowing how many operations were conducted would serve as a statistical baseline for determining the magnitude of Federal dollars spent and would begin to allow for comparative studies that would lead to determining the extent of over-utilization in Medicaid, including unncessary procedures.

With respect to public accountability of Federal dollars underwriting Medicaid, the Subcommittee determine that SRS did not know how many surgical procedures were disallowed for payment as a result of review activities. Svahn testified that he did not know how many Medicaid recipients who died as a result of surgical complications were paid for by the Title XIX program.[184]

The Subcommittee finds such lack of accountability on the part of HEW highly distressing. By not compiling baseline data concerning the outcome of measures of care, there is no way for HEW to determine the quality of care given to Medicaid recipients in spite of the fact that HEW is using taxpayer dollars for such care. This lack of baseline data totally contravenes the intent of Congress in enacting cost and quality control legislation. The program is geared to providing quality care comparable to mainstream medicine to Medicaid recipients. SRS is not able to tell Congress whether this goal is being met.

Mr. Svahn stated he was not aware that the Medicaid program continues to pay money to states that never required hospitals utilizing the Medicare, Medicaid programs to submit cost reports,[185] although this is, in fact, the case. These hospitals have never had an audit of their costs nor have any final settlements been made since the Medicaid program began in 1967. These findings were presented as part of a GAO study to Congress.[186] HEW has officially concurred with the findings of the GAO report, however.

This Subcommittee finds the fast that HEW cannot adequately account for monies that it authorizes to be paid under Medicaid to be irresponsible. Equally appalling is the lack of adequate data and information necessary to evaluate the Medicaid program.

IX. Conclusions

Second consultations before surgery could cut down signifiacntly on unnecessary surgical procedures. HEW should promptly institute a program of independent second professional opinions to confirm the need for elective surgery underwritten by Medicare and Medicaid. Such a program would save the Government millions of dollars.

Unnecessary surgery wastes lives and dollars. There were an estimated 2.4 million unnecessary surgeries performed in 1974 at a cost to the American public of almost $4 billion. These unnecessary surgeries led to 11,900 unnecessary deaths.

---

[183] *Id.* at 279.
[184] *Id.*
[185] *Id.* at 280.
[186] (GAO Report of May 9, 1975 at 4).

Evidence was compiled in the Subcommittee's investigation the fee-for-service mechanism of surgical payment encourages surgery in qustionable situations. An in-depth study of this should be undertaken by HEW.

In general, HEW has a totally inadequate data collection system—a situation that should be remedied immediately.

Professional Standards Review Organizations are being developed at too slow a pace and are not being encouraged to review the entire gamut of health care delivery. Their scope should be promptly broadened but for the indefinite future, they cannot be expected to substitute utilization review controls.

The Secretary of HEW is not fulfilling his obligations under the mandatory provisions of the Social Security Act that call for providing incentives for establishment of quality standards of care. This situation should be corrected immediately. Flaunting of the law by HEW means that millions of unauthorized dollars are being paid to States when Congress intended those dollars to provide quality health care to consumers.

Index

A

ABBOTT Laboratories (Chicago)—75, 117
ABORTION & Abortion Laws—1-2, 5, 7-39, 40-1, 131
Abortion use & impact—17-8, 33, 41, 46; death rate drop—10, 19, 40-1; illegal abortions—12, 26-7. Advertising law—36. Anti-abortion efforts—7, 10, 15, 21-33, 39; religious opposition 39 40 (see also specific denomination by name)
Congressional views & actions—5, 21-33. Court actions—11, 20-1, 33-7
Definition—8
Fetal rights controversy—1-2, 22-8, 64, 69-71
International developments—8
Legalization—7-11
Medicaid funds controversy—25, 30-5
State actions—See under 'S,' also specific state names
ABRAMSON, Dr. Harold A.—66
ABZUG, (former) Rep. Bella (D, N.Y.) —23-4, 26-8
ACETOHEXAMIDE (Dymelor)—121
ACUPUNCTURE—131
ADVERTISING—36, 124
AGRICULTURE, Department of (U.S.)—113
AHART, Gregory J.—155-6
AIR Force, Department of (U.S.)—62-3
ALABAMA: Human experimentation—61-2, 65, 67. Mental health care & the law—87-8.
ALASKA: Abortion—12
AMERICAN Association of Planned Parenthood Physicians (Boston)—44
AMERICAN Cancer Society—129
AMERICAN College of Surgeons—145
AMERICAN Diabetes Association—117
AMERICAN Federation of State, County & Municipal Employees (AFSCME)—144
AMERICAN Hospital Association—162
AMERICAN Medical Association (AMA)—15-6, 96, 105, 112-3, 120-3, 127-8
AMERICAN Psychiatric Association —81, 89
AMERICAN Surgical Association—145
AMINOREX—126
AMPHETAMINES—78, 118-20
AMYGDALIN (laetrile)—110-2
ANDY, Dr. O. J.—84-7
ANTIBIOTICS—123, 127
ARIZONA—112, 150
ARMSTRONG, Paul W.—101
ARMY, Department of (U.S.)—67-9
ASKEW, Gov. Reubin (Fla.)—14
ASLAN, Dr. Ana—131
ASPARTAME—117
ASSOCIATION for Voluntary Sterilization (N.Y.)—56
ATOMIC Energy Commission (AEC) (U.S.)—69

AVENTYL—78
AYERST Laboratories—108-9, 123

B

BAILAR 3d, Dr. John—128-9
BAIRD, William R—44
BALL, Dr. Phillip—53
BALTIMORE, Dr. David—73
BAPTISTS, Southern—40
BARBER, Mrs. Mary—144
BARRETT, Elizabeth—68-9
BARTER, Dr. Robert—15-6
BARTLETT, Sen. Dewey F. (R, Okla.) —31
BAYEV, Dr. A. A.—74
BAYH, Sen. Birch (D, Ind.)—33
BEAL V. Doe (law case)—34
BEALL Jr., Sen. J. Glenn (R, Md.)—83-4
BEARD Memorial Foundation, John —111
BEECHER, Dr. Henry K.—99
BEHAVIOR Modification—3-4, 77-83. Treatment for physical ills—82-3. Psychosurgery—85-7. Soviet political-psychiatric abuses—79-82
BEHRMAN, Dr. Richard—71
BELIN, David W.—65
BELLOTTI V. Baird (law case)—36
BERG, Dr. Paul—73-4
BERNARDIN, Archbishop Joseph L.—38
BIOMEDICAL Research Panel (U.S.)—82-3
BIRTH & Birth Defects (including birth control)—2-4, 7, 13-4, 21, 25, 71
Abortion—See under 'A'
Birth control & family planning—1-2, 5, 43-4, 46-51. Birth rate—15, 17, 27, 41, 48-50, 57-8
Contraceptives—44-6; DES & cancer—113-5; IUD dangers—58-60; oral contraceptives—51-6; British report—51-2, 54-5; Depo-Provera—59; drug experimentation—62; morning-after pill—44, 54; religious opposition—18, 57-8
Genetic engineering—2-4
Sterilization—3-4, 17, 56-7
Thalidomide—7, 126
BLACK, Justice Hugo L.—16
BLACK, Peter McL.—83
BLACKMUN, Justice Harry A.—16, 20, 35-6, 45
BLACKS—29, 61-2, 65, 88-9
BLACK Women Organized for Action (BWOA)—29
BLAUER, Harold—68-9
BLEICH, Rabbi J. David—26
BLOOM Dr. William H.—97
BLUE Cross-Blue Shield of Greater N.Y.—145-6
BOHANON, Judge Luther—111
BORISOV, Vladimir—80
BOSTON: Abortion—40
BOWMAN, Ralph S.—113
BOYD V. United States (law case)—24
BRADFORD, Robert W.—113
BREGGIN, Peter—85
BREITEL, Judge Charles B.—11
BRENNAN Jr., Justice William J.—17, 35, 45
BRICKNER, Rabbi Balfour—26
BRIDGETON Hospital (N.J.)—34
BROWN, Dr. Bertram S.—84-6
BROWN Jr., Gov. Edmund (Calif.) —100-1
BROWN, Dr. M. Hunter—86-7
BUCKLEY, Sen. James L. (R, N.Y.)—21, 26, 31, 33
BUKOVSKY, Vladimir—81
BUNDY, McGeorge—44
BUNKER, J. P.—135, 142
BURGER, Chief Justice Warren E—16, 21, 36-7, 45, 90
BURGESS, Anna—59-60
BURNS, Gov. John A. (Hawaii)—8-9
BUTZ, Earl L.—114
BYRN, Prof. Robert M.—11
BZ (3- uinuclidinyl benzilate)—68

C

CALIFANO, Joseph A.—75-6, 121-2
CALIFORNIA: Abortion—14-5. Death issue & transplants—96. Laetrile drug—110-1. Psychosurgery—87. 'Right to die' & mercy killing—100-1
CALIFORNIA, University of (at Los Angeles) (UCLA): Brain Research Institute & Department of Psychiatry—87
CAMDEN County (N.J.) Psychiatric Hospital—91
CANCER—52-4, 59, 63, 108-9, 111-6, 118, 123. DES action—113-5. Krebiozen ban—128. Laetrile controversy—110-3. X-ray hazards —128-9
CANADA—110, 116-8, 130
CAPRON, Alexander Morgan—100
CAREY 3d, Walter Burton—96-7
CAREY V. Population Services International (law case)—45

CARROLL, Rev. Charles Patrick—23
CARTER Jimmy—37-9
CATHOLICS, Roman: Abortion—7-11, 15, 17, 19, 20-1, 26, 38-40. Birth control—7, 18, 43, 57-8
CENSUS Bureau—47-9
CENTER for Disease Control (CDC)—130
CENTRAL Intelligence Agency (CIA)—65-7
CHALIDZE, Valery N.—81
CHINA, Peoples Republic of—50-1
CHLORPROPAMIDE (diabinese)—121
CHRYSLER Corp.—88
CHURCH, Sen. Frank (D, Ida.)—97
CIANFRANI, State Sen. Henry J. (D, Philadelphia)—92
CIBA-Geigy Corp.—121
CINCINNATI: Abortion—38
CLARIE, Judge T. Emmett—14
CLARK, Dr. Kenneth B.—78-9
COALITION for a National Population Policy—47
COBB, Capt. W. C.—69
COBURN, Daniel R.—104
COCA-Cola Co.—117-8
COHEN, Dr. Sidney—119
COHEN, Dr. Stanley H.—73
COLD Spring Harbor (N.Y.) Laboratory—73
COLLESTER Jr., Donald G—101
COLUMBIA University (N.Y.)—71
COMMERCE, Department of—75
COMMISSION on Population Growth (U.S.)—48
COMMISSION on Professional & Hospital Activities (CPHA)—163, 166
CONGRESS (U.S.): Abortion—22-33. Behavior modification & drug abuse—78. Birth control—43-4, 52-3. Death—97-101. Drugs & drug abuses—119, 125-8; DES action—114; testing regulations—107-10. Genetic research—75. Human experimentation—61-4. Laetrile controversy—112. Mental health—92. Psychosurgery—83-7. Unnecessary surgery report—133-73
CONNECTICUT: Abortion—14, 34-7
CONNELL, Dr. Elizabeth—53
COOKE, Terence Cardinal—9-10, 21
COOPER, Dr. T.—151, 169-70
CORDAY, Dr. Eliot—95-6
CORD Laboratories—123
COSMETICS—118, 121, 124
COURT Actions: Abortion—11-7, 20-1, 36-7, 40; federal funds—31, 33-4. Birth control—44-5, 58-9; sterilization ruling—56-7. Death—96-7, 101-5; mercy killing case—105. Drugs & drug abuses—114, 128, 130; FDA powers—126. Laetrile—111-2. Mental health—87-91. Psychosurgery—84-7
COUSINS, Most Rev. William E. (Milwaukee)—11
CRICK, Francis—73
CRILE Jr., Dr. George—147
CUMBERLAND Packing Corp.—117
CYCLAMATES—115-6

D

DALKON Shield—58-9
DALMANE—130
DANFORTH V. Planned Parenthood (law case)—36
DAVI, Richard—9
DAVIS, Dr. Hugh J.—52
DAVIS, Kingsley—15
DBI (phenformin)—121-2
DEATH & 'Right to Die' Problems—3-5, 9, 22-3, 25, 95-102, 105. Court action on Quinlan—101-5
DEEMER, Connie L.—58-9
DEFENSE, Department of (U.S.)—16, 62-3, 65-9
DELAHUNT, Rep. William (R, Mass.)—71
DELAWARE: Laetrile—112
DELLUMS, Rep. Ronald V. (D, Calif.)—28-9
DEMOCRATIC Party—19
DES (diethylstilbesterol)—54, 113-5
DEXEDRENE—78
DIABETES—76, 117, 120-2
DIABINESE (chlorpropamide)—121
DIET Drugs—126
DIETHYLSTILBESTEROL (DES)—54, 113-5
DISTRICT of Columbia: Abortion—16-7
DNA (deoxyribonucleic acid) Research—3, 71-6
DONALDSON, Kenneth—89-90
DONNELLY, Dr. Joseph P.—23
DOOLING Jr., Judge John F.—33
DOUGLAS, Justice William O.—14, 45
DOW Corning Corp. (Midland, Mich.)—124
DOWNEY, Rep. Thomas J. (D, N.Y.)—68
DOWN'S Syndrome (Mongolism)—71
DRUGS & Drug Abuses:
Amphetamines—78, 118-20. Antibiotics—123, 127

Behavior modification—3-4, 77-82
Cancer: Krebiozen ban—128; laetrile controversy—110-3. Cold remedies—124-5
DES action—113-5. Diabetes drugs—120-2
Gerovital—131. Government experimentation—62-3, 65-9
L-dopa—123
Oral contraceptives—see under BIRTH & Birth Defects. Other FDA action & powers—123-7
Polio vaccine—130. Prescription drugs—128, 130-1
Soviet political-psychiatric abuses—79-82
Tests & regulation—107-10. Thalidomide—7, 126. Tranquilizers—129-30 Uncertified & combination drugs—123-4
See also specific drug or drug firm by name
DULLES, Allen W.—67
DUMONT, Rene—50
DuVAL, Dr. Merlin K.—65
DYMELOR (acetohexamide)—121

E

EDELIN, Dr. Kenneth C.—40
EDUCATION—78
EDWARDS, Charles C.—51, 54, 113, 116, 119, 123-4
EFSTRATIADIS, Dr. Argiris—73
EGYPT—1
EISENHOWER, Milton S.—47
EISENSTADT, Marvin—117
ELI Lilly & Co.—75, 115
ENERGY Research & Development Administration (ERDA)—69
ENRIGHT, Judge William B.—113
ERVIN, Dr. Fran—86
EUTHANASIA—9, 100, 105

F

FAINBERG, Viktor—79-80, 82
FARVIEW State Hospital (Waymart, N.J.)—91-3
FATTEH, Dr. Abdullah—96
FEDERAL Employees Health Benefit Program Utilization Study—145
FEDERAL Food, Drug & Cosmetic Act—111
FEINBERG (Fainberg), Viktor—79-80, 82
FENNELLY, Dr. Joseph F.—104
FERRE, Gov. Luis A. (Puerto Rico)—57
FINCH, Robert H.—53
FINKBINE, Sherri—7
FINLEY, Dr. Joanne—90
FLOOD, Rep. Daniel (D, Pa.)—154
FLOREZ, Luis de—67
FLORIDA: Abortion—14. Mental health—89-90. Mercy killing—25. Unnecessary surgery—143
FOOD & Drug Administration (FDA)—51, 54-6, 58-60, 78, 107-18, 120-7
FORD, Betty—129
FORD, Gerald R.: Abortion—30, 32, 37-8
FORD Foundation—44
FOUNTAIN, Rep. L. H. (D, N.C.)—123
FOYE Jr. Dr. Laurance F.—98-9
FRASER, Rep. Donald M.—29
FREDERICKSON, Donald S.—75
FREEDMAN, Dr. Alfred M.—81
FREEDOM of Choice in Cancer Therapy, Committee for—112-3
FRIEDAN, Betty—50
FRIEDMAN, Milton—126
FUCHS, V. R.—147

G

GALLAGHER, Rep. Cornelius (D, N.J.)—78
GALLESE, Liz Roman—63
GEIS, Prof. Gilbert—7
GENERAL Accounting Office (GAO)—79, 107-9, 135, 155-60, 172
GENERAL Electric Co.—75
GENETIC Engineering—2-4, 71-6
GEORGIA: Abortion—20. Human experimentation—67
GEROVITAL (GH3)—131
GESELL, Judge Gerhard A.—17, 56-7
GIBSON, Campbell—49
GIMINEZ-Jimeno, Enrique—40
GITTLESON, A.—135
GOLDIN, Harrison J.—65
GOODMAN, Dr. Howard M.—76
GOODRICH, William W.—116
GORNICK, Marian—148-9, 168
GOTTLIEB, Sidney—66-7
GRISWALD V. Connecticut (law case)—102
GREAT Britain—8, 51-5, 105
GREELEY, Rev. Andrew—57
GREER, Germaine—50
GREENWALD, Dr. Peter—54
GREYSTONE Park Psychiatric Hospital (N.J.)—91

GRIGORENKO, Gen. Pyotr—81
GRISWOLD V. Connecticut (law case)—24
GUTTMACHER, Dr. Alan F.—21, 53
GUTTMACHER Institute, Alan—46

H

HAHNEMANN'S Hospital (Philadelphia)—86-6
HAMMURABI'S Code—1
HANDSCHIN, R.—135
HARRIS, Dr. David—10
HARVARD University—73, 75
HAWAII: Abortion—7-9
HAYWARD, Lisa—65
HEALTH & Hospitals Corp. (N.Y.)—33
HEALTH, Education & Welfare, Department of (HEW)—20, 32-3, 51-3, 56-7, 64-5, 69-70, 75-6, 116, 120-1, 133-73
HEALTH Maintenance Organizations (HMOs)—148
HEALTH Research Group—115
HEALTH Resources Administration (HRA)—162
HEART Disease & Transplants—2-4, 82, 95-6, 120-2
HELLER, Jean—65
HELMS, Sen. Jesse (R, N.C.)—26, 33
HEPATITIS—62, 64-5
HERBST, Dr. Arthur—114
HERESIES (book)—83
HERTZ, Dr. Roy—44, 52
HEXACHLOROPHENE—125
HEXOBENDINE—109
HIPPOCRATES & Hippocratic Oath—1-2
HIRSCHMAN, G. C.—148
HODGSON, Dr. Jane—13
HOFFMANN-La Roche Corp.—75
HOGAN, Rep. Lawrence J. (R, Md.)—21
HOLLAND, Dr. James G.—77
HOLTON, Gov. Linwood (Va.)—12
HOMOSEXUALITY—89
HORN, Justice Herbert—34
HOSPITAL Discharge Survey (HDS)—162
HOSPITALS & Other Health Institutions—104, 112. Abortion—9, 16-7, 34, 36-7. Family planning services—46. Human experimentation—63-4, 68-9. Mental health treatment & care—62, 64-5, 68-9, 79, 83-93. Psychosurgery—83-7. Soviet political-psychiatric abuses—79-82. Unnecessary surgery study—133-73. See also specific hospital by name
HUANG Shu-tse—50-1
HUGHES, Dr. Edward E. X.—135, 147, 149-50, 153
HUGHES, Chief Justice Richard J.—101
HUMAN Experimentation—4-5, 61-71
Biomedical research law—64.
Birth control drugs—62
CIA drug tests—65-7.
Congressional views & actions—61-4
Defense Department—62-3, 67—9
Fetal research—64, 69-71
Hepatitis experiment on retarded—62, 64-5
Nerve gas—68
Radiation tests—63, 69
Prisoners & psychosurgery—62, 64
Syphilis experiment—61-2, 65
HUMAN Resources Research Organization—77
HUMAN Rights Committee (U.S.S.R.)—80-1
HUME, Dr. David—96
HUTCHESON Jr., Dr. Robert—59
HYDE, Rep. Henry J. (R, Ill.)—33
HYLAND, William—105

I

IDAHO: Abortion—22
ILLEGITIMACY—19
ILLINOIS: Abortion—13
INDIANA: Abortion—37. Laetrile—112
INGERSOLL, John E.—119
INGRAHAM, Dr. Hollis S.—113
INMAN, William P.—117
INSULIN—76
INTERNAL Revenue Service (U.S.)—39
INTERNATIONAL Federation of Catholic Medical Associations—9
ISRAEL—130
ITALY 130

J

JAIN, Dr. Anrudh K.—55-6
JAPAN—8
JAVED, Arshad—104
JAVITS, Sen. Jacob K. (R, N.Y.)—75
JENNING, Robert—92
JENNINGS, Dr. John—112
JESUITS—39
JICK, Dr. Hershel—130
JOHNSON Jr., Judge Frank M.—87
JOHNSON, James—88
JOHNSON & Johnson Pharmaceutical Corp.—55

JUDAISM—26, 28
JUSTICE, Department of—33, 88–9, 109, 119, 122

K

KAIMOWITZ, Gabe—85–7
KAIMOWTZ V. Department of Mental Health (law case)—85–7
KALLEN Jr., Morris N.—85–6
KALUGA Psychiatric Hospital (U.S.S.R.)—80
KAPIOLANI Maternity & Gynecological Hospital (Honolulu)—9
KASSOUF, Dr. Edmond—53
KEATING, Rep. William J. (R, Ohio)—24–5
KEFAUVER-Harris bill—107–8, 110
KEKILOVA, Annasoltan—80
KELLEN, Robert M.—117
KELLER, R. F.—155
KELLOGG Foundation, M. K.—46
KENNEDY, Dr. Donald—110, 118
KENNEDY, Sen Edward M. (D, Mass.)—4–5, 61–4, 75, 114
KENNEDY, John F.—111
KHORANA, Dr. H. Gobind—72
KING, Judge Michael P.—91
KISTNER, Dr. Robert W.—55
KLAGSBRUN, Dr. Samuel C.—112
KLEIN, Ann—90
KOPOLOW, Dr. Louis E.—90
KOSTANTINOV, Lev—82
KRATTER, Marvin—131
KREBIOZEN—128
KREBS Sr., Dr. Ernst T.—111
KREBS Jr., Ernst T.—111
KRISTNER, Dr. Robert W.—52–3
KROL, John Cardinal—21, 26
KRUGMAN, Dr. Saul—64–5
KUCHERA, Dr. Lucile K.—54

L

LABOR, Department of—30, 32
LAETRILE—110–3
LANGLEY Porter Neuropsychiatric Institute (San Francisco)—86
LASHBROOK, Robert—66–7
LAW Enforcement Assistance Administration—79
LEDERLE Labs—109
L-DOPA (levo-dihydroxy-phlenlalanine)—123
LEFKOWITZ, Louis J.—75
LEMON Pharmacal Co. (Sellersville, Pa.)—123
LEWIS, E. M.—135
LIBRIUM—130
LIFSHITS, Dr. Alexander Y.—80
LINDEN Laboratories—123
LIVESTOCK—114
LOUISIANA—112
LOWER, Dr. Richard—96
LSD (lysergic acid diethylamide)—65–9
LUMBARD, Judge J. Edward—14
LYING-In Hospital (Chicago)—115

M

MAHER V. Roe (law case)—34
MAHONEY, Dr. Maurice J.—70–1
MALCOTTI, Dr. Marvin M.—88
MANDEL, Gov. Marvin (Md.)—12–3
MANIATIS, Dr. Thomas—73
MARK, Dr. Vernon—86
MARKS, Dr. Lawrence—109–10
MARSHALL, Justice Thurgood—14, 35, 45
MARTINEZ, Most Rev. Luis Aponte—57
MARYLAND: Abortion—12–3, 21–2. Human experimentation—67–8. Mental health—88–9
MARYLAND, University of: Psychiatric Institute—67
MASSACHUSETTS—71, 75, 145. Abortion—35–6, 40. Birth control—44
MASSACHUSETTS General Hospital—83, 86
MASSACHUSETTS Institute of Technology (MIT)—47–8
MATHEWS, Dr. F. David—160–1
MAXAM, Dr. Allen—73
McCARTHY, Dr. Eugene G.—135, 142, 144, 146, 163–4
McGUIRE, Judge James P.—40
McHUGH, Msgr. James T.—39
McNAUGHTON, Andrew R. L.—113
McNAUGHTON Foundation—111
McNEAL, Barbara—26
MEAD, Margaret—50
MEAD-Johnson Co.—55
MEADOWS, Dennis L.—48
MEDICAID & Medicare—25, 31–5, 131–73. Unnecessary surgery—133–73
MEDICAL Services Administration (MSA)—140, 149
MEDVEDEV, Roy A.—80
MEDVEDEV, Zhores A.—80
MELTROL-50 (phenformin)—121–2

MENTAL Health Planning Committee (N.J.)—90
MENTAL Illness & Health Care—2-4, 68-9, 77-83, 85-8, 91-3. Homosexuality—89. Hospitals probed—88, 91-3. Soviet psychiatric abuses—79-82. Treatment & care—87-93
MENTAL Retardation & Health Care—23, 59, 71, 87-9. Hepatitis experiment—62, 64-5
MERCK & Co. (West Point, Pa.)—123
MERKEL, Kenneth—11
MERCK, Sharp & Dome Research—109
MERRELL National Laboratories—109
MESOPOTAMIA—1
METCALFE, Rep. Ralph (D, Ill.)—79
METHODIST Church, United—40
MEXICO—110-1
MEYER V. Nebraska (law case)—24
MICHAELS, George M.—9
MICHIGAN: Abortion—12, 21, 36. DES experiments—115. Mental health care—88. Psychosurgery—85-7
MICHIGAN, University of: Health Service—54
MILLER, Gov. Keith (Alaska)—12
MILWAUKEE, Wis.—11
MINNESOTA: Abortion—13, 36
MINK, Patsy—115
MISSOURI: Abortion—34-6
MONDALE, Walter F.—2-4
MONTANA: Abortion—22
MORGAN, Dr. Arthur E.—97-8
MORGAN, Dr. Karl Z.—128
MORREALE, Mrs. Carol—39
MORRIS View Nursing Homes (Morris Township, N.J.)—104
MORSE, Robert—104
MOSS, Rep. John E. (D, Calif.)—136, 160

N

NADER, Ralph—115
NARCOTICS & Dangerous Drugs, Bureau of—120
NATIONAL Academy of Sciences and National Research Council—40-1, 75-6, 116, 123-5
NATIONAL Advisory Council for the Protection of Subjects of Biomedical & Behavioral Research—64
NATIONAL Cancer Institute—110, 112, 114, 118, 128-9
NATIONAL Center for Health Statistics (NCHS)—1, 48-50, 162
NATIONAL Center for Social Statistics (NCSS)—149, 171
NATIONAL Commission for the Protection of Human Subjects of Biomedical & Behavioral Research (U.S.)—70, 85, 87
NATIONAL Conference of Catholic Bishops—38-9
NATIONAL Fertility Study—57-8
NATIONAL Institute of Arthritis & Metabolic Diseases—121
NATIONAL Institute of Mental Health—77, 79, 84-7, 90-3, 119
NATIONAL Institutes of Health—69-70, 74-6, 108, 115, 164
NATIONAL Opinion Research Center—57
NATIONAL Research Act—64
NATIONAL Research Council—See NATIONAL Academy of Sciences, etc.
NATIONAL Welfare Rights Organization—56-7
NAVY, Department of (U.S.)—69
NEBRASKA: Abortion—22. Behavior modification—78
NELSON, Dr. Alan R.—132
NELSON, Sen. Gaylord (D, Wis.)—52, 69, 126
NEVADA: Acupuncture—131. Laetrile—112
NEWCOMB Hospital (N.J.)—34
NEWELL, Dr. Guy—112
NEW JERSEY: Abortion—13-4, 22, 34-5. Death—101-5. Mental health—90-3
NEWMAN, Judge John O.—14
NEW York Psychiatric Institute—67
NEW York State—132, 144. Abortion—9-11, 17, 19, 21-2, 27, 33-5, 41. Birth control—45. Death—96-7. Human experimentation—64-5. Laetrile—111-2. Mental health—69, 90
NEW York University (& Medical Center)—64, 72-3
NEW Zealand—130
NITTO, Judge Harold M.—91
NIXON, Richard M.—64. Abortion—10-1, 16, 19, 20-1. Birth control & family planning—43-4
NORTH Dakota: Abortion—21. Human experimentation—67
NORTHVILLE State Hospital (Mich.)—86

O

OBERSET, Dr. Byron B.—78
O'CALLAGHAN, Gov. Mike (D, Nevada)—131

OCHBERG, Frank M.—90
O'CONNOR V. Donaldson(law case)—89
O'GRADY, Mrs. Dorothy—143
OKLAHOMA: Abortion—22. Laetrile—112
OLMSTEAD V. United States (law case)—24
OLSON, Alice—67
OLSON, Eric—65-7
OLSON, Frank R.—65-6
OMAHA, Neb.—78
ORINASE—121
ORNEX—123
O'ROURKE, Rev. Joseph—39
ORTHO Pharmaceutical Corp.—55
OXMAN, Dr. Michael N.—71
OXPRENALOL Hydrochloride—109

P

PACKWOOD, Sen. Bob (R, Ore.)—32
PARROTT, Max—127
PAUL VI, Pope—9, 39, 58
PENICILLIN—62-3
PENNSYLVANIA—46. Abortion—15, 34, 36, 41
PEPSICO, Inc.—117-8
PERROTT, George S.—145
PETERSON, Dr. William—41
PFIZER Co.—123
PHARMACEUTICAL Industry—52-5, 58-60, 75, 107-10, 115, 119, 123, 125, 127-8
PHARMACEUTICAL Manufacturers Association (PNA)—127-8
PHENFORMIN (DBI)—121-2
PIERCE, Judge Lawrence W.—45
PIERCE V. Society of Sisters (law case)—24
PLAGER, Dr. John E.—64
PLANNED Parenthood, Inc.—21, 27, 33, 36, 46, 53, 58
PLUNKETT, Judge J. Jerome—13
PLYUSHCH, Leonid—81-2
POELKER, John H.—34
POELKER V. Doe (law case)—34
POLIOMYELITIS—130
POLLET, Michael N.—45
POMROY, Karen Ann—96-7
POPULATION—17, 46-7. See also 'Birth control' under BIRTH & Birth Defects
POPULATION Council (U.S.)—44
POPULATION Growth, Commission on—17, 19
POTTINGER, J. Stanley—88
POWELL, Jr., Justice Lewis F.—21, 34-5
POWERS, Galen D.—159-60
PRISONS & Prisoners—62, 64. Behavior modification—79. Psychosurgery—85-7. Soviet political-psychiatric abuses—79-82
PROFESSIONAL Standards Review Organizations (PSROs)—131-3, 137, 139, 145, 151-4, 168-70, 173
PSYCHOSURGERY—83-7
PUBLIC Citizen Inc.—115, 122
PUBLIC Health Association—10
PUBLIC Health Service (PHS) (U.S.)—65, 141
PUERTO Rico—57
PURE Food & Drug Act—125

Q

QUAKERS—40
QUEENS Medical Center (Hawaii)—9
QUINLAN, Joseph—101-4
QUINLAN, Julia—101, 104
QUINLAN, Karen Anne—101-5

R

RADIATION—128-9
RAND Corp.—78
RAUCH, Thomas N.—119
RAUSCHER Jr., Dr. Frank J.—114, 129
REAGAN, Gov. Ronald (Calif.)—87
REHNQUIST, Justice William H.—20, 36-7, 45
REID Jr., Judge Clarence A.—12
RELIGION—2, 7-11, 38-40, 43, 57-8. See also specific denomination
RELIGIOUS Society of Friends (Quakers)—40
REPUBLICAN Party—37-8, 71
RHINELANDER, John B.—154, 160-1
RIBICOFF, Sen. Abraham A. (D, Conn.)—107, 109
RICHARDSON, Dr. John A.—113
RITALIN (methylphenidate hydrochloride)—78
ROBINS Co., A.H.—58
ROCKEFELLER 3d, John D.—51
ROCKEFELLER, Margaretta—129
ROCKEFELLER, Gov. Nelson A. (N.Y.)—9-11
ROCKEFELLER Commission—65-6
ROE V. Wade (law case)—27

ROETHE, James—66
ROSENBERG, Morton—32
ROSENHAM, Dr. David L.—88
ROSEWOOD State Hospital (Md.)—88-9
ROUMELL, Judge Thomas—115
ROUSSIN, Rev. John J.—39
RUTTER, Dr. William J.—76
RUWET, Col. Vincent—66

S

SABIN, Dr. Albert—130
SACCHARIN—112, 115-8
SACKETT, Dr. Walter W.—99
St. CLARE's Hospital (Denville, N.J.)—104
SAKHAROV, Andrei D.—81
SALEM County Memorial Hospital (N.J.)—34
SALK, Dr. Jonas—130
SALK Institute—122
SAMMONS, Dr. James H.—122-3
San FRANCISCO—89
SANGER Research Bureau, Margaret (N.Y.)—56
SCHMICKEL, Bert W.—88
SCHREIBER, Justice Sidney M.—34
SEARLE & Co., G. D.—51, 54
SEIDOVA, Ogulsakhat—80
SERAX—130
SERC (vertigo drug)—125
SESSA, Dr. Grazia—72-3
SEWELL, Dr. David—96
SHAFAREVICH, Igor—81
SHAPP, Gov. Milton J.—15
SHCHELOKOV, Col. Gen. Nikolai A.—79
SHERWIN-Williams Co. (Cleveland)—117
SHIRKEY, Dr. Harry C.—127
SHOSTAKOVICH, Boris V.—80
SHUMWAY, Dr. Norman—96
SIM, Dr. Van M.—68
SIMMONS, Dr. Henry E.—119-20, 127
SINGLETON V. Wulff (law case)—36
SLEE, Dr. Virgil—166-7
SLOAN-Kettering Cancer Center, Memorial (N.Y.)—112
SMITH, Louis—85-6
SMITH, Kline & French Laboratories—119, 123, 125
SOCIAL Security Act—34, 45, 91-2, 133-4, 137, 141, 152-4, 157, 161, 173
SOCIAL & Rehabilitation Service (SRS) (of Department of Health, Education & Welfare)—135, 154, 157-60, 171-2
SOCIAL Services Department (N.Y.)—33-4, 132
SOLOMON, Dr. Neil—88
SOMATOSTATIN—122
SOUTH Dakota: Abortion—35
SQUIBB & Sons, E. R.—109-10
STAHL, Dr. William M.—146-7
STANFORD University—88
STANLEY V. Georgia (law case)—24
STATE Actions: Abortion—7-15, 20-2, 34-7, 41. Acupuncture legalized—131. Behavior modification—78. Birth control developments—44-5. Birth rate—41. Death—96-7, 100-5. Fetal research curb—71. Laetrile controversy—111-2. Mental health—87-8, 90-1. Psychosurgery—87. See also specific state by name
STERILIZATION—3-4, 36, 56-7
STEVENS, Justice John Paul—36
STEWART, Justice Potter—45, 89-90
STOKES, Rep. Louis (D, Ohio)—85
STOREWORKERS Union Welfare Fund—163
STUDY on Surgical Services for the United States (SOSSUS)—135, 145-6, 150
SUGIURA, Dr. Kanematsu—112
SULLIVAN, Gerald—97
SUPREME Court—11, 85-7, 89-90, 126, 128, 130. Abortion—13-5, 20-5, 27, 31, 33-5. Birth control rulings—44-5. Quinlan case—101-5
SURGEONS & Surgical Procedures: Abortion—See under 'A.' Acupuncture legalized 131. Mastectomy 129. Professional Standards Review Organizations—131-3. Sex-change operation—132. Unnecessary surgery—133-73; hysterectomies & tonsillectomies—143-5
SVAHN, John A.—171-2
SWEDEN—7
SWEET, Dr. William—86
SYNTEX Laboratories—52, 55
SYPHILIS—61-2, 65
SZASZ, Thomas S.—83

T

TAEUBER, Conrad F.—46-7
TAYLOR, Rev. Eamon—39

TECHNOLOGY Assessment, Office of—118
TEMIN, Dr. Howard—73
TENNESSEE—59-60
TERRY V. Ohio (law case)—24
TEXAS: Abortion—13, 20. Laetrile—112
THALIDOMIDE—7, 126
THOMAS, Dr. Lewis—112
THOMPSON Jr., Judge Gordon—111-2
TIETZE, Dr. Christopher—17-8
TODD, Dr. Malcolm C.—105
TOFRANIL—78
TOLAZAMIDE (Tolinase)—121
TOLBUTAMIDE—120-2
TOLINASE (tolazamide)—121
TRANXENE—130
TRAVIS, Alice—28-9
TRIFLOCIN—109
TUCKER, Bruce O.—96
TULANE University: Department of Neurology & Psychiatry—67
TUMMERMAN, Alexis—82
TUSKEGEE, Ala.—61, 65
TVERDOKHLEBOV, Andrei N.—81
TYDINGS, Sen. Joseph D. (D, Md.)—43, 47

U

UNION Pacific R.R. Co. V. Botsford (law case)—24
UNION of Soviet Socialist Republics—51. Political-psychiatric abuses—79-82
UNITED Auto Workers Union—47
UNITED Nations: World Population Conference—50-1
UNIVERSITY of Chicago—115
UNIVERSITY Group Diabetes Program—120-1
UPJOHN Co.—60, 75, 120, 123
UPSTATE Medical Center (Syracuse, N.Y.)—83
UTAH—45, 67. Abortion—22

V

VACAVILLE Prison (San Francisco)—86
VACCINES—130
VALENZUELA, Mrs. Marie—143-4
VALIUM—130
Van HOEK, Robert—151-2, 154, 168
VERMONT: Abortion—11-2, 22. Surgery & health care—145, 148, 167-8
VERTIGO drug (serc)—125
VIRGINIA: Abortion—11-2, 22
VUITCH, Dr. Milan—17

W

WARNER-Lambert Pharmaceutical Co. (Morris Plains, N.J.)—123
WASHINGTON: Laetrile—112
WASHINGTON, University of: Medical School—67
WATKINS, R.N.—135
WATSON, Dr. James D.—2, 73
WEIKEL, Dr. Keith—158-9
WEINBERGER, Caspar—50, 69-70
WEISSMANN, Dr. Gerald—72-3
WENNBERG, J. E.—135, 142, 145, 148, 167
WEST Germany—130
WESTOFF, Charles F.—48, 58
WEST Side Community of the Society of Jesus (N.Y.)—39
WEST Virginia: Abortion—22
WHITE, Justice Byron R.—20, 36-7
WIDMER, G.W.—135
WIESNER, Dr. Jerome—4
WILKE, Dr. J.C.—24
WILKINS, Roy E.—47
WILLIAMSON, Robert George—91
WILLOWBROOK State School (N.Y.)—64-5
WIMMERSHOFF-Caplan, Sue—29
WISCONSIN—44. Abortion—11
WISCONSIN, University of—67, 71-2
WOLFE, Dr. Sidney—146, 166
WOMEN—56-7. Abortion—See under "A." Birth control drug experiment—62; see also 'Birth control' under BIRTH & Birth Defects. Breast cancer & X-rays—128-9. DES action—113-4.
WOMEN's Caucus of the California Democratic Council (CDC)—28-9
WOMEN'S Lobby, The—39
WORKING Organization for Retarded Children—90
WORLD Health Organization (WHO)—8, 96
WORLD Population Conference (UN)—50-1
WORLD Psychiatric Association Congress—80-1

X

X-RAY Hazards—128–9

Y

YAKOVSON, Anatoly—82
YANO, State Sen. Vincent H. (Hawaii)—9
YOON, Dr. InBae—57

Z

ZERO Population Growth (ZPG)—46–7
ZICARELLI, Joseph—113
ZIGLER, Dr. Edward E.—78
ZUIDEMA, Dr. George—143–8, 150
ZWACH, Rep. John M. (R, Minn.)—26
ZYGMANIAK, George—105
ZYGMANIAK, Lester—105

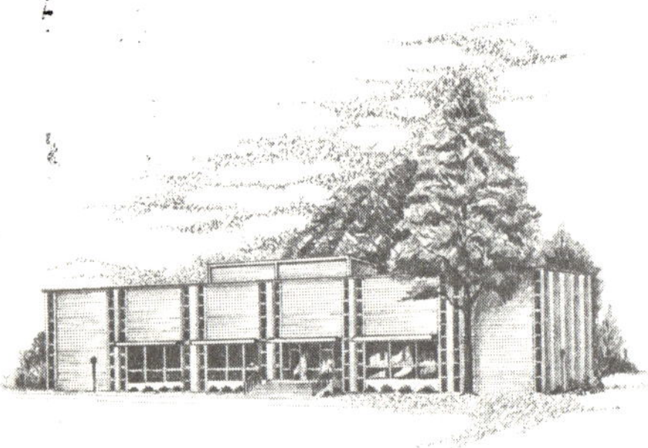